FOOD AND NUTRITIONAL TOXICOLOGY

STANLEY T. OMAYE

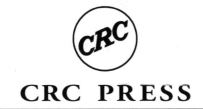

CRC PRESS

Boca Raton   London   New York   Washington, D.C.

FOOD AND NUTRITIONAL TOXICOLOGY

STANLEY T. OMAYE

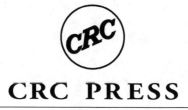

CRC PRESS

Boca Raton   London   New York   Washington, D.C.

Library of Congress Cataloging-in-Publication Data

Omaye, Stanley T.
   Food and nutritional toxicology / Stanley T. Omaye.
      p. ; cm.
   Includes bibliographical references and index.
   ISBN 1-58716-071-4
   1. Food—Toxicology. I. Title.
   [DNLM: 1. Food—adverse effects. 2. Food Additives—adverse effects. 3. Food
Analysis—methods. 4. Food Contamination. 5. Food Hypersensitivity. 6. Food Poisoning.
WA 701 O54f 2004]
RA1258.O46 2004
615.9′54—dc22   2003065211

This book contains information obtained from authentic and highly regarded sources. Reprinted material is quoted with permission, and sources are indicated. A wide variety of references are listed. Reasonable efforts have been made to publish reliable data and information, but the author and the publisher cannot assume responsibility for the validity of all materials or for the consequences of their use.

Neither this book nor any part may be reproduced or transmitted in any form or by any means, electronic or mechanical, including photocopying, microfilming, and recording, or by any information storage or retrieval system, without prior permission in writing from the publisher.

The consent of CRC Press LLC does not extend to copying for general distribution, for promotion, for creating new works, or for resale. Specific permission must be obtained in writing from CRC Press LLC for such copying.

Direct all inquiries to CRC Press LLC, 2000 N.W. Corporate Blvd., Boca Raton, Florida 33431.

Trademark Notice: Product or corporate names may be trademarks or registered trademarks, and are used only for identification and explanation, without intent to infringe.

Visit the CRC Press Web site at www.crcpress.com

© 2004 by CRC Press LLC

No claim to original U.S. Government works
International Standard Book Number 1-58716-071-4
Library of Congress Card Number 2003065211

Preface

Food can be defined as the nutritive material taken into an organism for growth, work, or repair and for maintaining the vital processes. Food sustains life, and, as such, many individuals view food as an uncomplicated, pure source of nutrition. Therefore, such individuals are often bewildered to learn that food is comprised of an array of natural chemicals, and not all the chemicals are nutrients or enhance nutritive value, but in fact may decrease nutritional value or, worse still, are toxic (e.g., naturally occurring toxicants). Also, chemicals can be added to food, either intentionally or unintentionally, during production and processing. Cooking, storing, and preparing food in our kitchens create new components and different chemical compounds, which may have a toxic effect, an improvement or enhancement effect, or no effect at all on the meal quality.

Food and nutritional toxicology is the field devoted to studying the complexity of the chemicals in food, particularly those that have the potential of producing adverse health effects. One begins to appreciate the complexity of the field when one recognizes that food chemicals can interact with body fluids and other components of the diet and that such interactions may have a multitude of effects, beneficial or harmful. For example, the endogenous secretions of the stomach have the ability to inactivate or break down many chemicals; however, chemicals such as nitrate can be reduced to nitrite, which has the potential of reacting with proteins in the stomach to produce carcinogenic nitrosamines. This may be inconsequential if vitamin C or E is present in the stomach, because of its capacity to inhibit the nitrosation process. Thus, interactions between food components and other chemicals are complicated but have dire implications as regards health and adverse effects.

Overall, because of the diversity of the field, food and nutritional toxicology spans a number of disciplines, such as nutrition, toxicology, epidemiology, food science, environmental health, biochemistry, and physiology. The field includes studies of human health impacts of food containing environmental contaminants or natural toxicants. The field includes investigations of food additives, migration of chemicals from packaging materials into foods, and persistence of feed and food contaminants in food products. Also, the field covers examining the impact of contaminants on nutrient utilization, adverse effects of nutrient excesses, metabolism of food toxicants, and the relationship of the body's biological defense mechanisms to such toxicants. Finally, because the study of food and nutritional toxicology has obvious societal implication, one must examine the risk determination process, how food is regulated to ensure safety, and the current status of regulatory processes.

This book is intended as a text for advanced undergraduate or graduate students in nutrition, food sciences, environment, or toxicology, and professionals in the areas of nutrition, environmental health and sciences, and life or health and medical sciences. The objective of this text is to present an in-depth study of toxicants found in foods by (1) providing the general principles of toxicology, including methods for food safety assessment and biochemical and physiological mechanisms of action of food toxicants; (2) developing an understanding of foodborne intoxications and infections and of diseases linked to foods; (3) applying the principles to the prevention of foodborne disease; and (4) providing a background about the regulation of food safety.

For nearly a decade, I have been working with students, in and out of the classroom, on many facets of this evolving area of toxicology. This textbook has evolved from my experiences while conducting a course on food and nutritional toxicology and is designed to be a teaching tool.

Stanley T. Omaye

Acknowledgments

This book is dedicated to students of food and nutritional toxicology — past, present, and future. Special thanks go to C.C. Bjerke for his contributions in writing Chapters 4 and 5. I am indebted to the encouragement from my mentors and colleagues and grateful for the support and understanding of my family and friends.

Contents

SECTION I Fundamental Concepts

Chapter 1 An Overview of Food and Nutritional Toxicology 3

Defining the Terms and Scope of Food and Nutritional Toxicology 3
    Toxicology 3
    Food and Nutritional Toxicology 4
Toxicants in Foods and Their Effects on Nutrition 5
    Nutrients 5
    Naturally Occurring Toxicants 7
    Food Additives and Contaminants 7
Impact of Diet on the Effects of Toxicants 8
Study Questions and Exercises 9
Recommended Readings 9

Chapter 2 General Principles of Toxicology 11

Phases of Toxicological Effects 11
    Exposure Phase 11
    Toxicokinetic Phase 13
    Toxicodynamic Phase 14
Dose–Response Relationship 14
    Frequency Response 15
    Potency and Toxicity 19
    Categories of Toxicity 20
    Reversibility of Toxicity Response 21
    Hypersensitivity vs. Hyposensitivity 22
Study Questions and Exercises 23
Recommended Readings 23

Chapter 3 Factors That Influence Toxicity 25

Diet and Biotransformation 25
    Effect of Macronutrient Changes 26
        Protein 26
        Lipids 28
        Carbohydrates 28
    Effect of Micronutrient Changes 30
        Vitamins 31

Minerals	32
Gender and Age	32
Species	34
Study Questions and Exercises	34
Recommended Readings	35

Chapter 4 Food Safety Assessment Methods in the Laboratory: Toxicological Testing Methods 37

Analysis of Toxicants in Foods	38
Oral Ingestion Studies	40
Acute Toxicity Testing	41
Toxicology Screen	42
Dose-Range-Finding and Dose–Response Curve for Lethality	47
Subchronic Toxicity Testing	48
Chronic Toxicity Testing	50
Genetic Toxicity	51
Ames Tests	52
Host-Mediated Assays	52
Eukaryotic Cells, *In Vitro*	53
DNA Damage and Repair	53
Forward Mutations in Chinese Hamster Cells	54
Mouse Lymphoma Cell Assay	54
Sister Chromatid Exchanges	54
Eukaryotic Cells, *In Vivo*	54
Drosophila melanogaster	54
Micronucleus Test	55
Specialized Oral Ingestion Studies	55
Developmental Toxicity — Teratogenesis	55
Reproductive	56
Metabolic — Toxicokinetics	56
Study Questions and Exercises	58
Recommended Readings	58

Chapter 5 Food Safety Assessment: Compliance with Regulations 59

Good Laboratory Practices (GLPs)	59
General Provisions: Subpart A	60
Section 58.1 — Scope	60
Organization and Personnel: Subpart B	60
Personnel	60
Testing Facility Management	61
Study Director	61
Quality Assurance Unit	62
Facility: Subpart C	63
Section 58.41 — General	63

- Equipment: Subpart D 65
  - Equipment Design 65
  - Maintenance and Calibration of Equipment 65
- Testing Facilities Operation: Subpart E 65
  - Standard Operating Procedures 65
  - Reagents and Solutions 66
  - Animal Care 66
- Test and Control Articles: Subpart F 67
  - Test and Control Article Characterization 67
  - Test and Control Article Handling 67
  - Mixtures of Articles with Carriers 68
- Protocol for and Conduct of a Nonclinical Laboratory Study: Subpart G 68
  - Protocol — Section 58.120 68
  - Conduct of a Nonclinical Laboratory Study — Section 58.130 69
- Records and Reports: Subpart J 69
  - Reporting of Nonclinical Laboratory Study Results — Section 58.185 70
  - Storage and Retrieval of Records and Data — Section 58.190 70
  - Retention of Records — Section 58.195 71
- Good Manufacturing Practices 73
- Regulatory Agencies 73
  - The Food and Drug Administration 74
  - Centers for Disease Control and Prevention 74
  - U.S. Department of Agriculture 74
  - U.S. Environmental Protection Agency 75
  - Occupational Safety and Health Administration 75
  - The National Marine Fisheries Service 76
  - Local and State Agencies 76
  - International Agencies 76
- U.S. Food Laws 77
- Study Questions and Exercises 78
- Recommended Readings 80

Chapter 6   Risk 81

- Risk–Benefit 81
- Hazard Identification, Dose–Response, and Exposure Assessment 85
  - Dose–Response Assessment 86
  - Exposure Assessment 86
- Risk Characterization 87
  - Threshold Relationships 88
  - Nonthreshold Relationships 90
  - Risk Put into Perspective 91
- Study Questions and Exercises 92
- Recommended Readings 93

Chapter 7 Epidemiology in Food and Nutritional Toxicology 95

Descriptive Strategies 96
    Ecological Studies 96
    Case Reports 97
Analytical Strategies 97
    Cross-Sectional Studies 98
    Prospective Studies 98
    Retrospective Studies 99
    Meta-Analysis 100
Molecular Epidemiology 100
    Exposure–Dose Studies 102
    Physiological Studies 102
    Gene–Environment Interactions 102
Foodborne Diseases and Epidemiology 103
Study Questions and Exercises 103
Recommended Readings 104

Chapter 8 GI Tract Physiology and Biochemistry 105

Anatomy and Digestive Functions 105
Gut Absorption and Enterocyte Metabolism 110
    Passive Diffusion 110
    Carrier Mediated 111
    Endocytosis and Exocytosis 111
    Movement of Substances across Cellular Membranes 112
        Lipid-to-Water Partition Coefficient 112
        Ionization and Dissociation Constants 113
Transport into the Circulation 114
    Delivery of Toxicant from the Systemic Circulation to Tissues 114
    Storage Sites 115
        Plasma Proteins 115
    Liver and Kidney 116
    Bone 116
    Lipid Depots 117
    Physiologic Barriers to Toxicants 117
Fluid Balance and Diarrhea 118
    Treatment 119
Study Questions and Exercises 120
Recommended Readings 120

Chapter 9 Metabolism and Excretion of Toxicants 121

Metabolism of Toxicants 121
    Conversion with Intent to Excrete 121
    Biotransformation Enzymology 123
        Phase I or Type I Reactions 124

Reduction Reactions	130
Hydrolysis	131
Phase II or Type II Reactions	132
Oxidative Stress	134
Cellular Reductants and Antioxidants	138
Enzymatic Antioxidant Systems	139
Targets of Oxidative Stress Products	139
Excretion	140
Urinary Excretion	141
Biliary and Fecal Excretion	142
Pulmonary Gases	142
Other Routes of Excretion	143
Milk	143
Sweat and Saliva	143
Principles of Toxicokinetics	143
Design of a TK Study	144
One-Compartment TK	145
Volume of Distribution	146
Multicompartment Models	149
Study Questions and Exercises	150
Recommended Readings	150

Chapter 10 Food Intolerance and Allergy 151

Allergy and Types of Hypersensitivity	152
Primary Food Sensitivity	152
Nonimmunological Primary Food Sensitivities	155
Secondary Food Sensitivity	157
Symptoms and Diagnosis	157
Treatment	158
Study Questions and Exercises	159
Recommended Readings	159

SECTION II   Toxicants Found in Foods

Chapter 11 Bacterial Toxins 163

Intoxications	164
Bacillus cereus	164
Mode of Action	164
Clinical Symptoms	165
Clostridium botulinum	165
Mode of Action	166
Clinical Symptoms	166

Staphylococci ... 167
    Mode of Action ... 168
    Clinical Symptoms ... 168
Infections ... 168
  Salmonella ... 168
    Clinical Symptoms ... 169
  Campylobacter jejuni ... 170
    Clinical Symptoms ... 170
  Clostridium perfringens ... 171
    Clinical Symptoms ... 171
  Escherichia coli ... 171
    Enteropathogenic *Escherichia coli* (EPEC) ... 172
    Enteroinvasive *Escherichia coli* (EIEC) ... 172
    Enterotoxigenic *Escherichia coli* (ETEC) ... 173
    Escherichia coli O157:H7 (Enterohemorrhagic *E. coli* or EHEC) ... 173
  Listeria monocytogens ... 175
    Clinical Symptoms ... 175
  Shigella ... 175
    Clinical Symptoms ... 176
  Vibrio ... 176
    Clinical Symptoms ... 176
  Yersinia enterocolitica ... 177
    Clinical Symptoms ... 177
Study Questions and Exercises ... 177
Recommended Readings ... 177

Chapter 12 Animal Toxins and Plant Toxicants ... 179

Marine Animals ... 180
  Scombroid Poisoning ... 181
    Mode of Action ... 181
    Clinical Symptoms ... 181
  Saxitoxin ... 182
    Mode of Action ... 182
    Clinical Symptoms ... 182
  Pyropheophorbide-A ... 183
    Mode of Action ... 183
    Clinical Symptoms ... 183
  Tetrodotoxin ... 183
    Mode of Action ... 184
    Clinical Symptoms ... 184
  Ciguatoxin ... 184
    Mode of Action ... 185
    Clinical Signs ... 185

Plants 185
    Goitrogens 185
    Cyanogenic Glycosides 186
    Phenolic Substances 188
    Cholinesterase Inhibitors 192
        Clinical Symptoms 192
    Biogenic Amines 193
        Clinical Symptoms 193
Study Questions and Exercises 193
Recommended Readings 194

Chapter 13 Fungal Mycotoxins 195

Ergot Alkaloids and Ergotism 196
    Mode of Action and Clinical Symptoms 197
Aflatoxin 197
Trichothecenes 198
Penicillia Mycotoxins 201
    Rubratoxin 201
    Patulin 202
    Yellow Rice Toxins 202
Other Mycotoxins 202
Study Questions and Exercises 203
Recommended Readings 203

Chapter 14 Toxicity of Nutrients 205

Macronutrients 205
    Carbohydrates 205
    Lipids 206
    Protein 207
Micronutrients 207
    Vitamins 207
        Fat-Soluble Vitamins 208
        Water-Soluble Vitamins 209
    Minerals and Trace Elements 209
        Magnesium 210
        Iron 210
        Zinc 210
        Copper 210
        Manganese 211
        Selenium 211
Antinutrients 211
    Antiproteins 211
    Antiminerals 212
    Antivitamins 212

Study Questions and Exercises 213
Recommended Readings 213

Chapter 15 Parasites, Viruses, and Prions 215

Protozoa 215
    E. histolytica..215
    Giardia lamblia 216
    Toxoplasma gondii 216
Worms 216
    Roundworms 216
        Trichinella spiralis 217
        Ascaris lumbricoides 217
        Anisakids 217
    Tapeworms 218
Viruses..218
Prions (Proteinaceous Infectious Particles)..223
    Diagnosing for BSE...225
Study Questions and Exercises 226
Recommended Readings 227

SECTION III   Food Contamination and Safety

Chapter 16 Residues in Foods 231

Insecticides..231
    DDT (1,1'-(2,2,2-Trichloroethylidene)bis(4-Chlorobenzene)......................232
    Organophosphates 234
    Carbamates 235
    Cyclodiene Insecticides..236
Herbicides 237
    Chlorophenoxy Acid Esters (Phenoxyalipatic Acids) 237
        Bipyridyliums..238
Fungicides...238
Industrial and Environmental Contaminants.......................................239
    Halogenated Hydrocarbons..239
        Polychlorinated Biphenyls 239
        Dioxins 241
    Heavy Metals 242
        Mercury 242
        Lead..244
        Cadmium 245
        Arsenic 246
Study Questions and Exercises 247
Recommended Readings 247

Chapter 17 Food Additives, Colors, and Flavors 249

Preservatives 251
    Benzoic Acid and Sodium Benzoate (Figure 17.1) 251
    Sorbate (Figure 17.2) 251
    Hydrogen Peroxide (Figure 17.3) 252
    Nitrite and Nitrate 252
Antioxidants 252
    Ascorbic Acid 252
    Tocopherol 253
    Propyl Gallate 253
    BHT and BHA 253
Sweeteners 254
    Saccharin 254
    Sodium Cyclamate 254
    Aspartame 255
    Acesulfame 255
    Sugar Alcohols 256
    Alitame 256
    D-Tagatose 256
    Sucralose 256
Coloring Agents 256
    Red No. 2 (Amaranth) 257
    Red No. 3 258
    Yellow No. 4 (Tartrazine) 258
    Methyl Anthranilate 258
    Safrole 258
    Monosodium Glutamate (MSG) 259
Study Questions and Exercises 259
Recommended Readings 259

Chapter 18 Food Irradiation 261

History of Food Irradiation 262
Types of Irradiation 265
Effectiveness of Irradiation 267
By-Products of Irradiation 268
Misconceptions 269
Regulations 269
Study Questions and Exercises 271
Recommended Readings 271

Chapter 19 Polycyclic Aromatic Hydrocarbons and Other Processing
                 Products 273

Benzo(α)pyrene and Polycyclic Aromatic Hydrocarbons 273
Hetrocyclic Amines 275

Nitrates, Nitrites, and Nitrosamines 279
Products of the Maillard Reaction 281
Study Questions and Exercises 283
Recommended Readings 283

Chapter 20 Emerging Food Safety Issues in a Modern World 285
HACCP 285
    Developing an HACCP Plan...287
        Assemble the HACCP Team..287
        Describe the Food and Its Distribution 287
        Describe the Intended Use and Consumers of the Food 287
        Develop a Flow Diagram Describing the Process 287
        Verify the Flow Diagram 288
    Principle 1: Hazard Analysis 288
    Principle 2: Determine Critical Control Points (CCPs)...............................288
    Principle 3: Establish Critical Limits for Preventive Measures..................289
    Principle 4: Establish Procedures to Monitor CCPs 289
    Principle 5: Corrective Action When a Critical Limit Is Exceeded 290
    Principle 6: Effective Record-Keeping Systems 291
    Principle 7: Verify That the HAACP System Is Working...........................291
Antibiotic Resistance...293
    Scope of the Problem..295
GMOs...296
    Pest Resistance..298
    Herbicide Tolerance 298
    Disease Resistance..298
    Cold Tolerance 298
    Drought Tolerance and Salinity Tolerance 298
    Nutrition 299
    Pharmaceuticals...299
    Phytoremediation 299
    Environmental Hazards...300
        Unintended Harm to Other Organisms...300
        Reduced Effectiveness of Pesticides..300
        Gene Transfer to Nontarget Species..300
    Human Health Risks 301
        Allergenicity...301
        Unknown Effects on Human Health..301
    Economic Concerns 301
    GMO Foods and Labeling 303
    Conclusion...304
Study Questions and Exercises 305
Recommended Readings 305

Index..307

Section I

Fundamental Concepts

1 An Overview of Food and Nutritional Toxicology

DEFINING THE TERMS AND SCOPE OF FOOD AND NUTRITIONAL TOXICOLOGY

TOXICOLOGY

In essence, toxicology is the science of poisons, toxicants, or toxins. A poison, toxicant, or toxin is a substance capable of causing harm when administered to an organism. Harm can be defined as seriously injuring or, ultimately, causing the death of an organism. This is a rather simplistic definition, because virtually every known chemical or substance has the potential for causing harm. The term *toxicant* can be a synonym for *poison*, or the term *poison* might be more appropriate for the most potent substances, i.e., substances that induce adverse effects at exposure levels of a few milligrams per kilogram of body weight (see later discussion). The term *toxin* usually refers to a poison derived from a protein or conjugated protein produced by some higher plant, animal, or pathogenic bacteria that is highly poisonous for other living organisms, e.g., botulinum toxins. Toxicologists study the noxious or adverse effects of substances on living organisms or on *in vitro* surrogate models, such as cell and tissue cultures. The substances toxicologists study are usually chemical compounds but may be elemental or complex materials. Radioactive elements, heavy metals (e.g., mercury or lead), or the packing materials used in food processing are examples of such substances. Food toxicology deals with substances found in food that might be harmful to those who consume sufficient quantities of the food containing such substances. On rare occasions, common foods are contaminated with unacceptably high levels of toxicants. Such substances can be inherent toxicants, substances naturally found in foods, or contaminants, which are substances that find their way into food either during the preparation or processing of such foods.

Nutritional toxicology is the study of the nutritional aspects of toxicology. Nutritional toxicology is related to and might even overlap but is not synonymous with food toxicology. Food toxicology emphasizes toxicants or toxins found in foods, whereas nutritional toxicology targets the interrelations that toxicants or toxins have with nutrients in the diet, which affect nutritional status. Nutritional toxicology can refer to the means by which the diet or components of the diet prevent against the adverse effects of toxicants or toxins.

It is likely that the first experience humans had with toxicology was with a toxicant found in food. The science of toxicology has been studied since antiquity,

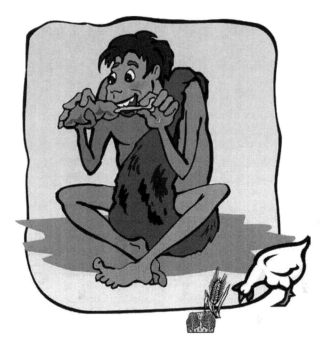

FIGURE 1.1 Early humans: What to eat?

starting when humans first realized that they had to be cautious with food selection or suffer dire consequences. Our ancestors probably learned from trial and error and by observation about which food sources satisfied hunger and which led to illness or death. As illustrated in the cartoon in Figure 1.1, early humans were quick to either learn or suffer the consequences of deciding whether to eat a plant where dead animals lay. Thus, our ancestors developed dietary habits that allowed for the survival, growth, and reproduction of the species.

Hemlock and various other poisons were known and studied by the ancient Greeks. The fundamental concept of toxicology — the dose determines the poison — was conceived by Paracelsus (1493 to 1541) and based on his commentary that all substances are poisons; there is none which is not a poison and the right dose determines the poison from a cure. Therefore, the premise that anything has the potential to be a poison if taken in a large enough dose dictates the scope of toxicology, which is to quantitate and interpret the toxicity of substances. Most toxicologists deal with exogenous compounds, or those compounds that are not part of the normal metabolism of organisms, i.e., xenobiotic or foreign compounds. Food and nutritional toxicologists deal with toxicants in food, the health effects of high nutrient intakes, and the interactions between toxicants and nutrients.

FOOD AND NUTRITIONAL TOXICOLOGY

Development of toxicology as a distinct science has been slow as compared with the sciences of pharmacology, biochemistry, and nutrition. Many toxicologists were trained in other disciplines and subsequently were rich in diversity. Food and nutritional toxicology can be considered an emerging subdiscipline of toxicology. The area of food and nutritional toxicology bridges traditional sciences and can be regarded as a branch of either nutrition, food science, or toxicology. In addition, there are significant contributions from other sciences, both new and emerging, to food and nutritional toxicology, e.g., behavior sciences, epidemiology, molecular biology, environmental sciences, public health, immunology, and microbiology. In the following chapters we will discuss some current research that deals with the effects, both good and bad, of food components on the modulation of the immune response or alterations of behavior.

Food safety is another area that can be encompassed within food and nutritional toxicology. Within the food safety arena we deal with the regulatory and consumer or economic implications of toxicity issues related to our food supply. Our concerns about food safety are not new. Around the time of the Civil War, W.O. Atwater warned in *Harper's Weekly* that city people were in constant danger of buying unwholesome meat and finding meat coated with glycerine to give it the appearance of freshness. It was common at that time to find milk diluted with water, coffee adulterated with charcoal, or cocoa mixed with sawdust. Upton Sinclair's *The Jungle* was a startling wake-up call and prompted the start of governmental controls on the food industry. Even at present, it seems that there are reports almost daily of a food or food constituent whose safety has come under scrutiny. So sometimes it is hard not to succumb to the belief that a food safety crisis exists; however, when these concerns and claims are put into perspective, one can understand why the U.S. still has the safest, cheapest, and most varied food in the world.

TOXICANTS IN FOODS AND THEIR EFFECTS ON NUTRITION

Potential sources of toxicants in food include nutrients, natural food toxicants, contaminants, and chemicals or substances intentionally added to food (food additives).

NUTRIENTS

One usually does not relate the ingestion of a specific nutrient with concerns about the toxicity of that nutrient. However, intakes of essential dietary chemicals from zero to excessive produce responses, from lethal because of nutrient deficiency to an optimal health response and back to lethal because of intolerably high concentrations. Thus, as the solid line in Figure 1.2 illustrates, an organism cannot tolerate either of the two extremes over an extended period. The figure illustrates that there will be intakes, both low and high, associated with lethality. Also, there will be minimum low and maximum high intakes associated with good health and a valley associated with optimal health. The valley of the curve for optimal health will vary, depending on a number of physical, biochemical, or physiological effects of the nutrient. For example, the intake level of vitamin E for optimal health has a rather wide valley compared with that for intake levels of vitamin D, vitamin A, or various essential metals for optimal health.

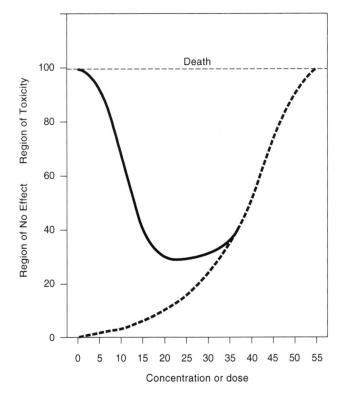

FIGURE 1.2 Concentration (dose) effect of nutrients (solid line) compared with a typical dose–response curve (dashed line).

With the exception of vitamin D, vitamin A, and some minerals, the intake of nutrients from natural food sources will not pose any significant health problems. However, one can argue that the health problems associated with high intakes of protein, fats, or energy are really manifestations of nutrient toxicity, i.e., cardiovascular diseases, cancers, and eye diseases such as macular degeneration and other chronic diseases. The other potential means whereby nutrient intakes can present health problems is the abuse of nutrient supplementation. A nonfood source of a nutrient can produce pharmacological actions at concentrations well above normal dietary amounts.

Over the last few years, dietary reference intakes (DRIs) have been developed by the Food and Nutrition Board of the National Academy of Sciences. The premise for developing DRIs is that such values reflect the current knowledge of nutrients, particularly with respect to their role in diet and chronic diseases. Similar to recommended dietary allowances (RDAs), DRIs are reference values for nutrient intakes to be used in assessing and planning diets for healthy people. A vital component involved in the development of DRIs is the value for tolerable upper level (UL). UL may be defined as the point beyond which a higher intake of a nutrient could be harmful. UL is the highest level of daily nutrient intake that is likely to pose no risk of adverse health effects in almost all individuals in a specified life stage group. The

An Overview of Food and Nutritional Toxicology

interest in developing ULs is partly in response to the growing interest in dietary supplements that contain large amounts of essential nutrients; the other concern is the increased fortification of foods with nutrients. For example, for vitamin C and selenium, the UL refers to total intake from food, fortified food, and nutrient supplements, whereas for vitamin E it might refer only to intakes from supplements, pharmacological agents, or their combination. Often, ULs apply to nutrient intake from supplements because it would be extremely unusual to obtain such large quantities of a specific nutrient in food form.

A risk assessment model was used to derive specific ULs, which included a systematic series of scientific considerations and judgements. The ULs were not intended to be recommended levels of intake because there are little established benefits for healthy individuals if they consume a nutrient in amounts greater than the RDA. Also, the safety of routine long-term intakes above the UL is not well established. The objective of ULs is to indicate the need to exercise caution in consuming amounts greater than the recommended intakes. It does not mean that high intakes pose no risk of adverse effects.

NATURALLY OCCURRING TOXICANTS

The notion that potentially toxic substances can be commonly found in conventional foods is difficult for the layperson and some well-educated people to accept. On an emotional level, food is regarded as that which sustains life, should be pure, unadulterated, and sometimes has a spiritual aura. Thus, many individuals are astonished to find that plants and some animals that are sources of food can produce an array of chemicals that can be harmful. There are some notable examples. A well-acknowledged naturally occurring toxicant is the toxin produced by the puffer fish, *Fugu rubripes*, which is popular in Japanese cuisine. Another example is the poisonous mushroom *Amanita muscaria*. The production of toxicants is more common than one might first realize. Plants produce both primary and secondary metabolic products. In the plant kingdom, many phytochemicals are produced as secondary metabolites, e.g., metabolic by-products of metabolism, excretion, and elimination. Through evolution, some of these secondary metabolites have become important defense chemicals used by the plant against insects and other organisms. The plant's weapons are not as technological as the one shown in the cartoon in Figure 1.3, but many are quite sophisticated biochemically. Primary metabolites are chemicals that have key roles in important physiological plant processes such as photosynthesis, lipid-energy and nucleic acid metabolism, and synthesis. It is likely that secondary metabolites evolved in response to and interaction with organisms of the animal and plant kingdoms or certain herbivores and pathogens. Recent advances in genetically modified foods have used such knowledge for developing plants with the ability to better defend themselves against disease and predators.

FOOD ADDITIVES AND CONTAMINANTS

A wide variety of chemicals enter foods during processing either because they are intentionally added or the food becomes contaminated with various substances. Food

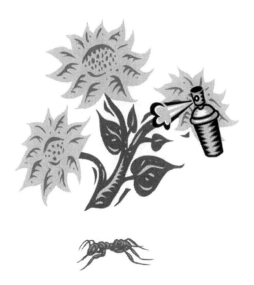

FIGURE 1.3 Plants have natural weapons.

additives include chemical preservatives such as butylated hydroxytoluene (BHT) and nitrite and microbial retardants such as calcium propionate. The food industry adds chemicals as texturing agents and flavors. Various chemicals may enter the food chain at different stages of processing, such as residues from fertilizers, pesticides, veterinary pharmaceuticals and drugs, and environmental chemicals such as lead or polychlorinated biphenyl (PCB). Some additives are generally recognized as safe (GRAS) items and require no testing for safety. Others require a battery of tests to ensure their safety for use in consumer foods.

Food additives can provide many benefits for the consumer and the food producer. Longer shelf life is advantageous not only to the producer but also to the consumer, for whom a longer shelf life means lower prices, reduced spoilage and waste, and fewer trips to the grocery store to stock up. However, some may argue whether such convenience is a benefit or a ploy by the industry to use more of their products. There are a multitude of reasons for using additives, some less meritorious than others (green catsup, anyone?). The bottom line is whether the product is safer with the additive present. Does the product have nutritional negatives, i.e., is it less nutrient dense or higher in saturated fats?

IMPACT OF DIET ON THE EFFECTS OF TOXICANTS

For several decades, nutritional research was concentrated on establishing a better understanding of macronutrients and micronutrients. The lack or deficiency of any specific nutrient will have devastating health ramifications. The lack of any specific nutrient in the diet may affect protein synthesis. It may produce membrane alteration, resulting in the loss of cellular structural integrity and changes in membrane permeability or various functional abilities of various macromolecules, which can subsequently affect the ability of the organism to metabolize various toxicants.

Several nutrients have been recognized for their roles in protecting against the toxic effects of noxious chemicals such as alcohol and free radicals. Recent research has directed our attention to studying other chemicals in the diets, studying phytochemicals, and reexamining how macro- and micronutrients may modulate our response to various toxicants. Specific phytochemicals have been found to act as anticancer agents and antioxidants, and to have other potential health benefits.

However, with these exciting advances in nutrition and health will arise concerns about safety and efficacy that must be addressed. Thus, with such advances, we can expect to see the field of food and nutritional toxicology at the forefront, addressing issues of mechanisms of action, risk, and safety and what is appropriate for optimal health.

STUDY QUESTIONS AND EXERCISES

1. Define toxicology, food toxicology and nutritional toxicology, phytochemical, and toxin.
2. Describe how toxicants might affect nutrition and health.
3. How might an organism's diet impact on the effects of a toxicant?

RECOMMENDED READINGS

Hatchcock, J.N., *Nutritional Toxicology*, Academic Press, New York, 1982.
Institute of Medicine, Food and Nutrition Board, *Dietary Reference Intake*, National Academy Press, Washington, D.C., 1997, 1998, 2000, 2001, and 2002.
Jones, J.M., *Food Safety*, Egan Press, St. Paul, MN, 1992.
Ottoboni, M.A., *The Dose Makes the Poison*, 2nd ed., John Wiley & Sons, New York, 1997.
Shibamoto, T. and Bjeldanes, L.F., *Introduction to Food Toxicology*, Academic Press, San Diego, CA, 1993.

2 General Principles of Toxicology

PHASES OF TOXICOLOGICAL EFFECTS

The genesis of toxicological effects, or biological effects, is an inordinately complex process involving many parts or steps. It is useful to categorize toxicological effects into three phases (Figure 2.1): (1) the exposure phase, which covers those factors that are responsible for determining the concentration of a toxic substance that effectively comes in contact with an organism; (2) the toxicokinetic phase, which includes the physiological processes that influence the concentration of the toxic substance or its active metabolite at the active site or receptors in the organism; and (3) the toxicodynamic phase, which includes interactions of the toxic substance with its molecular site of action and the biochemical or biophysical events that finally lead to the toxic effects observed. The details of each phase are discussed in this chapter.

Exposure Phase

For absorption, a toxic substance must be present in a molecular form that can be dispensed and be relatively lipophilic to penetrate biological membranes. The degree of ionization of the substance and the pH at the site of absorption are critical factors that affect the bioavailability and absorption of a toxic substance. Bioavailability is a measure of the degree to which a substance becomes available to the body after ingestion and is therefore available to the tissues. Many interactions between the toxic substance and various components in food influence the absorption of compounds. Therefore, various factors contribute to the exposure profile of a toxic substance's ability to be available to the organism.

In many situations, the uptake and elimination of a toxicant is mostly by passive diffusion processes, and a bioaccumulation factor, K_b, can represent a partition coefficient for the toxicant substance between the organism and its environment, i.e., a reversible partition between the two compartments of oil (representing the membrane) and water (representing the aqueous or cytosol). For example, an octanol–water model system can be used as an index of the relevant lipophilicity of a toxic substance. Therefore, if C_o is the aqueous concentration and C_i is the concentration in the lipid membrane of the organism, the reversible partition between the two compartments is described as:

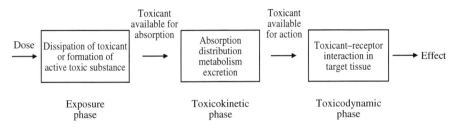

FIGURE 2.1 The three phases of toxicological effects.

$$C_o \underset{k_2}{\overset{k_1}{\longleftrightarrow}} C_i$$

The influx can be described as:

$$\frac{dC_t}{dt} = k_1 C_o - k_2 C$$

where k_1 and k_2 are first-order rate constants. Therefore, at equilibrium:

$$k_1 C_o - k_2 C_i \quad \text{or} \quad \frac{k_1}{k_2} = \frac{C_i}{C_o} = K_b$$

If C_o is virtually zero, then:

$$\frac{dC_t}{dt} = -k_2 Ci$$

For C_{i1} and C_{i2} and t_1 and t_2, respectively, the following is true:

$$\ln C_{i1} - \ln C_{i2} = k_2(t_2 - t_1)$$

For the half-life ($t_{1/2}$) of the toxicant, the following is derived:

$$\frac{C_{i2}}{C_{i1}} = 2 \quad \text{and} \quad (t_2 - t_1) = t_{1/2} = \frac{\ln 2}{k_2}$$

The partition coefficient of agents in an octanol–water system, as a rule, can be used as an index of the relevant lipophilicity of the substance. If the lipophilicity (log$P$) is plotted against the bioaccumulation factor (logK_b) for a number of compounds

General Principles of Toxicology

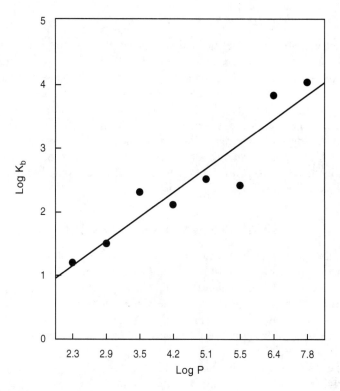

FIGURE 2.2 The linear relationship between lipophilicity (log$P$) and bioaccumulation factor (logK_b).

with varying lipophilicities, a linear relationship, as expected, is obtained. Figure 2.2 shows an example of this linear relationship taken from the literature.

TOXICOKINETIC PHASE

All of the physiological processes and factors involved in absorption, distribution, biotransformation, and excretion of a toxicant comprise the toxicokinetic phase. For the concentration of toxicant that is ingested by an organism, a fraction of the dose reaches the general circulation or becomes available systemically. The remaining dose is eliminated as waste in the feces. If the toxicant is ingested only once, availability will depend on the dose, rate of absorption, and rate of elimination. In a chronic exposure, the plasma concentration eventually reaches a steady-state level, i.e., the quantity absorbed is equal to the quantity eliminated per unit of time. Usually, elimination increases as plasma concentration increases. The amount of toxicant that reaches the target or receptor sites is designated as toxicologically available or bioavailable. However, the situation is complicated by the fact that toxicants may be converted to other products or metabolites that results in bioactivation or biotoxification. Bioactivation occurs when the metabolite is bioactive and biotoxification occurs when the metabolite is biologically inactive.

Toxicodynamic Phase

The processes involved in the interaction between the toxicant and its molecular sites of action constitute the toxicodynamic phase. Molecular sites of action include receptors for reversibly acting substances or sites that are responsible for the induction of chemical lesions for nonreversibly acting toxicants. The origin of toxicodynamics is pharmacodynamics, the beginning of which can be traced back to the early 1800s. Students in pharmacology were taught that the mode of action of drugs should be investigated by scientific means in order to introduce a more rational basis for therapy (a revolutionary approach for the time). The study of metabolism and statistical methods raised pharmacology to the level of an exact discipline equal in status to that of chemistry and physiology.

DOSE–RESPONSE RELATIONSHIP

No chemical agent is entirely safe and no chemical agent should be considered entirely harmful. The single most important factor determining the potential harmfulness or safeness of a compound is the relationship between the concentration of the chemical and the effect produced on the biological mechanism. A chemical can be permitted to come in contact with a biological mechanism without producing an effect on the mechanism, provided the concentration of the chemical agent is below a minimal effective level.

If one considers that the ultimate effect is manifested as an all-or-none response, or a quantal response such as death, and that a minimal concentration produces no effect, then there must be a range of concentrations of the chemical that will give a graded effect somewhere between the two extremes. The experimental determination of this range of doses is the basis of the dose–response relationship.

Toxicologists attempt to determine the cause-and-effect relationship between a given compound and an organism to establish what is considered a safe level for humans. Human exposure data are usually limited or not available, and a toxicologist often has to use animal models. Some people are against the use of animals, but it is unethical to test potentially toxic compounds on humans, and it is generally agreed that the benefits to society, such as safer consumer products and improvement in health from food and pharmaceutical development, far outweigh the objections for using animals as surrogates. The tragic event of thalidomide, which was used by mothers to prevent morning sickness, causing unfortunate deformities in newborns could have been avoided with proper animal toxicity studies. This catastrophic history also highlights the limitation of surrogates or alternative toxicity methods such as cell cultures or computer simulations. Toxicity studies provide systematic ways to measure the adverse effects of compounds, and to understand the relationship between a dose and the route of exposure and metabolism is vital. Toxicity testing must inevitably be performed largely on laboratory animals. It is advisable to use at least two phytogenetically different species for this purpose. Rats and dogs are most commonly used, but particular effects may have to be examined on a wider variety of animals, including nonhuman primates. Although the reactions of animal models are often surprisingly similar to those exhibited by humans, it is known that

General Principles of Toxicology

some substances (e.g., amphetamines) are metabolized along different routes in humans and dogs. Thus, a toxicant may not reproduce in humans the effects recorded in the animal species, and when assessing the potentiality of a new food substance care has to be taken to not assume too close a parallelism between the reactions of the two species.

Toxicity testing, no matter how carefully performed, cannot be expected to reveal all the potential adverse effects. Apart from the difficulty of predicting the responses of humans from the results of animal experiments, some toxic effects appear in only a minority of subjects. For example, antibiotics are among the safest of drugs; however, rarely, penicillin administration initiates a fatal anaphylactic reaction. The purpose of toxicity tests is to make a realistic assessment of the potential hazards in relation to the benefits likely to follow after use of the compound. In the final analysis, it is impossible to make this assessment with any assurance until the substance has been in actual use for many years.

Dose–response refers to the relationship between the exposure dose of a substance and the response of the organism ingesting the substance. A dose–response relationship is determined by experiments, usually done with laboratory animals, in which groups of individuals are dosed with the substance over a range of concentration. The animals are observed for symptoms for an endpoint, which must be measurable and quantifiable. The endpoint can be a physiological response, a biochemical change, or a behavior response. It is important to keep in mind that, when measuring the toxicity of a substance, the endpoint selected is relevant to organisms of the same species as well as among different species. Endpoints often selected for toxicity studies include, among others, the effective dose (ED) and the lethal dose (LD). ED endpoints are usually therapeutic efficacies, such as the dose to produce anesthesia or analgesia. For acute toxicity studies, a measure of LD_{50} is often used. The calculated LD_{50} is the statistically estimated dose that when administered to a population will result in the death of 50% of the population. Figure 2.3 graphically represents this concept. The relationship between dose and response is typically sigmoid in shape. Some individuals within a population show an intense response whereas others show a minimal response to the same dose of the toxicant. For a lethal compound at a particular dose, some animals will succumb to the dose whereas others will not. There are variations among a homogeneous population, be it animals or cells, and there are a range of responses depending on the endpoint measured. Basically, the dose–response curve will be the familiar Gaussian curve (bell-shaped, see later) describing a normal distribution in biological systems. The deviation of response around an otherwise uniform population is a function of biological variation in the population itself. Thus, it is difficult to predict beforehand what effect a compound under study will have on an individual within a population. Some animals respond at low doses whereas others do at high doses, with the majority responding at around the median dose.

FREQUENCY RESPONSE

Under practical conditions, differences exist between the individual members of a supposedly homogenous population of cells, tissues, or animals. Differences are

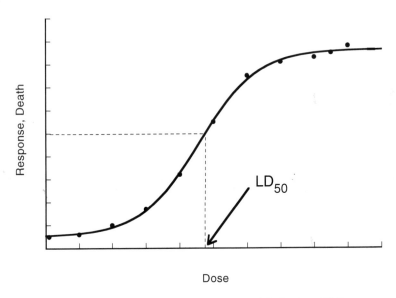

FIGURE 2.3 A typical sigmoidal dose–response curve and derivation of LD_{50}.

seldom obvious but become evident when a biological mechanism is challenged, such as by exposure to a chemical agent.

If a chemical is capable of producing a response (such as death), and the response is quantitated, not all members of the group will respond to the same dose in an identical manner. What was considered as an all-or-none response applies only to a single member of the test group and is actually found to be a graded response when viewed with respect to the entire group. Such deviations in the response of apparently uniform populations to a given concentration of the chemical are generally ascribed to result from biological variation. In response to a toxicant, biological variation within members of a species is usually low compared with variation between species. The species population differences reflect metabolic or biochemical variations within the species itself. Testing a toxicant's effect on a homogeneous animal population eliminates the potential causes of high variation that might occur in a heterogeneous population, if gender and age are controlled. Homogeneity of test subjects allows for valid comparisons between members of a population, and they share common characteristics. Thus, toxicity studies often use inbred strains of rodents or organisms.

Figure 2.4 illustrates the response of any given population to a range of doses. The criteria of an experiment for toxicity testing are that the response is quantitated and that each animal in a series of supposedly uniform members of a species may be given an adequate dose of the chemical to produce an identical response. Such data can be plotted in the form of a distribution or frequency–response curve, which typically follows a bell-shaped or Gaussian distribution. The frequency–response curve plots identical response vs. dose (quantal response curve) and represents the range of doses required to produce a quantitatively identical response in a large population of test subjects. In a large population, a large percentage of the animals

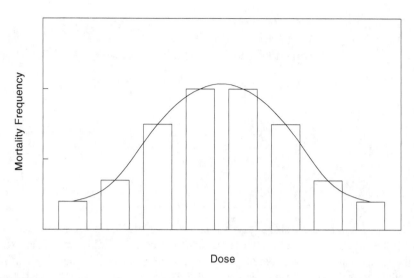

FIGURE 2.4 A typical bell-shaped frequency response for mortality, comparing death with dose.

that receive a certain dose will respond in a quantitatively identical manner, such as a particular response, e.g., death. If the dose is varied between low and high, some animals will exhibit the same response to a low dose whereas others will require a higher dose. The curve indicates that a large percentage of the animals receiving a given dose will respond in a quantitatively identical manner. As the dose varies in either direction from the x-axis, some animals will show the same response to a lower or higher dose.

In practical applications, the frequency distribution is skewed toward the low- or high-dose side when the data is applied to methods seeking the best-fitting curve. In a Gaussian distribution, one typically finds that 66% of the responses are within one standard deviation of the mean dose. Eighty-six percent of the individuals will respond to a dose within two standard deviations of the mean and 95% within three standard deviations. Thus, toxicological data may be analyzed in a manner that allows one to use acceptable statistical methods in evaluating the results. In practice, the toxicologist usually analyzes the data from an experiment by first transforming the results into cumulative distribution. Frequency response curves are not commonly used. The convention is to plot the data in the form of a curve relating the dose of the chemical to cumulative percentage of animals showing the response (death). Defining the dose–response curves involves doing an experiment by using groups of homogenous species given a substance at different doses. The dose to give to each group is found experimentally and should be at a level that does not kill all the animals in a group. The initial dose may be very low so as not to kill most of the animals. The intermediate doses can be multiples (logarithmic basis). Plotting the data in the form of a curve relating the dose of the toxicant to a cumulative percentage of animals demonstrating the response gives the sigmoid dose–response curve shown in Figure 2.3.

TABLE 2.1
Percent Response, NEDs, and Probits

Percent Response	NED	Probit
0.1	−3	2
2.3	−2	3
15.9	−1	4
50.0	0	5
84.1	+1	6
97.7	+2	7
99.9	+3	8

The plot can be divided into several important areas. First there is a linear area, where the incidence of the quantal response is directly related to the concentration of the compound. It is also apparent that the compound may be considered as harmful or safe, depending on the dose given. The LD_{50} is a statistically obtained visual value, which is the best estimation of the dose required to produce death in 50% of the population. This value is always accompanied by an estimate of the error of the value. The LD_{50} can be derived graphically by drawing a horizontal line from 50% and dropping a vertical from intersection. The LD_{84}, LD_{16}, etc., values can be similarly determined. In practice, a normal distribution is more likely to occur if the scale of the abscissa is logarithmic rather than linear. If a plot of the actual doses against the response gives a normal distribution, a similar distribution will emerge if the logarithms of the doses are used in the graph. There is no disadvantage in basing calculations on the logarithms of doses even in situations in which the doses themselves could have been used.

Because quantal dose–response phenomena are usually normally distributed, one can convert the percent response to units of deviations from the mean, the so-called normal equivalent deviations (NEDs), or convert to probit units. The NED is defined for any value of the log (dose) as $(x - \bar{x})/\delta$; it represents the distance, in multiples of the standard deviation, of the point x from the mean $\bar{x}$. For values of x less than $\bar{x}$, the normal equivalent deviation is a negative quantity and for arithmetical convenience the negative values of the deviation are eliminated by adding 5 to the normal equivalent deviation. This gives the probit (a contraction of probability unit). The quantity 5 is chosen because it brings the zero of the probit scale to a point located five standard deviations below the mean. For example, the normal equivalent unit for a 50% response is zero, which equals a probit unit of 5. Table 2.1 lists other conversions.

Note that probits are related to mortality in the same way as the doses themselves. Thus, the relationship between probits and doses is a straight line.

In an NED or probit transformation, an adjustment of quantal data to an assumed normal population distribution is accomplished, which results in a straight line. The LD_{50} is obtained by drawing a horizontal line from the NED of zero or a probit of 5, which is the 50% mortality point, to the dose–effect line. At the point of intersection, a vertical line is drawn and at its intersection of the x-axis is the LD_{50} point.

General Principles of Toxicology

Such transformations of the data can be useful to determine lethal doses for 90% or for 10% of the animals. In addition, the slope of the dose–response curve can be obtained, which can be useful for comparisons.

Tables are available that enable percentages to be converted directly into probits. Alternatively, it is possible to use a special graph paper (probit paper) in which the ordinates are ruled on a probit scale and the abscissa on a logarithmic scale.

POTENCY AND TOXICITY

As Figure 2.5 illustrates, the relative toxicities of two compounds can be compared provided the slopes of the dose–response curves are roughly parallel. If the LD_{50} for B is greater than that of A, B is less potent than A. An example is comparing the relative toxicities of two compounds in relation to the doses required to produce an equal effect — death. However, the LD_{50} for one may be in micrograms and for the other in grams. Two or more compounds having approximately the same slopes suggest similar mechanisms of toxic action. Compound C in Figure 2.5 is likely not to have the same mechanism of action as compounds A and B. Note that the LD_{50} of C is more than the LD_{50} of A and B, but the reverse is true for LD_5s of compounds C and B. Compound C is less toxic than A or B at LD_{95}.

The relative toxicity of similarly shaped curves shifts to the right as toxicity decreases. A higher concentration of a toxicant is needed to evoke the same response as that of a toxicant that is more toxic. As the curves get closer to the y-axis, the toxicant becomes more potent, i.e., the higher-potency toxicant is required at lower concentrations to evoke the same response. As the curve moves farther from the y-axis to the right, there is a decrease in toxicity, i.e., more toxicant is required to get

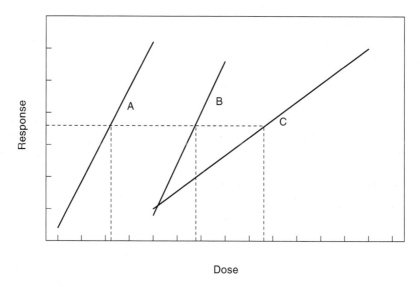

FIGURE 2.5 Dose–response curves: different slopes for different mechanisms of action. Compound A has the same slope as compound B, but the slopes of both compounds A and B are different from that of compound C.

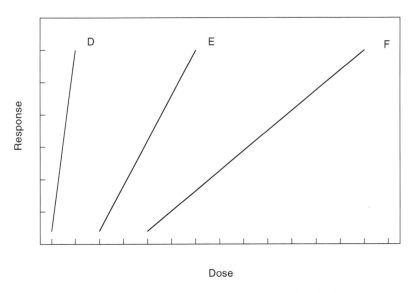

FIGURE 2.6 Slopes of dose–response curves influence the margin of safety.

an equal response. Therefore, potency of a compound is related to its toxicity. A more potent toxicant elicits a toxic response at lower concentrations, and vice versa. As shown in Figure 2.5, for two compounds, a variety of slopes are possible when the dose–response data for different compounds are plotted. Every compound has an identifiable slope for its dose–response relationship.

The slope of a curve can be used as an index of the "margin of safety," which is defined as the magnitude of the range of doses involved in progressing from a noneffective dose to a lethal one. The dosages range between the dose producing a lethal effect and the dose not producing a lethal or desired effect. In Figure 2.6, compound F has a higher margin of safety than compound E. If the slopes are parallel, the margin of safety might not be different.

Death is the ultimate extreme in toxicity; however, other effects are possible, from desirable through just undesirable to harmful. Examples can be found with drugs, because drugs have side effects. As a rule, a chemical is a drug if undesirable actions are not significant in comparison with desirable actions. Morphine produces analgesia but also respiratory depression, and antihistamines or penicillin may initiate undesirable immunological actions. Undesirable effects are dose-related too. Thus, in the board view, any adverse effect or potentially undesirable side effect can be used to determine a dose–response curve.

CATEGORIES OF TOXICITY

When classifying compounds as toxic, extremely toxic, or nontoxic, a practical and useful consideration is where to draw the line in toxicity classification. It is apparent that toxicity is relative and must be described as a relative dose–effect relationship between compounds. However, it is also clear that the concept of toxicity as a relative

TABLE 2.2
Categories of Toxicity

	Dose	
	Metric Concentration (Per kg of Body Weight)	U.S. Standard Weight (Per 150 lb) (oz.)
Extremely toxic	≤1 mg/kg	0.003
Highly toxic	1–50 mg/kg	0.003–0.1
Moderately toxic	50–500 mg/kg	0.1–1.2
Slightly toxic	0.5–5 g/kg	1.2–12.4
Practically nontoxic	5–15 g/kg	12.4–37
Relatively harmless	>15 g/kg	>37

phenomenon is true only if the slopes of the curves of the dose–response relationship for the compounds are essentially identical.

Table 2.2 is a useful guide that categorizes toxicity on the basis of amounts of a substance necessary to produce harm, i.e., a lethal dose, based on metric or U.S. standard weights. This information helps classify substances based on weights.

Another way to categorize lethal doses is by comparing compound ratios of minimal toxic level to the minimal adequate level, as might be done for nutrients. For example, when comparing biotin (toxic dose of 50 mg) and vitamin A (a toxic dose of 5 mg), it is observed that it takes 10 times more of the toxic oral dose of biotin to produce an adverse effect. Toxicity is relative and must be described as a relative dose–effect relation among compounds.

REVERSIBILITY OF TOXICITY RESPONSE

Any consideration of the relative safety of a chemical must also take into account the degree to which the response to the toxicant is reversible. In other words, as the concentration of the substance decreases in the tissues and it is eliminated from the body, will the effects of the toxicant be reversed? It is known that after a single exposure (a one-time ingestion of a toxicant), the body will in time eliminate the substance. But will the biological (adverse) effects diminish over time? Reversal of adverse effects depends on the type of effect. The reversibility of a toxicity response can be categorized as readily reversible, not readily reversible, or nonreversible. Most chemical-induced effects short of death are reversible in time if the chemical subsides over time. However, once an effect is produced, it may outlast the presence of the original chemical. An example is the compound organophosphate and its target site choline esterase. Organophosphate toxicity results in an inactivated esterase, meaning that the effects are essentially irreversible (not readily reversible), at least till the time it takes to synthesize more esterase. The body must synthesize new esterase, which might take as long as a few weeks.

In reversible toxicological effects, once the chemical has been removed, the deranged system will return to its normal functional state either immediately or later, after some regeneration has occurred. Specific toxicological effects that are irreversible (nonreversible), particularly when they are life threatening, include teratogenesis, mutagenesis, and carcinogenesis. Because of the consequences, exposure to such xenobiotics must be limited. However, many substances do not clearly fall under or out of these categories; thus, toxicologists rely on a battery of *in vivo* and *in vitro* tests to determine whether a compound produces toxicity.

HYPERSENSITIVITY VS. HYPOSENSITIVITY

In some situations, no fixed dose can be relied on to produce a given response in a population. Therefore, a distribution curve can show a normal response, a hypersensitive response, and a hyposensitive response.

Figure 2.7 is a plot of a theoretical compound in which each point represents one item of contributing data. The mean dose–response relation exists, shown by line B. Lines A and C are extreme responses to the toxicant. Subjects who deviate from the mean in the direction of line A are hypersensitive and those that deviate from line B toward line C are hyposensitive. Factors responsible for such sensitivities will be discussed later.

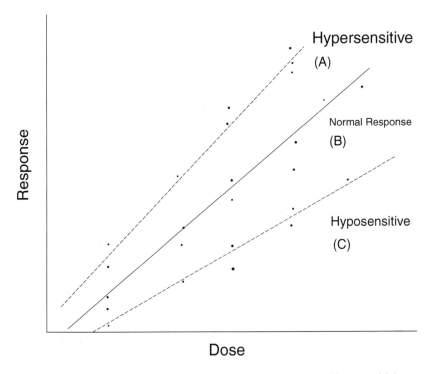

FIGURE 2.7 Mean-dose relationships illustrating hypersensitivity and hyposensitivity.

STUDY QUESTIONS AND EXERCISES

1. Can there be a dose–response curve that is completely vertical or parallels the abscissa?
2. What factors might contribute to species differences seen in the results of toxicity testing?
3. Describe the key points of a dose–response curve and the significance of broad and narrow plateaus or valleys in such curves.
4. Discuss how one can assess whether two toxicants act on a species by a similar biologic mechanism, and provide a rationale for your assessment.

RECOMMENDED READINGS

Klaasen, C.D., Amdur, M.O., and Casarett, L.J., *Casarett and Doull's Toxicology: The Basic Science of Poisons*, 6th ed., McGraw Hill, New York, 2001.

Loomis, T.A. and Hayes, A.W., *Loomis's Essentials of Toxicology*, 4th ed., Academic Press, New York, 1996.

Omaye, S.T., Safety facet of antioxidant supplements, *Top. Clin. Nutr.* 14, 26-41, 1998.

Ottoboni, M.A., *The Dose Makes the Poison: A Plain Language Guide*, John Wiley & Sons, New York, 1997.

Timbrell, J., *Principles of Biochemical Toxicology*, 3rd ed., Taylor & Francis, London, 2000.

3 Factors That Influence Toxicity

DIET AND BIOTRANSFORMATION

The biotransformation of a toxic compound usually, but not always, results in detoxification. It can, however, lead to the metabolic activation of foreign compounds. The effect of dietary constituents on the metabolism of foreign compounds has been the subject of intensive study for many years. More than two decades ago, the term *toxicodietetics* was coined for the study of dietary factors in the alterations of toxicity — a term that was perhaps ahead of its time.

There are a multitude of dietary factors that can affect toxicity. Dietary factors can be associated with the exposure situation, ranging from factors such as palatability of the food to the physical volume or rate of food ingestion. Dietary factors can be responsible for producing changes in the body composition, physiological and biochemical functions, and nutritional status of subjects. These factors, and others, can have marked influences on the toxicity of substances. For example, it is customary to fast laboratory animals for toxicity studies, usually 2 h before killing them at the end of the study. Fasting the animals has been shown to increase catabolic effects and decrease liver glycogen stores. Laboratory animals are fasted to decrease their liver glycogen, which interferes with the preparation of microsomal enzyme fractions. Also, fasting is done because the presence of food in the stomach impedes gastric absorption. Fasting is a traditional procedure practiced by physicians on their surgical patients to prevent regurgitation of fluids into the airways. Fasting animals and patients is, for most purposes, considered normal. However, there is ample evidence that fasting affects mechanisms of drug metabolism, toxicokinetics, and toxicity. Fasting for as long as 8 h has been shown to reduce blood glucose and produce changes in the activity of several toxicant-metabolizing enzymes. In addition, fasting induces the activity of cytochrome P450 in the liver and kidneys of rats, and results in glutathione depletion and generation of reactive oxygen species (ROS), oxidative stress, lipid peroxidation, decreased glucuronide conjugation, and overall decreased detoxification.

Also, investigators need to be concerned about the composition of the diet affecting the outcome of their toxicity studies. Reduced caloric intakes increase the toxicity of caffeine and dichloro diphenyl trichlorotethane (DDT) in rats, and low-protein diets have been shown to increase the toxicity of several pesticides and other toxic agents. In contrast, low-protein diets have been found to protect rats against the hepatotoxicity of carbon tetrachloride and dimethylnitrosamine exposure. Protective effects of low-

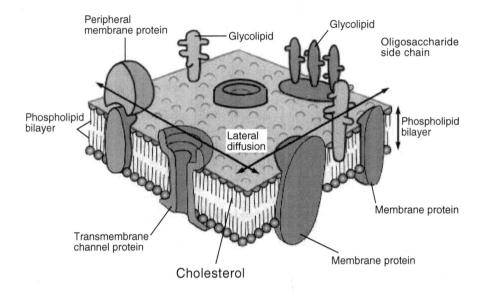

FIGURE 3.1 Biomembrane structure is influenced by a variety of nutrients.

protein diets are likely due to a decrease in microsomal enzyme systems, i.e., depressed protein availability for enzyme synthesis in protein-deficient animals.

Diet can affect enzymatic mechanisms of detoxification in several ways. Dietary deficiencies of essential macro- or micronutrients that are required by metabolizing systems can lead to decreased activities of such enzyme systems. Enzyme systems can be localized in the membrane or the soluble fractions of cells. As illustrated in Figure 3.1, the importance of dietary factors in toxicant metabolisms is evident by the diverse composition nature of membranes that harbor such detoxification enzyme systems.

Effect of Macronutrient Changes

Protein

Essential amino acids are the building blocks for proteins. For mammalian organisms, amino acids are the only dietary source of nitrogen for protein synthesis. Malnutrition due to protein-calorie insufficiency is one of the major nutritional problems worldwide. In young children, protein-calorie malnutrition is the world's most important and devastating nutrition problem. Included are diseases such as kwashiorkor, which is caused by a deficiency of protein or certain amino acids, and marasmus, which is essentially a lack of calories but also affects protein. Protein intakes vary widely in various parts of the world. The wide range in total protein intakes is probably because of differing consumptions of meat protein, which is linked to the economy of different regions in the world. In addition to individuals suffering from a lack of protein, or those who may have variations in intakes of dietary protein either because of choice or due to physiological impairment or disease, protein deficiencies may be seen in chronic alcoholics with abnormal diets, those who abuse drugs, those with various behavior abnormalities, or those dealing with food fads.

Protein deficiencies affect many aspects of metabolism. Foreign substances, together with endogenous compounds, e.g., steroid hormones, all may be metabolized *in vivo*. Subsequently, hormonal balance, pharmacological activity of substances, acute toxicity, and carcinogenesis all may affect the metabolism of toxicants. Lack of protein affects enzymes, including enzymes responsible for toxicant metabolisms. The reactions that these enzymes catalyze are affected, because of the amino acids quality or quantity required for protein synthesis that goes into the production of metabolizing enzymes. Lack of protein may lead to changes in amino acid composition of enzymes, which, in turn, may affect substrate binding or interaction with the enzyme. Cytochrome P450-dependent mixed-function oxidase, primarily located in the liver, is generally considered to be the predominant enzyme involved in detoxification. Also important are various conjugation enzymes, which help form products that are more water soluble and excretable.

Protein deficiency can lead to a reduction of NADPH cytochrome P450 reductase and certain cytochrome P450 isoenzymes. Uridine diphosphate glucuronic acid (UDPGA)-glycuronyl transferases, glutathione (GSH) S-transferases, and numerous enzymes of the antioxidant defense can be compromised by a lack of protein in the diet. UDPGA-glycuronyl transferases are involved in the conjugation of drugs with UDPGA. Dietary protein is crucial for the biosynthesis of glutathione, which is an intracellular reductant and has a vital role in protecting cells against the toxic effects of ROS. The amino acids glycine, glutamine, cysteine, and taurine also are involved in the conjugation of foreign substances. A reduction in enzyme quantity often, but not always, results in a lower ability to detoxify certain toxicants. The activity of mixed-function oxidase enzymes is inversely correlated with barbiturate sleeping times in several animal models. In rats, the decrease of serum pentobarbital is directly related to dietary protein concentration ranging from 0 to 50%. On the other hand, protein deficiency decreases the toxicities of substances such as heptachlor, because such substances are metabolized to more toxic products by mixed-function oxidases. Thus, low-protein diets depress cytochrome P450, and the outcome may be either more or less toxicity of the toxicant, depending on whether the products are less or more toxic.

Protein intakes are variable in different parts of the world. Industrial nations consume twice the recommended levels. The answer to the question of whether such consumption is detrimental to health is still being debated. Some stress concern that high-protein diets may increase renal stress and subsequently impair function. Bone demineralization, increased colon cancer because of changes in lower gut bacteria, and obesity are other concerns that may be related to high-protein diets. Also, there is the fear that amino acid supplements may result in amino acid imbalances.

High-protein diets enhance oxidative drug metabolism in humans. Hepatic mixed-function oxidase activities increase with increase in dietary protein. High-protein diets may result in lower toxicity of chemicals. Some studies have reported that high dietary protein fed to rats decreases the 7,12-dimethylbenz(alpha)anthracene-induced incidences of breast cancer, and a high-protein diet markedly decreases the incidence of gastric cancer induced by the direct-acting carcinogen N-methyl-N'-nitro-N-nitrosoguanidine (MNNG).

Lipids

Dietary fats serve various needs. They are sources of concentrated energy. Fats provide the building units for biological membranes. Fats or lipids are sources of essential unsaturated lipid and lipid-soluble vitamins. Animals cannot synthesize fatty acids containing double bonds in either the omega-3 (n-3) or the omega-6 (n-6) position. Both linoleic acid (derived from omega-6, 18:2) and linolenic acid (derived from omega-3, 18:3) are usually consumed with plant products. Linoleic acid is converted by animals to arachidonic acid (20:4, n-6) and linolenic acid to eicosapentaenoic acid (EPA, 20:5, n-3). EPA and arachidonic acid can eventually be converted by various tissue lipoxygenases and cyclooxygenases (COX) to a family compound identified as eicosanoids, e.g., prostaglandins, prostacyclins, thromboxanes, and leukotrienes. Eicosanoids have profound physiological effects (hormone-like) at extremely low concentrations as well as pharmacological effects at higher concentrations. There appears to be a Yin–Yang relationship between eicosanoids produced from EPA vs. those derived from arachidonic acid. Thus, as shown in Figure 3.2, the oxygenation products of essential fatty acids serve as important communication mediators between cells of the organism. About 30 to 55% of the dry weight of the hepatic endoplasmic reticulum is lipid, comprising cholesterol esters, free fatty acids, triglycerides, cholesterol, and phospholipids. Phosphatidylcholine content is important because enzymatic degradation of such components with phospholipase C decreases the metabolism of drugs and depresses binding of substrates of mixed-function oxidases. Phosphatidylcholine probably has a role in maintaining membrane integrity, and it is suggested that lack of this substance causes changes in the membrane integrity. Lipid substances, such as steroids and fatty acids, may occupy cytochrome P450–binding sites, thereby displacing exogenous substrates and interfering with their metabolism. Feeding diet deficient in linoleic fatty acids depresses the activities of certain toxicant-metabolizing enzymes, and therefore lipid quality is an important factor.

High-fat diets promote the spontaneous incidence of cancer. This may be due, in part, to a low dietary intake of lipotropes. Choline, methionine, glycine, folate, vitamin B12, pyridoxal, polyunsaturated fatty acids, and phosphate make up the dietary lipotropes, which are required for the synthesis of phospholipids and biological membranes. This synthesis is crucial for components of the microsomal mixed-function oxidase system. Dietary deficiencies in the lipotropes choline and methionine lead to a decrease in some cytochrome P450 isomers and to enhanced tumorigenic effects of chemical carcinogens.

Carbohydrates

Well-known sources of carbohydrates in the diet are the starches, such as cereals, potatoes, and pulses. A specific role for carbohydrates in biotransformation is not

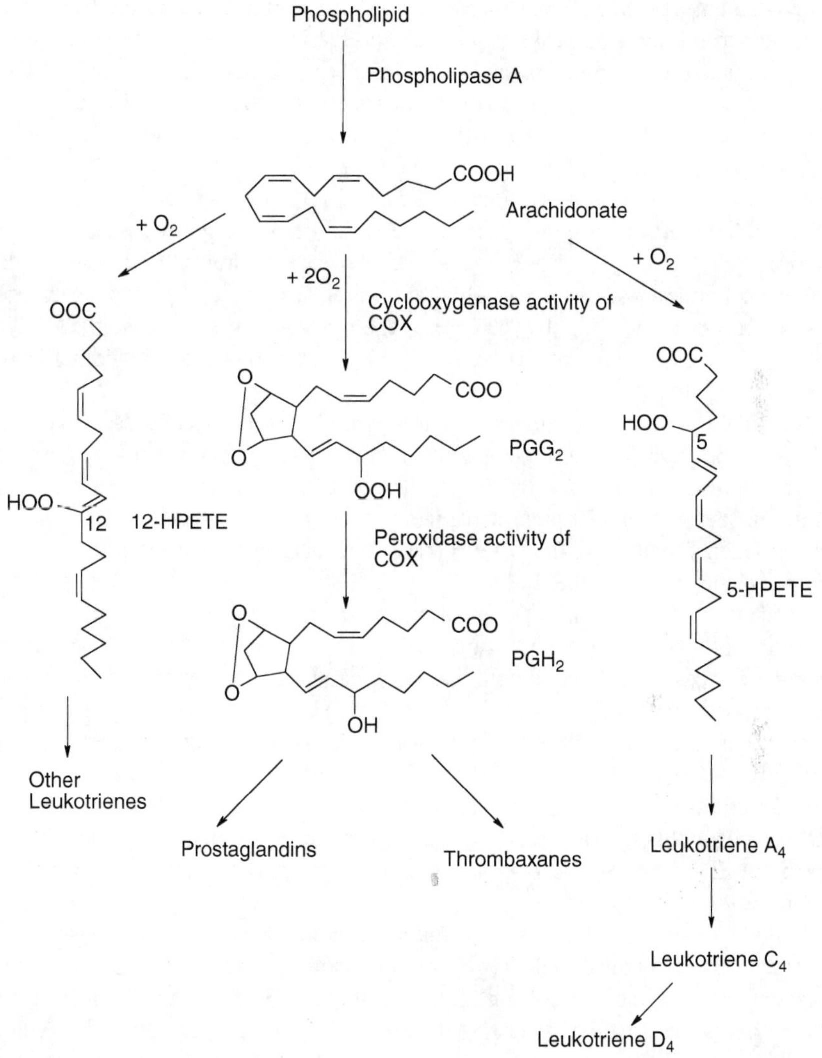

Factors That Influence Toxicity

FIGURE 3.2 Oxygenation products of fatty acids.

likely. The effects of dietary carbohydrate manipulation are likely because of generalized effects on intermediary metabolism, such as caloric effects and hormonal alteration effects. Animals use glucose as the principal carbohydrate and the level of blood glucose and amounts available to the animal's organs are closely regulated. It is well known that when carbohydrate intakes are high, any excess glucose is first converted to glycogen for storage, and when those stores are filled, it is converted to fat, in which form the storage is probably unlimited. When energy is required, glycogen stores are utilized, followed by gluconeogenesis concomitant with mobilization of fat stores.

High intakes of sugars, such as glucose, sucrose, or fructose, increase the duration of phenobarbital-induced sleep in rodents, and the longer sleeping times are correlated with a decreased metabolism of the barbiturate. Other studies have found that high-sucrose diets as compared with starch potentiate the lethal reaction to benzylpenicillin because of lower rates of conversion of its toxic products. Also, rats fed high sucrose or glucose plus fructose have lower levels of biphenyl 4-hydroxylase activity, which is correlated with lower levels of cytochrome P450.

Carbohydrates affect genes because the structure of the genetic material, deoxyribose (DNA) and ribose (RNA), is derived from carbohydrates. Portions of specific biological membranes contain carbohydrate components, such as part of the structure of some receptor sites. Finally, glucose as the precursor of glucuronic acid plays a role in Phase II detoxification reactions, which are crucial to the detoxification process (see later).

In addition, diets contain other carbohydrates such as celluloses and other polysaccharides derived from plant walls. Fiber plays an important role in maintaining gastrointestinal tract function and health. Dietary fiber plays a role in the metabolism and deposition of lipids, and dietary fat and fiber affect chemical-induced colon cancer. Usually, fat has little effect when dietary fiber is high but increases tumor incidences when fiber is low.

Rodents and other animals fed a calorie-restricted diet have a much lower incidence of spontaneous and chemically induced tumors than *ad libitum* fed animals. For example, 7,12-dimethylbenz(alpha)anthracene failed to induce mammary tumors in calorie-restricted rats, even when such diets were high in fat content. Some drug-metabolizing enzymes, such as 4-nitrophenol hydroxylase, are markedly increased (110%) by diet restriction compared with *ad libitum* fed animals. In addition, calorie restriction increases several phase II enzymes, such as UDP-glucuronyltransferases, glutathione S-transferases, and N-acetyltransferase, which are speculated to be responsible for the decreased incidence of chemical carcinogenesis.

Calorie restriction also has been found to exhibit lower oxygen consumption, increased insulin binding, and alter energy metabolism through changes in enzymes of glycolysis, gluconeogenesis, and lipid metabolism. The combined effect of metabolic effects and lowered oxidative stress has led to the speculation that calorie restriction may decrease age-associated enzyme degradation. Dietary studies have shown that unrestricted feeding decreases hepatic cytochrome P450, increases aflatoxin B1 activation, increases aflatoxin binding to DNA, and decreases *in vivo* detoxification of this carcinogen.

EFFECT OF MICRONUTRIENT CHANGES

Many vitamins and minerals have been examined for their effects on the metabolism of foreign chemicals by microsomal systems. Most studies reported have found that the effects of deficiencies of micronutrients on microsomal enzymes are not as striking as those observed for protein deficiency. Activities of toxicant metabolism enzymes are affected to some degree, particularly if the deficiency of the micronutrient is severe.

Vitamins

Ascorbic Acid

Depressed microsomal oxygenation of many xenobiotics is an essential function of vitamin C. In addition, vitamin C facilitates the elimination of Phase I products by UDPGA-mediated conjugation to glucuronides. Vitamin C deficiency reduces toxicant metabolisms in guinea pigs. Ascorbic acid deficiency affects the liver contents of cytochrome P450 isoforms, CYP1A and CYP2E, which are pivotal in the activation of food carcinogens, aflatoxin B1, and heterocyclic amines. Ascorbic acid decreases covalent binding of reactive intermediates, eliminates free-radical metabolites, and inhibits the formation of nitrosamines from the nitrosation of secondary amines.

Other physiological effects of vitamin C deficiency include poor wound healing and capillary integrity, probably related to the vitamin's role in collagen formation; decreased immunity; skeletal muscle atrophy; and nervous disorders.

In contrast, there is little information available on the effects of excess ascorbic acid on toxicant metabolism. There is considerable controversy over the efficacy of megadoses beyond the requirement or dietary reference intake (DRI) of ascorbic acid for the prevention and treatment of diseases.

Riboflavin (Vitamin B2)

Because riboflavin is an essential component (prosthetic group) of NADPH–cytochrome P450 reductases, such as the cofactors FAD and FMN, a deficiency will adversely affect toxicant metabolism. Also, a lack in riboflavin can result in uncoupling of electron transport and subsequent ROS generation. Deficiencies of riboflavin are associated with symptoms such as dermatitis (alopecia, seborrheic inflammation, epidermal hyperkeratosis, and atrophy of sebaceous glands), ocular problems (cataracts, conjunctivitis, blepharitis), and myelin degeneration (associated with paralysis).

Folate

Folate is required in toxicant metabolism and chemical detoxification, particularly during induction of oxidases (protein synthesis). Folate deficiency leads to loss of drug metabolism, loss of enzyme induction, hyperchromic anemia, and teratogenic effects in offspring. Birth defects (neural tube) associated with folate deficiency have led to the increased recommendation of the vitamin by the medical community for women of childbearing age. In rats, folate is required for increased turnover of toxicant-metabolizing enzymes during chronic drug administration.

Thiamin (Vitamin B1)

Increased cytochrome P450 activity, aminopyrine metabolism, and ethylmorphine metabolism are seen in dietary deficiency of thiamin. Thiamin deficiency is inversely related to increases in cytochrome P450 activity and an induction of ROS, lipid peroxidation, and destruction of cytochrome P450. Thiamin deficiency in humans and animals is characterized by anorexia, weight loss, cardiac involvement, and neurological involvement.

Vitamin E

Tocopherols act to protect microsomal membranes against lipid peroxidation. A lack of tocopherols results in a loss of cytochrome P450 and loss in drug metabolism. Vitamin E protects against chronic liver damage induced by carbon tetrachloride and increases hepatic CYP2C11 and CYP3A2. Also, there is strong evidence that vitamin E, particularly with selenium, inhibits dimethyl benzanthracene mammary tumors. Vitamin E deficiency has been shown to increase the susceptibility of laboratory animals to oxidative injury from a variety of air pollutants such as ozone and nitrogen dioxide. It is likely that the most important function of vitamin E is its ability to scavenge free radicals and prevent oxidative damage to crucial biomolecules.

Vitamin A

Retinoids have a protective function against chemical carcinogens, probably by inhibiting the bioactivation of carcinogens or binding of foreign compounds to microsomal proteins. Retinols decrease the mutagenicity of cooked food heterocyclic amines by preventing their activation. Although carotenoids are previtamin A compounds, they have their own unique property of inhibiting mutagenicity of aflatoxin B1 independent of vitamin A.

Minerals

Iron

Heme synthesis is dependent on iron, and heme is essential for cytochrome P450 and mixed-function oxidase activity. Iron deficiency results in anemia but has minimal effects on cytochrome P450. Iron excesses result in enhanced production of ROS, lipid peroxidation, and oxidative stress, which destroy cytochrome P450 and mixed-function oxidase activity. Dietary supplementation of iron has been shown to promote 1,2-dimethylhydrazine-induced colorectal cancer in rodents.

Selenium

Several enzymes (e.g., glutathione peroxidase) require selenium as an essential component. These enzymes have key roles in protecting biological membranes from lipid peroxidation and damage by ROS. Selenium deficiencies result in more lipid peroxidation, destabilization of the microsomal membrane, and decrease in heme synthesis and increase in heme catabolism, resulting in loss of cytochrome P450 and subsequent drug metabolism.

Zinc

Deficiencies of zinc seem to promote lipid peroxidation and thus decrease cytochrome P450 and mixed-function oxidase activity.

GENDER AND AGE

Toxicity can depend on sex, circadian rhythms, and age. Such dependence is well documented in both laboratory animals and humans. Diurnal variation is mostly related to eating and sleeping habits. Nocturnal animals usually have more food in their stomach in the morning than in the late afternoon. Agents that affect activity and are ingested by animals that normally eat at night exhibit a different effect compared with agents ingested by animals that sleep throughout the night.

The classical example of gender effects is the observation that the sleep time is longer in female rodents than in male rodents of the same age and weight following injections of barbiturate anesthetics, because female rats metabolize the drug slower. Nicotine, picotoxin, and warfarin are more toxic to female rodents than to their male counterparts. Ergot and epinephrine are more toxic to male rats than to female rats. Much of the difference can be explained by differences in phase I or II enzymes, which in turn cause differences in enzyme sensitivities to blood steroid levels in males and females or the indirect effect of sex steroid imprinting of sexually dimorphic patterns of growth hormone (GH) secretion by the pituitary. Males have periods with no GH secretion whereas females have a baseline of continuous GH secretion. In addition, testosterone and estrogen can directly stimulate expression of xenobiotic-metabolizing enzymes. Castration and hypophysectomy significantly reduce renal cytochrome P450 expression.

One of the most striking examples of gender differences in toxicity is the nephrotoxic effect of chloroform in male mice. Female mice of the same strain show no effect of chloroform exposures that are lethal to male mice. Castration or the administration of estrogens reduces the effect in males and providing androgens to females induces susceptibility to chloroform in them. In addition to chloroform, gender differences have been found for organophosphate insecticides. Overall, female rats are more susceptible to the toxic effects of parathion than are male rats, and the reverse occurs with methyl parathion. The latter situation is likely because those compounds require metabolic activation to inhibit cholinesterase. Again, castration and hormone treatment reverses the gender-related effects. Weanling male and female rats are equally susceptible to such agents.

In addition to the toxicity differences that can occur between genders, several other hormone-dependent effects influence the toxicity of compounds. Pregnancy markedly increases the susceptibility of animals to pesticides, and lactating animals are more susceptible to heavy metals. Hyperthyroidism and hyperinsulinism may alter the susceptibility of animals and humans to toxicants.

With age, our ability to metabolize foreign compounds reduces. Xenobiotic metabolism is low or absent in the fetus and neonates, develops rapidly after birth, and is highest in early adulthood. Before birth, the capacity for handling metabolism of foreign compounds is through the mother's metabolism. Clusters of different enzymes seem to develop rapidly during development periods, birth, weaning, and puberty. Many of the age-related differences, particularly between the young and old, can be explained by quantitative differences in detoxification processes. There is also a difference in hepatic and renal clearances of toxicants between newborn and adult animals. The necessity for dose adjustment is well recognized in pediatrics and in certain situations wherein patients have impaired kidneys.

Many phase II enzymes are expressed soon after birth. Enzymes for glucuronidation of steroids and bilirubin develop after birth, which explains the development of neonatal jaundice. Phase I and II enzymes can be expressed at higher levels during lactation and decline following weaning. This may be due to high fat intake and estrogen imprinting of the brain, related to reproductive physiology.

SPECIES

It is appropriate to consider the kinds of differences that can exist between animals from different species. This consideration is important in toxicology because the use of animal surrogates for humans is an important toxicological strategy and is the basis for almost all toxicological predictions. A completely accurate evaluation of the toxicity of a toxicant in a particular species can only be obtained by conducting toxicological studies in the desired species. For humans, such situations seldom occur, except for accidental poisoning or industrial exposures, and for ethical reasons the deliberate exposure of humans is out of the question. Even if the ethical considerations are overlooked, animals are still required to characterize the environmental hazard of the toxicant and its probable mechanism of action.

As one ascends through the different taxonomic levels, it can be assumed for comparison that the more closely related taxonomically the surrogate species, the more likely it is that the test will be predictive for humans. Species and strain differences in susceptibility to a toxic compound are generally greater than litter mate differences. Biological diversity is often taken advantage of when seeking to discover new pesticides or chemotherapeutic agents, such as the ability of the host to detoxify a compound compared with that of a pest or parasite, i.e., comparative or selective toxicity.

Mechanisms responsible for diversity include differences in metabolism, differences in renal and biliary excretion, plasma protein binding, tissue distribution, and response of target (receptor) sites. Understanding *why* there are differences can be important in the designing of toxicity studies to account for such differences. For example, if protein binding explains the difference between two species, then an appropriate modification of the toxicity study might include ensuring that the free plasma concentration of the toxic compound is identical for the two species.

STUDY QUESTIONS AND EXERCISES

1. Describe some common metabolic or endocrine considerations that may account for toxicity differences due to gender, age, and species.
2. Describe the metabolic pathways that are likely affected and which affect toxicity because of deficiencies in protein, carbohydrates, lipids, and micronutrients.
3. List the essential fatty acids and describe their metabolic roles and how the lack of such compounds might affect toxicity.

RECOMMENDED READINGS

Albert, A., *Selective Toxicity: The Physio-Chemical Basis of Therapy*, 6th ed., Chapman & Hall, London, 1979.

Combs, G.F, Jr., *The Vitamins: Fundamental Aspects in Nutrition and Health*, 2nd ed., Academic Press, New York, 1998.

Meydani, M., Impact of aging on detoxification mechanisms, in *Nutritional Toxicology*, Kotsonis, F.N., Mackey, M., and Hjelle, J., Eds., Raven Press, New York, 1994, pp. 49-66.

Netter, K.J., Toxicodietetics: dietary alterations of toxic action, in *New Concepts and Developments in Toxicology*, Chamber, P.I., Gehring, P., and Sakai, F., Eds., Elsevier, Amsterdam, 1993, pp. 17-26.

Parke, D.V. and Ioannides, C., The effects of nutrition on chemical toxicity, *Drug Metab. Rev.*, 26, 739-765, 1994.

Ronis, M.J.J. and Cunny, H.C., Physiological factors affecting xenobiotic metabolism, in *Introduction to Biochemical Toxicology*, 3rd ed., Hodgson, E. and Smart, R.C., Eds., John Wiley & Sons, New York, 2001, pp. 137-162.

4 Food Safety Assessment Methods in the Laboratory: Toxicological Testing Methods

Over the years, many tests have been devised to determine the adverse effects of chemicals in living organisms. Procedures are available for use with intact animals, laboratory-cultured single-cell organisms, isolated organs (perfused liver or lungs), or mammalian cell lines. Toxic endpoints used by investigators range from the traditional acute lethality, weight loss, and carcinogenesis to exciting new tests for effects of immunosuppression, behavioral aberrations, and genetic injury. Given this spectrum of procedures, an orderly and systematic approach to toxicity testing is undeniably needed. One of the first proposals in the U.S. for a systematic strategy involved the safety decision tree approach of the Food Safety Council Scientific Committee in 1980. In 1982, the publication titled *Toxicological Principles for the Safety Assessment of Direct Food Additives and Color Additives used in Foods* (also known as *Redbook I*) was developed by the U.S. Food and Drug Administration, Bureau of Foods (now the Center for Food Safety and Applied Nutrition, CFSAN). The draft for *Redbook II* was available in March 1993, followed by *Redbook 2000: Toxicological Principles for the Safety of Food Ingredients*, which is available electronically at http://vm.cfsan.fda.gov/~redbook/red-toct.html.

The overall strategy for assessing food additives has received strong endorsements from the scientific community, and only the details have been modified to keep pace with scientific advancements. Figure 4.1 gives a schematic representation of the safety decision tree protocol proposed by the U.S. Food Safety Council. The first step involves the careful selection and characterization of the substance to be tested. Preliminary evaluations of the substance are made by assessing physical and chemical properties of the test substance. A literature search is done to collect any available information regarding the toxicity testing of the substance. Exposure assessment involves gathering information on probable human exposure, i.e., estimated intake levels for the population as a whole or any subpopulation that might be vulnerable to significant levels of the substance. An example of a subpopulation is diabetic patients when the test substance is a new sugar substitute.

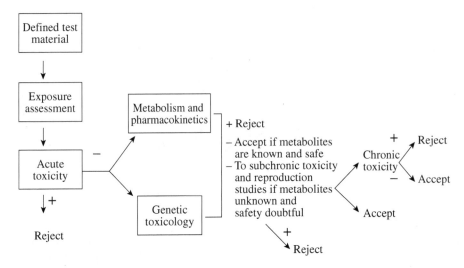

FIGURE 4.1 Safety decision tree protocol for food additives.

Testing begins with acute toxicity studies, starting with a single dose administered to a rodent species. Acute toxicity studies provide background information and guidance for subsequent tests to be used in the assessment. Unless the substance is found at this point to be too toxic for further study, the assessment moves further to gather information on genetic toxicology and toxicokinetics of the substance. Negative genetic toxicity results lead to metabolism, subchronic, and chronic toxicity testing.

ANALYSIS OF TOXICANTS IN FOODS

Chemical or other suitable methods to measure the toxic substance are critical for toxicity assessment. If the toxicant in question can be obtained as a pure substance, it can be relatively simple to establish procedures for the chemical identification of such a substance in food. Determining the safety of complex mixtures is more complicated, starting by establishing the composition of the mixture and followed by determining which components of the mixture are bioactive. For an effective analysis of toxicants in foods, both an assay for detecting the test substance and a method for separating the bioactive component from the rest of the chemicals in the food substance are required. Bioactivity is usually assessed by using an animal model system, linking some adverse effect, such as death, to the identified bioactive chemical. The initial step in identifying the bioactive chemical is to separate the food into its components, usually between lipid-soluble and water-soluble fractions, and testing each fraction for bioactivity. Active fractions are further separated into various components and tested until the pure toxicant is completely isolated. Thereafter, the pure bioactive chemical is structurally identified by various analytical spectroscopy techniques (ultraviolet, infrared, nuclear resonance, and mass spectroscopy). In addition to having analytical methods for the test substance, there are several pretest considerations a toxicologist should address (Table 4.1).

TABLE 4.1
Pretest Considerations

- Data in the literature, including purity and stability of the substance
- Species selection, age and gender for toxicity tests
- Mode of test substance administration
- Any toxicokinetic data
- Dose selection and frequency
- Housing and diet
- Quality control

It is essential to have all the available data on the chemical and physical properties of a substance in order to avoid duplication of effort in establishing such information in the laboratory. Gathering information about the quality and stability of the substance, species selection, test species age, and route of test substance is the important first step, and provides efficient and effective utilization of intellectual and physical resources. Having information about the stability of the test substance will determine whether the substance will be more viable by the intravenous route if the test substance is inactivated via the gastrointestinal route. If the test substance is new, data might be limited and caution must be used in extrapolating from chemicals with similar structures for toxicity properties. For example, the structural change of the reduction of one double bond in the aflatoxin molecule can reduce that compound's ability to induce tumors by a factor of 150. Limited information regarding the purity of a substance can lead to invalid assumptions, because impurities have, on occasion, been found to contribute to toxicological findings.

For species selection, the ideal species is one that metabolizes and excretes the test substance as humans would. The mouse, rat, and dog have become the human surrogates, mostly because such animals are economical, have an abundance of historical data, are amenable to frequent handing, and lack an appreciable vomiting reflex. Lack of a vomiting reflex ensures that the test substance is retained in the gut once it is ingested. One drawback of coprophagous animals such as rodents is the subsequent effect of a metabolite on toxicity. Metabolic processing may render the test substance more toxic than the original substance. Metabolic differences between humans and surrogate test animals can result in erroneous conclusions on how the substance might react in humans.

Throughout the toxicity literature and cited in Chapter 3 are numerous accounts of the influence of age and gender on the outcome of the assessment. It is common to use the rapidly growing or young male adult rodent for toxicity testing; however, caution is required because the findings from such studies might not apply to other age groups and there might be gender-dependent effects. Younger animals have a higher metabolism because of growth and hormone-related changes to the reproductive drive. Using younger animals provides the advantage of faster results because of their higher rate of metabolism, and thereby a more economical use of resources (younger animals usually cost less). From a practical standpoint, younger animals are often easier and safer to handle or manipulate: it takes a set of large hands to hold a 500-g old laboratory rat than to hold a 200-g young rat.

Gavage or gastric intubation (gavage) of the test substance can be advantageous because of the exactness and reduced variation of the method compared with adding the test substance to water or food. However, the method is somewhat artificial and the handling manipulation of the animal might induce other artifacts. The gavage technique is usually done after the animals have been fasted in order to decrease variation resulting from interaction with stomach contents. Putting the test substance in water or food may be more natural, but the test substance can be affected by exposure to air (oxidative breakdown), temperature variations, and the feeding habits of the test species.

Toxicokinetics or pharmacokinetics is the study of movement of a chemical within the body, i.e., absorption, distribution, metabolism, and excretion of a substance. Thus, aqueous- and lipid-soluble chemicals exhibit different toxicokinetics. Aqueous substances are absorbed into the portal system and immediately pass through the liver (first-pass effect), whereas lipid substances are transported via the lymphatic system and enter the systemic circulation via the superior cava and do not pass through the liver.

Dose selection can be extremely critical to the outcome of a toxicity test, particularly when the test duration increases. A high dose may exceed the homeostatic capabilities of the test species, i.e., ability to metabolize, transport, and excrete the substance. Ideal is a high dose that is sufficient to induce a toxic effect, and a low dose should be a reasonable multiple of the anticipated human exposure. In general, the dose should not exceed 5% of the diet. In addition, frequency of the dosing should not exceed levels anticipated to be experienced in a normal setting for humans.

Housing of animals and their diets are toxicity testing parameters that can induce serious variables. Chemical residues found on wood chips used for animal bedding can have profound effects on drug-metabolizing enzymes, which in turn can affect toxicity testing. Housing animals individually in stainless steel cages may induce stress in animals, because animals normally live in colonies and may become sensitized to living on the hard metal surfaces, e.g., induction of cutaneous dermatitis because of reactions to zinc-coated metal surfaces.

Quality control is essential to ensure that the data obtained are reproducible and accurate. Knowing the vendor's ability to assure quality animals is vital to the success of toxicity testing. Vendor control over the quality of animals is crucial, because diseased or weak strains can seriously compromise the outcome of studies.

ORAL INGESTION STUDIES

Under normal situations, the oral route is usually the means by which toxicants from food enter organisms. Through industrial exposures or other rare situations, toxicants from foods may enter organisms by inhalation as a dust or vapor suspension in the air or percutaneous (dermal) penetration, respectively. The toxicologist selects the experimental route to test the bioactivity of a chemical based on the common route of exposure for the substance. Selection of the route of exposure is important because the toxicant encounters various barriers during absorption, distribution, biotransformation, and elimination or excretion. The route of administration can influence the quantitative toxicological response to a bioactive compound, such as altering the slope and position on the dose–response curve.

The oral route may be viewed as providing entry of a bioactive substance to the body through a tube in the body, starting at the mouth and ending at the anus. As such, the tube is essentially exterior to the body fluids, because the gastrointestinal surface is a barrier to the contents of the tract, similar to the skin being a barrier. Therefore, ingested chemicals can impact systemically only after absorption through the gastrointestinal tract. Usually, food stays for too short a time in the mouth and esophagus to allow appreciable chemical absorption.

The bioactivity of a toxicant ingested varies with the frequency, presence of food, and the makeup of the food, such as amount of purified sugar, fiber, high protein, or high fat. The different pH conditions of the gastrointestinal tract affect the ionization of weak organic acids and bases. Following absorption in the gastrointestinal tract, the bioactive chemical is translocated to either the lymphatic system or the portal circulation. The portal circulation directs the chemicals to the liver, and many of the chemicals are excreted by the liver as bile. Because the bile empties back into the intestine, a cycle involving translocation of the chemical from the gastrointestinal tract to the liver and via the bile back to the intestine occurs. This cycle is known as enterohepatic circulation. Ingestion of chemicals from the gastrointestinal tract and enterohepatic cycle exposes the liver to those concentrations of the agent that would not be obtained by other exposure routes, such as intravenous or inhalation routes (first-pass effect). Thus, the hepatotoxicant is expected to be more toxic following oral ingestion on repeated situations but less hazardous when administered by other routes. A major function of the liver is to detoxify many natural and human-made chemicals that enter the body. The liver is able to handle many substances because of its large surface area and the high blood flow rate through this organ. The high blood flow to the liver provides nourishment and allows tissue repair and regeneration if there is no irreversible damage.

Toxicologists employ three types of ingestion toxicity studies: acute, subchronic, and chronic. Ingestion toxicity studies are differentiated by the length of time for which the test substance is administered via gavage, in the feed, or in the drinking water.

Acute Toxicity Testing

Essentially all chemicals of biological interest undergo acute toxicity testing. The purpose of the test is to determine the order of lethality of the substance. Lethality information can be used to give a quantitative measure of acute toxicity (LD_{50}) for comparison with other substances and to give a dose-ranging guidance for other tests. Acute toxicity testing represents the first line of toxicity testing for toxicity assessment, particularly in the absence of data from long-term studies. In addition, the acute toxicity test is useful for determining the symptoms consequent to administering the toxicant or to identify clinical manifestations of the acute toxicity. In pharmacology, these tests have been referred to as screening for the physiological

TABLE 4.2
Objectives of Acute Toxicity Testing

- Define intrinsic toxicity
- Predict hazard to nontarget species or toxicity to target species
- Identify target organs
- Provide information for risk assessment of acute exposure
- Provide information for the design and selection of dose levels for prolonged studies
- Provide valuable information for clinicians to predict, diagnose, and prescribe treatment
- Be useful for regulatory classification and labeling
- Develop clues on mechanism of toxicity

---

basis of toxicity. Careful evaluations of the symptoms produced by administering a bioactive chemical can provide significant information to help characterize the toxicant's mode of action, i.e., neurological, cardiovascular, respiratory, or others. Table 4.2 shows the objectives of acute toxicity testing.

Thus, the objectives of acute toxicity testing are to define the intrinsic toxicity of the substance, predict hazards to nontarget species or toxicity to target species, identify target organs, and provide information for risk assessment of acute exposure. In addition, the information derived from acute toxicity studies can be useful to design long-term studies, such as predicting, diagnosing, and prescribing treatment; providing information to support classification and labeling by regulatory authorities; and providing clues used by research to determine the underlying mechanisms of toxicity.

The test material is administered by gavage (gastric intubation) once or as a single bolus dose to test animals, and the animals are kept under observation for 2 weeks (14 days). Gastric gavage involves intubating the animal with a dosing tube (plastic or stainless steel) into the mouth and down the throat, through the esophagus into the stomach. Alternatively, in the bolus dose, a series of small doses may be administered during a 24-h period. Often, adverse effects are noticed within a short time, e.g., 24 h. The goal is to test multiple levels in groups with at least two species. Number of animal deaths, duration between the administration of the test material and death, and various symptoms before death and observed changes at necropsy are recorded. Thereafter, a second test may be performed in which the test substance is incorporated in the diet at various levels and includes at least one level found toxic in the prior test using at least two species.

If the substance does not demonstrate acute toxicity at levels that are comparable to expected normal intakes of the substance by populations, testing proceeds to the next stage.

Toxicology Screen

The basic premise of toxicological or pharmacological screening is not to allow true biological activity to go undetected. Screening has been a useful tool for pharmacologists to identify potentially useful therapeutic compounds. The use of toxicity screens during experimental determination of the acute toxicity of a compound in rodents can be extremely valuable to assess the site and mechanisms of action of a toxicant.

Screening involves scanning and evaluation. Scanning involves a test or a group of tests that permit the detection of physiological activity and is referred to as the multidimensional screening-evaluative procedure, blind screen, or the "Hippocratic screen." The Hippocratic screen for detecting physiological activity is analogous to a physician's Hippocratic diagnosis, a clinical situation in which the physician views the symptomatology of the patient. A patient's gross physical appearance, muscle tone, coordination, and even mental attitude are integrated with the physician's subjective impressions and clinical measurements, e.g., urinalysis or blood analysis. Diagnosis of a disease by this procedure can be rapid and provide clues, which can be verified by additional clinical and medical tests. Likewise, scanning can be followed by evaluation that involves other more refined or specialized tests designed to better remove the uncertainty of scanning tests. Thus, if the results from a scanning test suggest neurological toxicity, a more specific neurofunction test may be used in the evaluation.

Expensive equipment is not required for the Hippocratic screen or scanning tests; however, attentiveness and training to be unbiased is important. Because individuals differ in their abilities to observe, use of standardized work sheets with blanks to be filled in sequentially for either positive or negative observations is critical. Procedures are largely observational, qualitative, and use semiquantitative techniques utilizing standardized work sheets by trained researchers. The etiology of these procedures is that toxic compounds do not create new activity; these compounds can only modify existing physiological systems. Overall, compounds act by the basic mechanisms of stimulation, inhibition, or irritation of a biological system, or their combination. Irritation is an undesirable nonspecific type of response characterized eventually by necrosis if concentration is sufficiently high enough.

The Hippocratic screen is the initial screen, general in nature but carefully standardized to give reliable and reproducible results. Usually, the amount of test material needed for the scanning is less and can be either chemically pure or grossly crude material. Scanning can be a useful tool as crude material extracts during chemical fractionation can be followed pharmacologically.

Table 4.3 gives a standardized work sheet for the Hippocratic screen. A work sheet must be used for each animal and dose tested. Numbers used to fill in a blank are the actual measurements (rectal temperature, body weight), and subjective ratings are indicated by + and 0 (neutral) values. For example, decrease of motor activity is rated in the following manner: 0, animal is quiet, occasionally moves spontaneously; +, does not move spontaneously, but when handled moves rapidly; ++, when handled moves slowly; +++, when handled moves very sluggishly; ++++, when handled does not move at all. Observations for the Hippocratic screen or scanning may be elicited during experimental determination of the acute toxicity of a compound, including initial rough dose-range-finding and subsequent experiments to narrow the range of effective doses for measurement of lethality and to establish the dose–response curve for lethality.

TABLE 4.3
Hippocratic Work Sheet: Observational Examination of Animals

Date: Notebook Number:/Page: Project title:
Source of Sample:
Dosage: Test Concentration: Dosage Vehicle
Test Animal: Sex: Animal Source:
Animal Identification: Time of Fasting:
Weight: Volume of Sample: Time of Intubation:
Tested By: Evaluated By:

Symptom	Control	+5 min	+10 min	+15 min	+30 min	+60 min	+2 h	+4 h	+6 h	+24 h	+2 d	+4 d	+7 d
							Response[a]						
					Decreased Motor Activity								
Ataxia													
Loss of righting reflex													
Analgesia													
Anesthesia													
Loss of corneal reflex													
Loss of pinnal reflex													
Screen grip loss													
Paralysis, neck													
Paralysis, hind legs													
Paralysis, front legs													
Decrease in respiratory rate													
Decrease in respiratory depth													
Dyspnea													
Cheyne–Stokes respiration													

Increased Motor Activity

Fine body tremors
Coarse body tremors
Startle sensitivity
Clonic convulsions
Tonic convulsion
Fasciculation
Increase in respiratory rate
Increase in respiratory depth
Enopthalmus
Exopthalmus
Palpebral ptosis
Pupil size (mm)
Pupil size (mm) (to light)
Nystagmus
Lacrimation
Chromodacryorrhea
Skin blanching (ears)
Hyperemia
Cyanosis
Metachrosis
Salivation
Rales
Tail erection
Tail lashing
Tail grasping
Pilomotor erection
Robichaud test
Micturition
Diarrhea

TABLE 4.3 (Continued)
Hippocratic Work Sheet: Observational Examination of Animals

Symptom[a]	Control	+5 min	+10 min	+15 min	+30 min	+60 min	+2 h	+4 h	+6 h	+24 h	+2 d	+4 d	+7 d
Priapism/colpectasia													
Abdominal griping													
Temperature (Rectal, °C)													
Body weight (g)													
Head tap, aggressive													
Head tap, passive													
Head tap, fearful													
Body grasp, aggressive													
Body grasp, passive													
Body grasp, fearful													
Circling motions													
Status positions													
Excess curiosity													

Response[b]

Notes and other symptoms:

Death and autopsy notes:

[a] Subjective or quantitative intensity of the response after administration of the dose.

Dose-Range-Finding and Dose–Response Curve for Lethality

Methodical and rigid standardized procedures for the standard components of the screen are essential to produce reproducible and meaningful results.

Animals and Sample Administration

Nonfasted young albino rats weighing between 150 and 250 g are used, with doses assigned to both sexes randomly. Food and water are taken away for a period of 2 h after oral administration and returned subsequently, allowing *ad libitum* feeding. Test samples are dissolved or suspended in an aqueous vehicle or 0.25% agar. In situations where oily substances resist uniform dispersion by trituration, vegetable oils may be used; however, caution is recommended because of the potential of the solvent vehicle to interact with the test sample or produce its own physiological effects. The dosage volume should be constant; 5 ml/kg eliminates handling errors or aberrant effects due to too much or too little volume. Initially, one or two rats are used at each dosage level, ending with a minimum of five rats to an optimum of ten rats per dosage level. Approximately 200 mg of a pure chemical or 2 g of crude material is needed to complete the evaluation.

The goal of the acute toxicity study is to determine one lethal dose, one dose that is ineffective, and at least three log doses in between the lethal and ineffective dosages. The initial dosage given to the first animal is 100 mg/kg and depending on the effects seen in the first animal, the second animal receives either 10 mg/kg or 1 g/kg. For example, a lethal observation at 100 mg/kg results in reducing the dose to 10 mg/kg and no effect results in increasing the dose to 1 g/kg. Once the ineffective dose and the lethal dose are determined, the experimenter narrows down the range by dosing an animal with a log dose between the extremes. This scheme is continued until the dose elicits some symptoms but is neither ineffective nor lethal. The aim is to have one lethal dose, one ineffective dose, and three log doses in between that exhibit dose–response symptoms. Therefore, each injection is based on the result of the preceding animal. After each animal is injected, observations given in Table 4.3 are made at prescribed time intervals. Observations of the animals are made by placing the animal in a rink (65 × 54 × 8 cm^3) with normal animals to make comparisons. The listed format for observations facilitates evaluation; however, observations need not be determined in the order listed.

Autopsy is done immediately after an animal dies acutely from the effects of the test substance. Particular attention is given to whether death is due to cardiac or respiratory arrest. Whether the heart is in systole or diastole if the heart has stopped and whether the auricles are beating in normal rhythm should be noted. The color of abdominal wall, kidneys, liver, uterus, testes, and lungs; the degree of intestinal motility; dilatation or constriction of mesenteric vessels; and any unusual changes should be described.

It is extremely important that an acute toxicity test be standardized as much as possible. Table 4.4 summarizes factors that are likely to cause variations in the LD$_{50}$ values if serious consideration is not given during standardization. Use of subjective evaluations can introduce considerable amount of human variation if not controlled.

TABLE 4.4
Potential Factors Causing Variation in LD_{50} Values

Species	Health	Temperature
Strain	Nutrition	Time of day
Age	Gastrointestinal content	Season
Weight	Route of administration	Human error
Sex	Housing	

The acute toxicity data aid in designing subchronic toxicity tests. Researchers and regulatory people often review the data from acute toxicity testing in order to derive a starting point by which to set guidelines and design further testing. The information in the absence of long-term studies may help find ways to proceed for future work, give safety information, and help decide whether to proceed with the development of the food products or additive or to discontinue further research.

During the last decade, because of animal rights activism or humanitarian reasons, the issue of using alternative methods to animal testing for toxicity has been debated. The outcomes of such debates have been the recognition of the need to reduce the number of animals used in testing, refining existing testing methods to minimize suffering and pain of the animals, and setting a goal to develop replacement non-animal-based methodologies. Several *in vitro* strategies have been suggested to replace whole-animal toxicity testing, but, to date, none has been accepted by regulatory agencies. Thus, replacement of whole animals with test-tube methods for toxicity testing is more of a goal than a reality.

SUBCHRONIC TOXICITY TESTING

Experimental parameters for subchronic toxicity testing are based on the results of acute toxicity testing. Subchronic testing is usually for a prolonged period, ranging from several months to perhaps a year. The length of the testing period gives time to evaluate the possible cumulative effects of the substance on tissues or metabolic systems, or both. Dietary exposures of 90 days and for two test animal species are common subchronic testing protocols. Animals are monitored for changes in physical appearance, behavior, body weight, food intake, and excretion. Blood, urine, and excreta are routinely obtained and tested for hematological, urine and fecal alteration, and biochemical changes. Other tests may be used to measure specific functions (hepatic, eye, renal, gastrointestinal, and blood pressure and body temperature). Table 4.5 lists some commonly used analytical and functional tests used in conjunction with prolonged toxicity studies. Most tests are performed on the test species at 1- to 2-week intervals.

Observations are made on the animals, such as measuring animal activity levels, response to stimuli, general behaviors (eating and grooming), morbidity, and death. Other parameters include heart rate, blood pressure, nervous system function, and other tests required to answer specific questions, depending on the research design

TABLE 4.5
Prolonged Toxicity Tests: Clinical and Functional Evaluations

Blood Chemistry and Hematology	Urine	Function Tests
Electrolytes	pH	Liver function tests
Calcium	Specific gravity	Kidney filtration tests
Carbon dioxide	Total protein	RBC hemolysis
Serum glutamate (pyruvate/oxalacetic transaminase)	Sediment	
Serum alkaline phosphatase	Glucose	
Serum protein electrophoresis	Ketones	
Fasting blood sugar	Bilirubin	
Blood urea nitrogen		
Total serum protein		
Total serum bilirubin		
Serum albumin		
RBC and WBC		
Leukocyte, differential count		
Hematocrit and sedimentation rates		
Hemoglobin		

protocol. Because of limited time and resources, it is not uncommon for investigators to limit their observations to only those required by regulatory authorities.

At the completion of the study or when any animal becomes ill or moribund, all animals undergo necropsy, and tissues are examined for pathological changes and organ and major glandular weights are obtained. Table 4.6 lists common patho-

TABLE 4.6
Prolonged Toxicity Tests: Histology and Pathology

Weight	Histology
Total body weight	Liver
Heart	Heart
Liver	Adrenals
Thyroid	Gastrointestinal tract
Spleen	Spleen
Adrenals	Ovary
Testes and epididymis	Mesenteric lymph nodes
	Pituitary
	Thyroid
	Kidneys
	Pancreas
	Urinary bladder
	Testes
	All tissue lesions

logical and histological parameters measured in prolonged toxicity testing. The preparation of tissue slides is vital to assess pathological changes in tissues, such as lesions and other gross abnormalities that might occur. Histology is an integral part of the process of evaluating toxicity in tissue, and pathological interpretations are integrated into the final reports of findings for submission to publication, study sponsors, or review by regulatory authorities. These slides are typically archived and stored for possible review by researchers, contact research laboratories, sponsoring companies, and regulatory authorities.

The subchronic toxicity study usually involves the use of four groups of test animals, including a control group. Animals range from 10 to 20 per group per gender. The test diet is prepared by blending the test substance with a commercial stock or purified diet on a weight-to-weight basis. Caution is taken to ensure the stability of the test substance, which may require refrigeration of prepared test diets before feeding animals.

It is important that some form of toxic effect is exhibited in the high-dose test group. If, during the course of testing, the animals assigned to the high-dose group fail to develop signs of toxicity, the dose has to be adjusted such that some form of significant toxicity is exhibited.

The subchronic testing regimen seeks information about chronic effects but not necessarily with respect to cancer formation. These studies are often used to derive a dose regimen for long-term studies. Important information can be derived regarding effects on the target organ and the bioaccumulation of the test substance in the tissue. Such information can be useful to derive the no observable effect level (NOEL), discussed in Chapter 6.

Guidelines from regulatory agencies cover the spectrum of potential routes of exposure to toxic substances. For example, one may conduct tests based on other potential exposure routes, such as a 30-day dermal test or a 30- to 90-day inhalation test for compounds that may come in contact with the skin or be inhaled, respectively.

A company can investigate a compound more thoroughly than what may be required by regulatory agencies; however, the regulatory agency requirements must be satisfied so that the test substance qualifies for consideration by the regulatory agency with jurisdiction over its development and use.

Chronic Toxicity Testing

Chronic toxicity testing refers to long-term studies over the major duration of the animal's life span. The objective of such testing is to look for adverse effects that are not evident in subchronic testing, such as the propensity for carcinogenesis. This type of study is most valuable in terms of elucidating the biochemical mechanisms responsible for toxicity. The potential toxic effects from structure and function of the compound can be discovered and confirmed by results obtained through chronic toxicity testing.

Testing for cancer-producing substances usually requires 50 animals of each gender per dose level. Choosing the number required for the test group has been debated. The theoretical sizes of test groups based on the number required to determine toxicity at a frequency of 1 in 20 for a level of significance of 0.05 and

0.001 are 58 and 134 animals, respectively. The sizes increase for a frequency of 1 in 100 for a level of significance of 0.05 and 0.001 to 295 and 670 animals, respectively. High numbers of animals are needed to ensure adequate survivors at the end of the lifetime study to detect small percentage changes in histopathology and statistically evaluate the data.

In the past, large doses of the substances were used to reduce the group sizes as dictated by statistical theory; however, because test organisms respond differently to high and low doses, high-dose protocols are less commonly used. High doses of a substance are likely to produce toxic effects because the substance overburdens various systems of an organism that would normally dispose of at low doses. Systems include absorption via gastrointestinal tract, excretion by kidneys, hepatic metabolism, and DNA repair, which may be highly sensitive to concentration, particularly saturable substrate levels.

Chronic testing is costly and rats and mice are widely used to keep costs down. Besides cost, the advantage of using mice and rats as test species is the well-established volume of knowledge available on these species. Strain-specific species of rodents can be selected for susceptibility or sensitivity to organ-specific carcinogens or toxicity. Thus, if a substance is a carcinogen, the effect can be better shown in a particular stain sensitive to such compounds.

If a substance is found to be a carcinogen, then it is likely to be rejected as a substance for use in food. Thus, the chronic toxicity test is the final step of the overall risk assessment of a substance. Extra testing beyond chronic toxicity testing occurs in unexpected situations, e.g., when there are concerns about faulty data or inadequate test design.

GENETIC TOXICITY

Most cancers, as well as one tenth of the human diseases (e.g., sickle-cell anemia, cystic fibrosis, and Down's syndrome), are thought to occur by one or more mutations. Also, less than 10% of the substances shown to be mutagenic by various assays have not been shown to be carcinogenic in animal species. To be marked by bioassay as a mutagen strongly suggests that such substances are carcinogens. Hence, genetic tests are usually done early in the decision tree approach for toxicity screening. Positive mutagenic tests of a substance greatly reduce its further consideration for use in foods. Negative tests of a substance warrant further consideration for additional testing, including chronic carcinogen studies.

A mutation may be regarded as a disruption of the genetic code at any level of DNA organization, thereby changing the genetic information either in germ cells or in somatic cells. If the mutated cell is capable of reproducing itself — not all cells do — the cell will divide into two cells. The two cells formed will be made according to the new instructions provided by the mutated genetic code and will be different from the parent cells. The progeny cells will be different from the parent, but the differences might be so small that they go unnoticed or so great that the new cells are very different. Mutations that are produced in the germ cells of individuals before or during the reproductive period are capable of transmission to later generations. Changes in the genetic material of somatic cells and tissues can have implications by way of cancer or teratogenic effects. The mutation might be detrimental so that the progeny die, or might have no effect at all. Alternatively, the progeny cells survive and are competitive or compatible with neighboring cells and may group together with other cells with the same mutation and produce a benign or cancerous tumor. Cancer experts feel that a certain minimum number of cells in close proximity must undergo a similar mutation before a tumor can occur. Theoretically, one mutated cell can initiate the tumor process.

Mutagenic test batteries include point mutations in microorganisms (*Salmonella typhimirium*, Ames assay) and mammary cell lines (Chinese hamster ovary cells); chromosomal alterations in mammalian cell lines or intact animals species; and transformed cells, either animal or humans, implanted in animals.

AMES TESTS

The premise of the Ames tests is that carcinogens are initially mutagens that cause base-pair substitutions or frameshift mutations. Thus, carcinogenesis is the result of somatic mutations. The basis of the bacterial tests and others is either a reverse mutation from the nutrient-dependent strain to a wild-type capable of sustaining itself on minimal medium or a forward mutation whereby additional agent-induced changes in the genetics of the cell result in a new, easily identified and scored phenotype. The Ames tests are a rapid, inexpensive microbial assay used to screen substances for potential mutagenicity. Strains of *Salmonella typhimurium* are employed that are genetically defective for histidine, requiring the amino acid for survival. Different strains of the bacteria can be used to detect mutagens that cause base-pair substitutions (TA1535) or frameshift mutations (TA1538 and TA1537), causing the bacteria to produce the withheld nutrient. As shown in Figure 4.2, *S. typhimurium* (mutant tester-strain organism) is grown on nutrient agar and transferred to test tubes with low-nutrient agar with or without the suspected mutagen. The contents of the test tubes are decanted onto plates with minimal medium and incubated. A dose-related growth of colonies on the minimal medium indicates mutagenic action of the suspected mutagen. Other strains have been developed to increase the sensitivity for detecting weakly mutagenic agents. The Ames tests have been used to detect carcinogens from a variety of sources, such as blood, urine, saliva, air, soil, water, and food.

Because bacteria do not duplicate mammalian metabolism for activating chemicals, rat or human liver homogenates (supernatant fraction of the $9000 \times g$ centrifugation, S9) are added to the incubation mixture. This provides the necessary chemical-activating enzymes, which can be used to convert procarcinogenic agents into ultimate carcinogens.

HOST-MEDIATED ASSAYS

A host animal receives a dosage of the suspected mutagen, followed by an injection of the tester microbial strain into the peritoneal cavity. After a suitable incubation period of the microbial strain in the host, samples of the peritoneal fluid and microbial organisms are retrieved and applied to a medium-agar plate without nutrients. The assumption is that the suspected mutagen might be activated by the

Food Safety Assessment Methods in the Laboratory

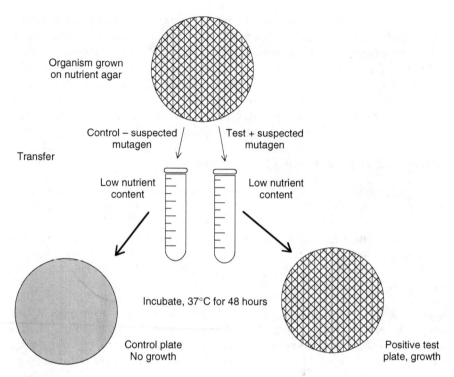

FIGURE 4.2 The Ames test protocol.

host's enzyme systems. Significant growth of colonies indicates mutagenic activity of the test compound.

Eukaryotic Cells, In Vitro

Tests for chromosomal damage require a more advanced organism than bacteria. Fungi have the advantage of having features similar to those of prokaryotic organisms, such as rapid growth, large test population, a genome that is organized into chromosomes, requiring a mitotic apparatus similar to that found in higher mammalian cells. Also, there are extensive studies done on yeast genetics, including detailed genetic maps of the organism and an understanding of biochemical markers. Tests include *Saccharomyces* forward-mutation assay and *Neurospora crassa* reverse- and forward-mutation assays. Although both yeast and fungal test systems have been around for some time, they are not very popular, mostly because fungal systems offer no clear-cut advantage over bacterial systems. Thus, there are a wide variety of assays that use various mammalian cells *in vitro* with both established cell lines and primary cultures of tissue cells derived from treated animals.

DNA Damage and Repair

When the nucleic acids of mammalian cells are damaged by chemicals, the cells' enzymatic repair systems are activated to repair the defect. The burst in synthesis of DNA can be monitored and reflects damage to DNA. Isolated primary-culture hepatocytes or lymphocytes, fibroblasts, etc., are grown on glass slides in a medium containing a range of doses of the suspected mutagen. Nonhepatic cells require the addition of the S9 fraction to encourage mutagen activation, if needed. Following incubation, the slides are washed to remove the unabsorbed chemical and are incubated with tritiated thymidine. If the test chemical has caused damage to the cellular DNA, repair mechanisms are initiated, with enzymes incorporating the radiolabeled thymidine into the nucleic acid, which in turn can be monitored.

Forward Mutations in Chinese Hamster Cells

The Chinese hamster ovary (CHO) grows rapidly in culture, doubling its number every 12 to 16 h. CHO cells contain the enzyme hypoxanthine-guanine phosphoribosyltransferase (HGPRT) and are sensitive to the cytotoxic agents 6-thioguanine and 8-azaguanine. Chemical test compounds cause mutations or produce HGPRT-deficient cells that are capable of growing in the presence of the guanine analogs.

Mouse Lymphoma Cell Assay

There is an established line of mouse lymphoma cells that are heterozygous for the enzyme thymidine kinase. Chemical-induced mutations at the locus of the enzyme site result in the loss of thymidine kinase activity or formation of a homozygous strain. Incorporation of 5-bromo-2-deoxyuridine into the medium results in cytotoxicity to the heterozygous line.

Sister Chromatid Exchanges

This test has been used to detect clastogenic chemicals, or substances that cause chromosome breakage. The assay can be employed with a variety of cell lines and primary cultures of cells. Cells are incubated with the test chemical (with or without the S9 fraction). Following a wash to remove excess test chemical, the cells are transferred to a medium containing 5-bromo-2-deoxyuridine and are allowed to pass through two DNA replications before adding colchicine to arrest the cells in the metaphase stage of chromosomal replication. Slides of the cells are prepared and stained. Damage (i.e., chromosomal pieces) caused by the test chemical can be seen under a microscope.

EUKARYOTIC CELLS, IN VIVO

The procedure usually involves treating animals with the test chemical and harvesting the desired cells for an *in vitro* assessment of the effects.

Drosophila melanogaster

Drosophila melanogaster (the fruit fly) has been used to screen large numbers of chemicals. A variety of endpoints can be used, ranging from effects on X and Y chromosomes, changes in body color, shape and color of the eyes, to bristles on the thorax.

Micronucleus Test

Micronuclei come from chromosomal fragments that are not incorporated into daughter-cell nuclei at mitosis because they lack a centromere. They are detached, broken segments seen as small bodies when appropriately stained and viewed under the light microscope. A variety of nucleated cells can be harvested from chemically treated animals and used for the assay. The mouse is the animal of choice but fetal hepatic cells, bone-marrow erythrocytes, and lymphocytes are also used.

SPECIALIZED ORAL INGESTION STUDIES

DEVELOPMENTAL TOXICITY — TERATOGENESIS

Some toxic substances exhibit toxicity by lethality whereas others are toxic because they are predominantly able to produce abnormalities of the fetus, i.e., cause embryotoxicity. The difference in type of embryotoxic effect induced by a toxic substance is a function of dose and the particular time during gestation when the fetus is exposed to the toxic agent. The stage of development of the fetus is an important determinant of teratogenic susceptibility, particularly during organogenesis. Introduction of the toxic substance to the mother before implantation of the fertilized ovum rarely induces fetus malformations. Likewise, few malformations occur when exposed cells of the fetus are undifferentiated in the early stages of cell multiplication. Day 7 of the fetus appears to be the earliest a teratogen can induce malformations. When organogenesis reaches completion, malformation susceptibility decreases; however, the fetus may be vulnerable to growth retardation.

The placenta often acts as a barrier in the transfer of substances between the mother and embryo. In addition, maternal protection to the fetus is given by the mother's ability to rapidly excrete or detoxify foreign substances. Enzyme induction may be an important factor, because pretreatment can defer teratogenicity of a substance. In addition, the fetus relies on its maternal link for growth and maintenance. Factors such as hormonal imbalance, dietary deficiencies, infections, diseases, and various stresses during pregnancy can cause the toxic substance to initiate abnormal development of the fetus.

Rodents are the most frequent test animals for teratogenicity tests because of prior experience with these species and cost effectiveness of the numbers required for statistical significance. A minimum of 10 female rats producing ca. 100 fetuses is needed; however, it is not unusual to see twice that number in teratogenicity studies. Tests for teratogenicity should be conducted by using two species with three dose concentrations per species, plus a negative control. Often, a positive control is added by using a reference test teratogen, e.g., a high dose of vitamin A or trypan blue. The highest dose tested should be one that does not cause serious maternal toxicity and the lowest dose tested should have no adverse effects on the mother. Regular estrus cycles of rodents should be monitored by checking their vaginal smears and mating permitted in the proestrus stage. Observation of sperm in the vaginal fluid is used to verify gestation, followed by development of a permanent diestrus. A fetal mass becomes palpable in the abdomen in ca. 15 days and gestation period is 21 to 22 days for rats and 21 days for mice.

For rodents, the teratogen, placebo, or positive control is administered by daily dosing from day 7 to day 15 of pregnancy. Pregnant females are housed separately to avoid aggressive interactions and weighed daily. Pups are removed by caesarean section on the day before the calculated date of delivery. Live and dead fetuses are counted and inspected in detail for abnormalities or malformations and the mothers undergo complete necropsy.

REPRODUCTIVE

Reproductive tests are usually fairly comprehensive. In addition to obtaining information on fertility and general reproductive performance, reproductive tests yield information about the effects of the substance on teratogenesis, mutagenesis, and neonatal morbidity and mortality. There are three facets to reproductive tests:

1. *Effects of the test substance on fertility.* Look for altered gonadal function, estrus cycles, changes in mating behavior, and changes in conception rates. Also look for effects of the substance on the early stages of gestation, such as implantation of the fertilized ovum.
2. *Effect of the substance on the developing fetus.* Look whether the developing fetus is normal and whether there are teratogenic or mutagenic effects.
3. *Effects of the substance on the mother and the offspring after birth.* Are there effects on lactation or nurturing of offspring, and do the offspring grow, develop, and mature sexually?

Reproductive testing for chemical toxicity should involve a study of animals exposed to the substance from the time of conception to the time they produce their own offspring and continuing of their progeny during development and growth, i.e., a three-generation study. The test substance is incorporated in the diet or drinking water. A large number of animals are involved, because at least three different levels of the test substance are studied, including the highest dose which represents a nearly maximally tolerated dose that produces no significant effect. Figure 4.3 illustrates a typical three-generation reproductive study. F_0 female rats are bred to males, which results in offspring F_{1a}, which are terminated at birth for examination. After resting the F_0 females, they are bred again to produce the F_{1b} offspring. F_{1b} females become the next (F_2) generation. F_{1b} have been exposed to the test substance transplacentally and via the milk and continue to be exposed at weaning and throughout maturation. F_{2a} litters are terminated at birth and F_{1b} females are rested and bred again to produce F_{2b} offspring, the females of which mature into the F_3 generation. Eventually, all animals in the reproductive test are terminated and pathologically examined.

METABOLIC — TOXICOKINETICS

The objective of metabolic toxicity tests is to find out qualitatively and quantitatively the effect of the test substance on the bodies of the species tested. An assessment

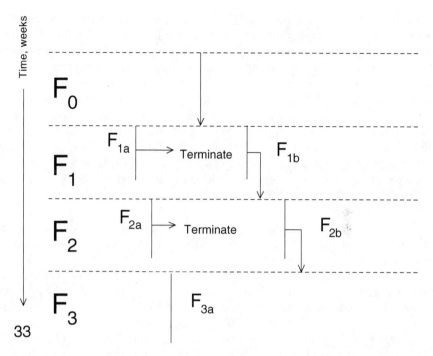

FIGURE 4.3 Typical three-generation study for reproductive toxicity testing.

of the toxicokinetics (pharmacokinetics) parameters of the compound, such as rates of absorption, tissue distribution, and elimination from the body is made in relation to variables such as dosage regimen and to time following administration. Thus, metabolic studies can provide significant information for designing prolonged feeding studies, including selection of test species, dose, frequency of test substance administration, and study duration.

Given the rather unconventional nature of metabolic toxicity tests, there are no routine procedures established. The overall purpose is to establish a metabolic fingerprint of the toxic substance, including identification and quantitation of metabolites. Therefore, investigations that use *in vitro* and *in vivo* models, including the use of radioactive or stable tracers, can be useful. The objective of the studies is to produce detailed analyses of metabolic pathways and the relationship of various metabolites to dose and time. Metabolic differences between species for the substance, potential species variation, and the usefulness of extrapolating the data to humans are assessed. Additional experiments are designed to identify chemically reactive metabolites and the target macromolecules or sites, technically the domain of toxicodynamics or pharmacodynamics. The toxicodynamic evaluation of toxic substances comprises the study of processes involved in the interaction between the bioactive substance and its receptor or molecular sites of action responsible for the chemical lesion. Toxicodynamics also encompasses the resultant sequence of biochemical and biophysical events that result in the toxic effects observed on ingesting the toxic substance.

Through toxicokinetic studies, mathematical models can be devised to describe the observations of other studies and to develop a better understanding about the dosage relationships to metabolism, transport, and excretion of the toxic substance. A measure of biological or systemic availability of a substance is the fraction of the dose that reaches general circulation. For a single bolus dose, the concentration depends on the initial dose and rates of absorption and elimination. For chronic exposure situations, the systemic concentration will reach a steady-state level, i.e., the concentration absorbed is equal to the concentration excreted per unit time. The biological system is more complex because the substance can undergo metabolic conversion, which may result in the compound's bioactivation or biotoxification. Through interspecies comparisons, toxicokinetics can provide a valuable guide to determine the dose range for prolonged studies and appropriate safeguards to consider in desired human metabolic studies.

In certain situations, specific studies, such as autoradiography, placental transfer, or neurological effects, may be designed to address critical observation results noted in previous acute toxicity screens.

When metabolic studies identify unique metabolites or demonstrate that the normal metabolism is altered, further testing is done. Additional metabolic and toxicokinetic studies are designed when the metabolic mechanisms become overwhelmed and the toxic substance or its metabolites persist in the body. If the test substance is found to be easily and entirely converted to normal metabolic intermediates and such intermediates are in a small proportion, no further testing is required.

STUDY QUESTIONS AND EXERCISES

1. Describe how you would perform a dose–response experiment using lethality as the endpoint. Calculate five log doses between 10 and 100 mg/kg body weight.
2. Describe the use of acute, subchronic, and chronic testing methods for assessing *in vivo* the toxicity of food toxicants.
3. What will an *in vitro* model system require before it is accepted by various federal regulatory agencies as an appropriate toxicity testing system?
4. Design a toxicity test for assessing potential adverse effects of a newly identified phytochemical isolated from tomatoes.

RECOMMENDED READINGS

Malone, M.H. and Robichaud, R.C., A Hippocratic screen for pure or crude drug materials, *Lloydia,* 25, 320-332, 1962.
Turner, R.A., *Screening Methods in Pharmacology,* Academic Press, New York, 1965.
Watson, R.R., *Trace Elements in Laboratory Rodents*, CRC Press, Boca Raton, 1996.

5 Food Safety Assessment: Compliance with Regulations

Toxicity research and testing are conducted in a variety of settings, including academia, government, and private industry. Some of this research is theoretically based and some is based on practical application. A university researcher might be interested in elucidating the biochemical mechanisms involved in a toxic effect of a certain compound or substance. A government researcher could be looking for answers to whether a particular food additive is safe for consumption by the general public. A clinical investigator could be looking at the effects of a certain dose range of a test article in order to evaluate the safety of a compound for human clinical trials.

This chapter deals with toxicity testing and reviews how testing procedures are managed and the quality aspects that are critical if one has to rely on the resultant data, which can be used to ensure product safety. The interaction of the food industry and various regulatory groups for the purpose of having safe foods is discussed.

GOOD LABORATORY PRACTICES (GLPS)

The conduct of nonclinical research is a highly regulated function. In the U.S., the substances tested, the manner in which they are tested, and who tests them is governed by guidelines promulgated by the regulatory branch of the federal government. The reasons for regulations are primarily to safeguard the public by ensuring that mechanisms to test food additives, drugs, and other substances adhere to a uniform standard that provides a way to consistently measure the risks and benefits they might pose to the public. Thus, good laboratory practices (GLPs) are regulations that define conditions under which a toxicology study should be planned, conducted, monitored, reported, and archived. Many agencies from the U.S. and other nations have adopted GLPs. In 1983, the U.S. EPA implemented GLP regulations under the mandate of the Federal Insecticide, Fungicide, and Rodenticide Act (FIFRA, see later) and the Toxic Substance Control Act (TSCA) for pesticide and toxic chemical registration and use.

The use of laboratory animals in nonclinical research is a necessity and the regulation and use of these animals is tightly controlled. Regulations, known as GLPs, set forth by regulatory agencies govern the manner in which nonclinical hazard assessment studies are to be conducted, documented, and reported. Such regulations are set forth in Chapter 21 of the "Code of Federal Regulations, Part 58

(21 CFR 58)." The Food and Drug Administration (FDA) promulgates and enforces these codes as interpreted by applicable laws passed by the U.S. legislative branch of the government. The scope of the GLPs is defined in 21 CFR 58.1 as follows (selected quotes or paraphrases).

General Provisions: Subpart A

Section 58.1 — Scope

This part prescribes GLPs for conducting nonclinical laboratory studies that support, or are intended to support, applications for research or marketing permits for products regulated by the FDA, including food and color additives, animal food additives, human and animal drugs, medical devices for human use, biological products, and electronic products. Compliance with this part is intended to assure the quality and integrity of the safety data filed pursuant to Sections 406, 408, 409, 502, 503, 505, 506, 507, 510, 512-516, 518-520, 721, and 801 of the Federal Food, Drug, and Cosmetic Act and Sections 351 and 354-360F of the Public Health Service Act.

Several professional organizations are dedicated to improving the quality of GLP studies. The most prominent is the Society of Quality Assurance (SQA), which is a professional organization founded to promote the quality assurance profession through the discussion and exchange of ideas and the promulgation and continued advancement of high professional standards. Members of the SQA are dedicated to promoting the highest quality and integrity in studies under their jurisdiction.

When a pharmaceutical firm, biotechnology company, or any other enterprise contracts work to a private research laboratory that will be submitted to or reviewed by the FDA, then the research laboratory is required to have its work adhere to GLPs while conducting the study. The FDA inspects the testing facility. The FDA must have access to the nonclinical research laboratory and the documents of the quality assurance (QA) unit. If access to the facility or the data is denied, then the material will not be accepted or considered by the FDA for an application for a research or marketing permit.

Organization and Personnel: Subpart B

Personnel

Individuals engaged in or who otherwise supervise nonclinical studies must have the proper education and experience to practice in their area of responsibility. Nonclinical research laboratories are required to maintain a current summary of education and experience of staff that conduct or supervise studies. The study protocol implicitly or explicitly indicates the necessary resources needed to complete a study. It is therefore the responsibility of the contract research laboratory to have adequate human resources to conduct the study in accordance with the written protocol.

A vital element of GLPs is the requirement to ensure that the test article under study is not advertently contaminated or otherwise compromised in the conduct of the study. The use of personal protective equipment is pivotal in the conduct of studies and it should be changed as often as necessary to ensure that there is no cross

Food Safety Assessment: Compliance with Regulations

contamination of the test method, procedures, or test article under study. The need to prevent microbial, chemical, and radiological contamination to the test system and test article is important so that the integrity of the results is not in doubt. Human safety, no less important, is not dealt with in the GLP regulations but is covered under the Occupational Health and Safety Administration (OSHA) regulations.

Medical surveillance of personnel is often conducted in the clinical research laboratory environment to exclude personnel who could alter the outcome of the study by an infection or other means. This is particularly important in research environments that use nonhuman primates, because of the particular susceptibility of the animals to diseases such as tuberculosis and other infections. The use of protective masks in the research environment is as much for the protection of the staff as for the animals under study.

The medical surveillance can be as simple as having employees notify their supervisors when they have a fever or other symptoms or it can be as elaborate as testing serum for viruses as is done when personnel working with rhesus monkeys are potentially exposed to the herpes B virus.

Testing Facility Management

The conduct of a nonclinical study is under the direction of a study director (SD), who is designated by management before the study to ensure adherence to the study protocol and lead the research in accordance with GLPs. Facility management also ensures that a QA unit is in place to audit the conduct of all aspects of the study. The importance of maintaining the integrity of the test article and testing procedures is a critical aspect that management, under the direction of the SD, is required to ensure. These aspects of the study require strict adherence to processing, storage, purity, strength, and consistency of the test article and test material as necessary in order to trust the results of the test. The QA unit's role is to verify that the study protocol is adhered to and that there are no deviations in the protocol during auditing and data review.

It is the responsibility of the SD to acquire and maintain adequate resources, including personnel, equipment, and materials. Scheduling and training to enable personnel to complete the study is required, and any deviations noted by the QA unit must be communicated to the SD. Actions taken by the study director to correct deviations must be documented.

Study Director

The SD is the primary point of contact for the sponsor (the representative or company placing the study). The level of education and experience of the SD must satisfy the requirements of the study protocol for the conduct of the study. The SD is often a scientist trained in biomedical sciences and holds a professional-level degree (i.e., Ph.D. or M.S.) from a university. It is unlikely that a sponsor will place a study with a nonclinical research laboratory whose SDs are not educationally or technically qualified. However, the GLP standards address these issues as a requirement to maintain high standards because of the importance of these studies to society.

Technical supervision is the responsibility of the SD as is data analysis and interpretation of results. The documentation and reporting of results are also the SD's responsibility. However, in addition to quality assurance review, senior scientists and peers normally review, comment on, and, in some cases, amend conclusions of the study. These reviews in themselves act as a quality check and often provide an extra pair of eyes to discover something that might have been overlooked. It is typical for the final product to be reviewed by all the different departments that have a stake in its outcome. This includes clinical chemistry, histology, pathology, and the SD and senior scientists.

The SD must approve the protocol and any changes to it. All testing systems and observations must be verified and documented by the SD. Any unusual circumstances, observations, or events must be documented in accordance with GLPs. On completion of the study, the SD must ensure that the study's raw data, documentation, protocols, specimens, and final reports are transferred to the archives during or at the close of the study.

Quality Assurance Unit

Every nonclinical contract research laboratory conducting GLP studies must have a dedicated QA unit. Each study should be monitored by the QA unit to assure management that the equipment, personnel, practices, and records comply with GLPs. It is necessary that the QA unit act as a stand-alone function, separate in management and supervision from the personnel engaged in the study. This way the QA unit can act independently and be theoretically less influenced by those managing and conducting the study.

The QA unit maintains the study master schedules for all nonclinical studies at the facility. These studies should be indexed by the test article and test system, kind of study, e.g., toxicokinetic (TK) studies, the date started, the status of any given study, the sponsor (e.g., company), and the SD. Copies of the nonclinical studies that the QA unit is responsible for are kept on the site.

Inspection mechanisms are left to the discretion of the QA unit, but must be at intervals adequate to ensure written and properly signed records documenting the time, location, inspector, phase of the study, and any negative findings. Items of concern that have the potential to negatively affect the integrity of the study are noted and brought to the attention of the SD and management. The documentation requirements include regular written reports summarizing the status of the study, and any unapproved deviations from the protocol or SOPs.

When the SD submits the final report, the QA unit must review it to determine whether it accurately reflects the methods and SOPs under which the study was conducted. This is accomplished by QA auditing the raw data and reviewing inspection findings as well as taking corrective actions to address any deviations from the protocol or SOPs. Attached to the final report is a statement describing the QA findings as reported during the course of the study.

The organizational management of the QA unit and the methods and procedures it uses to conduct inspections should be maintained in written SOPs. Records of its findings of studies at the facility, the dates of inspection, and the QA auditor conducting the inspection are to be maintained and available for review by management and the FDA. An FDA representative may require the QA unit to certify that it complies with these written guidelines, ensuring that inspections are completed and documentation requirements followed.

FACILITY: SUBPART C

Section 58.41 — General

Each testing facility should be of suitable size and construction to facilitate the proper conduct of nonclinical laboratory studies. The facility should be designed such that a degree of separation prevents any function or activity from having an adverse effect on the study.

Animal Care Facilities

Often, a variety of species are housed at a facility. Therefore, it is necessary that enough animal rooms are available to keep these species and testing systems separated. The isolation or quarantine of animals is often a real concern that must be considered. The need for specialized housing is often a consideration to address, depending on the species being studied and the social or behavioral considerations of the species.

The facility must often accommodate procedures for which precaution to animals and workers must be considered. Among these are adequate ventilation requirements for studies using volatile or reactive substances, infectious agents, radioactive isotopes, or aerosols. Special protective clothing and special precautions are often employed to safeguard animals and lab workers.

Areas designated for laboratory animal medicine, including diagnosis, treatment, and control of animal diseases or infections, must be provided as necessary. The need to isolate sick, injured, or otherwise diseased animals from other healthy animals is important. Typically, a nonclinical research laboratory has a dedicated laboratory animal medicine unit that cares for the health and general well-being of the animals in its care. Specialized facilities include surgical suites, x-ray rooms, and treatment rooms.

Biohazardous waste must be managed in accordance with GLPs where animals are housed. The collection, storage, and disposal of animal waste or biowaste refuse must be safe and sanitary. The management of vermin infestation, environmental contamination, odor, and disease is a primary consideration. The biowaste containers should be either incinerated on the site or contracted for disposal with a licensed disposal company. It is important that the biowaste stream be managed properly and the disposal and destruction of pathologic agents done correctly.

Large quantities of water and specialized cleaning and disinfecting products are used to sanitize a facility. As a result, wastewater discharges may pose a concern to local wastewater regulatory authorities. Also, standing water and poor housekeeping can lead to unsanitary conditions that favor vermin infestation. As a consequence, vector control must be an ongoing concern.

Animal Supply Facilities

Animal supplies and feed storage must be in a separate area away from the test system and should have safeguards in place for pest control or cross contamination.

Food items that need to be preserved should have adequate means to accomplish this. These methods can include refrigeration, freezing, humidity control, or other means that will prevent them from spoiling.

Separate access of food products is necessary to avoid cross contamination with chemicals or other products that could compromise the quality of the food sources. A food storage unit should be properly maintained, including records on inventory control and use to guarantee that food is cycled in and out and does not accumulate shelf life and expire.

Facilities for Handling Test and Control Articles

The test article must be preserved and processed reliably to ensure that it is not compromised or mistaken for another substance. There are requirements for a separate area for the receipt and storage of test articles. Other requirements include designated areas for mixing a test article with its carrier (i.e., solid food or liquid) and storage of the mixed article. These facilities must be separate from the areas where test systems and animal housing are located. Storage must maintain and preserve the test article so that it is not compromised before dosing in the animals.

The facility should be equipped with a variety of measurement and mixing equipment. The laboratory should have ventilation hoods used to prepare test articles that are thought to pose an undue risk to dose-preparation technicians. Refrigeration and storage of the test article material must be contained within the formulation lab so that technicians do not carry chemicals long distances. Exclusion zones for dose preparation of a test article are set up for batch mixing of test articles.

Laboratory Operation Areas

There must be separate laboratory areas for specialized tasks or procedures. The use of radioisotopes in studies requires a dedicated space for setting up a contamination zone and limiting access to authorized personnel only. These studies should be conducted by specially trained staff in rooms that can be easily accessed and provide room to move around without much difficulty.

Other studies require that the subjects be restrained for an extended period of time, which often requires the use of restraining devices that are suited to the species under study. Restraining harnesses and chairs are often used for this purpose. The use of these devices is necessary to minimize interference with the procedure and to reduce discomfort to the animal.

Specimen and Data Storage Facilities

There must be a designated archive facility to store raw data and specimens associated with the study. These facilities have humidity and temperature control requirements for data storage. Also, access should be limited to authorized personnel only. Every piece of data associated with the study in support of a research or marketing license should be archived for future retrieval as necessary. In addition to raw data, stored materials include pathology slides, fixed tissue, draft and final reports, and anything else necessary to support the application process.

EQUIPMENT: SUBPART D

Equipment Design

Monitoring equipment or equipment used to generate or assess data must be sufficient to achieve its intended function. The design requirements are met when the equipment is able to function in accordance with study protocols. The equipment must be located such that it can be easily monitored, inspected, calibrated, cleaned, and maintained.

Monitoring equipment can include telemetry equipment, dosimeters, freezers, data loggers or anything else used to generate data. Remote computers that use sophisticated software to monitor dosing instruments must meet validation requirements in order to satisfy internal and external customers. Calibrations to some primary or secondary standards recommended by the manufacturer are typically required.

Maintenance and Calibration of Equipment

Any equipment used to make measurements in support of a GLP study must be adequately tested and calibrated to an acceptable standard. Nonclinical research laboratories should have written SOPs that detail the schedule, means, and methods by which equipment is to be cleaned, maintained, tested, and calibrated. The SOPs should indicate the actions that need to be taken in the event of a deviation from normal operating procedures, including malfunctions or failures. In addition, the SOPs should detail the person responsible for the performance of each piece of equipment used to directly or indirectly generate data.

In addition to the aforementioned points, a written record is required for any equipment failure or malfunction, and the corrective action taken to rectify it. The data should include the times and dates, the maintenance performed, and any deviation from SOPs. Nonroutine maintenance and repairs must be documented and detail what happened and how it was corrected.

TESTING FACILITIES OPERATION: SUBPART E

Standard Operating Procedures

The testing facility must have written SOPs that define all aspects of the nonclinical study methods used. The SOPs must have enough detail to ensure that the management is confident that the quality and integrity of the studies conducted will be maintained. Any and all deviations from the SOPs must be authorized by the SD and documented in the raw data collection. Any deviations from the SOPs deemed to be significant must be authorized by the management.

The SOPs should cover the preparation of animal rooms, transfer of animals, identification of animals, placement of animals, animal care, test article or dose preparation, and observations made in the test system. Other SOPs include laboratory tests, discovery of moribund or dead animals on study, necropsy or postmortem examinations, and histopathology. SOPs are required for data handling, storage, and retrieval. Other SOPs cover maintenance and calibration of equipment, as mentioned previously.

A laboratory that supports GLP studies must have SOPs immediately available for review. Manuals or other material such as manufacturers' instructions can be used to supplement SOPs. A history of SOPs used must be maintained, with a notation of any changes or revisions made, when they were made, and by whom. This is essential because archived data can only be reviewed in the light of the SOPs under which it was conducted.

Reagents and Solutions

Laboratory reagents must have labels clearly identifying their content or concentration. Any storage requirements should also be listed, as should be the expiration date. Expired or otherwise deteriorated reagents should not be used. (Note that other regulatory requirements such as OSHA require labeling with much of the same information listed.) The disposal of expired reagents should be done in compliance with EPA waste disposal requirements under the Resource Conservation and Recovery Act (RCRA). Some expired reagents (such as some fixative products containing picric acid) can be extremely dangerous and should only be handled by qualified personnel.

Animal Care

The humane treatment of animals is not covered explicitly in the GLP requirements. However, the USDA has specific requirements for the humane treatment of animals. The Institutional Animal Care and Use Committee (IACUC) reviews and approves study protocols, and any changes to a protocol must be submitted to the IACUC coordinator for consideration. The main purpose of the IACUC is to ensure the humane treatment of animals in GLP studies. In addition, nonclinical labs should strictly enforce humane treatment to animals. Violations are to be reported to the management or a member of the IACUC, and violations of humane treatment policies routinely lead to severe employment sanctions, including termination.

All facilities housing, feeding, and handling animals should have detailed SOPs. Animals received from outside sources must be isolated from other animals and examined to ascertain their health status by accepted practices in veterinary medicine. This may require extended periods of quarantine for imported animals or those purchased domestically. Several levels of biohazard protection, ranging from 1 to 4, are associated with the risk of exposure to pathogenic agents. Level 1 is the least restrictive and requires minimal personal protective equipment and facility requirements, whereas level 4 is reserved for those infectious agents that can be spread by aerosols and require full encapsulation and elaborate safeguards because of the potential lethality to those exposed. A normal quarantine operation will likely have a level 2 protection.

Animals must be healthy before the start of the study. Any animal found ill with a disease during the study should be isolated as necessary to prevent other animals from contracting the disease. The animal can be treated for diseases if it does not interfere with the study. All diagnoses of illnesses and treatment and dates of treatment must be supervised by a veterinarian and recorded as appropriate. Animal treatment records must be maintained on the site and become a permanent part of the study record subject to review by the FDA.

Identification of warm-blooded animals (not including suckling rodents) that must be manipulated by hand, removed for any length of time, and returned to cages for any reason is mandatory. The animal housing unit must clearly identify each animal within a unit. Different species must be housed in different locations. Similar species used in different studies should not be housed with each other unless there is a good reason for doing so. The chance of cross contamination between subjects with different test articles is possible in mixed housing. If it is absolutely necessary to house these animals in the same room, detailed means for separating and identifying them must be implemented.

Cleaning and disinfecting cages and animal rooms is part of GLPs for general hygiene and health reasons. Also, feed and water must be analyzed for contaminants that may interfere with the normal metabolic processes. These analyses must be maintained by the facility as raw data. Any contaminant found in food or water above accepted regulatory guidelines should be noted in the QA reports to the SD and management.

Pest control measures used must also be documented. Any pesticides that can interfere with the study should not be used. This usually precludes the use of aerosol-based insecticides. Other means of vector control include adhesive traps for rodents, blue light with adhesive strips for flying insects, larvae-disrupting compounds for standing water and some wastewater applications, and other methods that generally do not require the use of chemical agents.

TEST AND CONTROL ARTICLES: SUBPART F

Test and Control Article Characterization

The test article is very important and as such must be tested for identification, strength, and purity. Each test article batch should be tested and documented in accordance with GLPs. The test article synthesis or the method by which it was derived must be documented by the sponsor company or the testing facility. When consumer products are used as test articles, either in whole or in part, the label can be used to characterize them. The sponsor or the testing facility must characterize the stability of the test article as well.

Depending on the SOPs, a periodic analysis of each batch must be completed before or at the beginning of the study. Name, chemical abstract or code number, batch number, and expiration date must be labeled on each storage container for a test article or control article. Storage containers for a test article are assigned to that test article for the duration of the study. Storage must be adequate to maintain purity and strength of the test article for the duration of the study. For studies that last longer than 4 weeks, reserve samples of test articles and control articles must be maintained.

Test and Control Article Handling

The proper procedures that create and maintain a system for handling and testing the test and control article must be detailed in the SOP. These include the storage, distribution, and identification. This is to prevent contamination or destruction of the test and control article. It is essential to properly identify the test article throughout the process. The distribution and the receipt of each batch include the date, time, and quantity, and the lab must document any returns.

Mixtures of Articles with Carriers

If a test article is to be mixed with a carrier molecule, then a test by an appropriate analytical method must be done. This is necessary to determine the concentration of the test and control article in the mixture. The stability of the test and control article can be done before or at the beginning of the study and as required, depending on the conditions of the study. If the test or control article has an associated expiration date, it must be clearly marked on the label. If more than one expiration date applies, then the earliest one should be listed.

PROTOCOL FOR AND CONDUCT OF A NONCLINICAL LABORATORY STUDY: SUBPART G

The protocol is the instrument by which objectives and methods about the study are presented. It varies in its requirements, depending on the type of animal studied and the particular requirements of the study. However, it is uniform and defines the specific criteria that must be followed in order to obtain the desired results. A protocol should contain the following information.

Protocol — Section 58.120

(a) Each study will have an approved written protocol that clearly indicates the objectives and all methods for the conduct of the study. The protocol will contain, as applicable, the following information:

(1) A descriptive title and statement of the purpose of the study.
(2) Identification of the test and control articles by name, chemical abstract number, or code number.
(3) The name of the sponsor and the name and address of the testing facility at which the study is conducted.
(4) The number, body weight range, sex, sources of supply, species, strain, substrain, and age of the test system.
(5) The procedure for identification of the test system.
(6) A description of the experimental design, including the methods for the control of bias.
(7) A description and/or identification of the diet used in the study as well as solvents, emulsifiers, and/or other materials used to solubilize or suspend the test or control articles before mixing with the carrier. The description will include specifications for acceptable levels of contaminants that are reasonably expected to be present in the dietary materials and are

known to be capable of interfering with the purpose or conduct of the study if present at levels greater than established by the specifications.
(8) Each dosage level, expressed in milligrams per kilogram of body weight or other appropriate units, of the test or control article to be administered and the method and frequency of administration.
(9) The type and frequency of tests, analyses, and measurements to be made.
(10) The records to be maintained.
(11) The date of approval of the protocol by the sponsor and the dated signature of the study director.
(12) A statement of the proposed statistical methods to be used.

(b) All changes in or revisions of an approved protocol and the reasons therefore shall be documented, signed by the study director, dated, and maintained with the protocol.

Conduct of a Nonclinical Laboratory Study — Section 58.130

(a) The nonclinical laboratory study will be conducted in accordance with the protocol.

(b) The test systems will be monitored in conformity with the protocol.

(c) Specimens shall be identified by test system, study, nature, and date of collection. This information shall be located on the specimen container or shall accompany the specimen in a manner that precludes error in the recording and storage of data.

(d) Records of gross findings for a specimen from postmortem observations should be available to a pathologist when examining that specimen histopathologically.

(e) All data generated during the conduct of a nonclinical laboratory study, except those that are generated by automated data collection systems, shall be recorded directly, promptly, and legibly in ink. All data entries shall be dated on the date of entry and signed or initialed by the person entering the data. Any change in entries shall be made so as not to obscure the original entry, shall indicate the reason for such change, and shall be dated and signed or identified at the time of the change. In automated data collection systems, the individual responsible for direct data input shall be identified at the time of data input. Any change in automated data entries shall be made so as not to obscure the original entry, shall indicate the reason for change, shall be dated, and the responsible individual shall be identified.

RECORDS AND REPORTS: SUBPART J

Record keeping and reports have defined requirements that vary by type but not content with respect to the final product. The format does not depend on the particular species being studied nor does it depend on the nuances of the study or the facility layout.

Reporting of Nonclinical Laboratory Study Results — Section 58.185

(a) A final report shall be prepared for each nonclinical laboratory study and shall include, but not necessarily be limited to, the following:

(1) Name and address of the facility performing the study and the dates on which the study was initiated and completed.
(2) Objectives and procedures stated in the approved protocol, including any changes in the original protocol.
(3) Statistical methods employed for analyzing the data.
(4) The test and control articles identified by name, chemical abstracts number or code number, strength, purity, and composition or other appropriate characteristics.
(5) Stability of the test and control articles under the conditions of administration.
(6) A description of the methods used.
(7) A description of the test system used. Where applicable, the final report shall include the number of animals used, sex, body weight range, source of supply, species, strain and substrain, age, and procedure used for identification.
(8) A description of the dosage, dosage regimen, route of administration, and duration.
(9) A description of all circumstances that may have affected the quality or integrity of the data.
(10) The name of the study director, the names of other scientists or professionals, and the names of all supervisory personnel involved in the study.
(11) A description of the transformations, calculations, or operations performed on the data, a summary and analysis of the data, and a statement of the conclusions drawn from the analysis.
(12) The signed and dated reports of each of the individual scientists or other professionals involved in the study.
(13) The locations where all specimens, raw data, and the final report are to be stored.
(14) The statement prepared and signed by the quality assurance unit as described in Section 58.35(b)(7).

(b) The final report shall be signed and dated by the study director.

(c) Corrections or additions to a final report shall be in the form of an amendment by the study director. The amendment shall clearly identify that part of the final report that is being added to or corrected and the reasons for the correction or addition, and shall be signed and dated by the person responsible.

Storage and Retrieval of Records and Data — Section 58.190

(a) All raw data, documentation, protocols, final reports, and specimens (except those specimens obtained from mutagenicity tests and wet specimens of blood, urine,

Food Safety Assessment: Compliance with Regulations

feces, and biological fluids) generated as a result of a nonclinical laboratory study shall be retained.

(b) There shall be archives for orderly storage and expedient retrieval of all raw data, documentation, protocols, specimens, and interim and final reports. Conditions of storage shall minimize deterioration of the documents or specimens in accordance with the requirements for the time period of their retention and the nature of the documents or specimens. A testing facility may contract with commercial archives to provide a repository for all material to be retained. Raw data and specimens may be retained elsewhere provided that the archives have specific references to those other locations.

(c) An individual shall be identified as responsible for the archives.

(d) Only authorized personnel shall enter the archives.

(e) Material retained or referred to in the archives shall be indexed to permit expedient retrieval.

Retention of Records — Section 58.195

(a) Record retention requirements found in this section do not supersede the record retention requirements of any other regulations in this chapter.

(b) Except as provided in paragraph (c) of this section, documentation records, raw data and specimens pertaining to a nonclinical laboratory study and required to be made by this part shall be retained in the archive(s) for whichever of the following periods is shortest:

(1) A period of at least 2 years following the date on which an application for a research or marketing permit, in support of which the results of the nonclinical laboratory study was submitted, is approved by the Food and Drug Administration. This requirement does not apply to studies supporting investigational new drug applications (INDs) or applications for investigational device exemptions (IDEs), records of which shall be governed by the provisions of paragraph (b)(2) of this section.
(2) A period of at least 5 years following the date on which the results of the nonclinical laboratory studies are submitted to the Food and Drug Administration in support of an application for a research or marketing permit.
(3) In other situations (e.g., where the nonclinical laboratory study does not result in the submission of the study in support of an application for a research or marketing permit), a period of at least 2 years following the date on which the study is completed, terminated, or discontinued.

(c) Wet specimens (except those specimens obtained from mutagenicity tests and wet specimens of blood, urine, feces, and biological fluids), samples of test or control articles, and specially prepared material, which are relatively fragile and differ markedly in stability and quality during storage, shall be retained only as long as the quality of the preparation affords evaluation. In no case shall retention be required for longer periods than those set forth in paragraphs (a) and (b) of this section.

(d) The master schedule sheet, copies of protocols, and records of quality assurance inspections, as required by Section 58.35(c) shall be maintained by the quality assurance unit as an easily accessible system of records for the period of time specified in paragraphs (a) and (b) of this section.

(e) Summaries of training and experience and job descriptions required to be maintained by Section 58.29(b) may be retained along with all other testing facility employment records for the length of time specified in paragraphs (a) and (b) of this section.

(f) Records and reports of the maintenance and calibration and inspection of equipment, as required by Section 58.63(b) and (c), shall be retained for the length of time specified in paragraph (b) of this section.

(g) Records required by this part may be retained either as original records or as true copies such as photocopies, microfilm, microfiche, or other accurate reproductions of the original records.

(h) If a facility conducting nonclinical testing goes out of business, all raw data, documentation, and other material specified in this section shall be transferred to the archives of the sponsor of the study. The FDA shall be notified in writing of such a transfer.

Many regulations govern toxicology testing in the nonclinical research environment, such as the GLPs in support of application for research or marketing permits. It is important to remember that GLP regulations in support of a nonclinical research also apply to university and private research labs that may be directly or indirectly involved in the support of an application to the FDA.

It should be remembered that the results from research conducted under GLP studies is not necessarily better or worse than that under non-GLP studies. The GLP guidelines give regulators, researchers, and pharmaceutical and biotech companies a frame of reference from which to plan, conduct, and compare results. It also lays out steps that need to be taken in order to bring new products and drugs to the market. The guidelines were meant to create a level playing field for researchers and companies and to eliminate guesswork about what may or may not be acceptable. The GLP guidelines provide a frame of reference about what is required to bring a product to the market, how to organize studies in a way acceptable to regulators, how to represent findings of these studies, and how to address concerns in a methodical way.

GOOD MANUFACTURING PRACTICES

For manufacturers and industry, good manufacturing practices (GMPs) are analogous to GLPs for toxicologists. GMPs were based on the FDA's proposed regulation in the 1967 Federal Register, indicating that food is adulterated if it has been prepared, packed, or held under unsanitary conditions. The code of GMPs, which defines conditions for acceptable sanitary practice in the food industry, went into effect in 1969. GMPs cover aspects of building and facilities, production and processing, equipment and temperatures, maximum allowances for contamination, and action levels for defects in the manufacturing practices. Also, quality of water used for manufacturing and limits for environmental substances are documented, including recall procedures for when food is found to be in violation of the Pure Food Law.

GMP regulations are used by manufacturers of pharmaceuticals, medical devices, and food, as they produce and test products that people use. FDA has issued these regulations as the *minimum* requirements. GMPs are regulations that describe the methods, equipment, facilities, and controls required for production. GMPs define a quality system that manufacturers use as they build quality into their products. For example, approved drug products developed and produced in accordance with GMPs are safe, properly identified, of the correct strength, pure, and of high quality. Originally, GMPs were based on the best practices of the industry. As technology and practices improved, GMPs evolved as well.

GMPs can change formally and informally; for example, the U.S. drug GMPs are currently undergoing significant changes. The U.S. medical device GMPs have been completely rewritten. In fact, device GMPs were renamed by the FDA as the Quality System Regulation. In addition to the formal changes, expectations that inspectors have for quality have evolved over time. Such formal changes are communicated to stakeholders by presentations and papers presented by FDA personnel and through agency guides and guidelines.

GMPs of various nations are very similar to those of the U.S. Most have the following requirements: (1) equipment and facilities to be properly designed, maintained, and cleaned; (2) SOPs to be written and approved; (3) an independent quality unit (like quality control or quality assurance, or both); and (4) well-trained personnel and management.

REGULATORY AGENCIES

Toxicology and regulation are intertwined in distinct ways. Those who are regulators rely on toxicological experiments and studies to provide the data, which may be used by them to reach a decision to protect health and the environment. The decision may be to approve a new substance or to restrict the use of a substance being currently used. Because such substances under investigation may be used by consumers, toxicological findings are likely to be influential if not conclusive on items important to our daily lives. In addition, in being a consumer of the experimental results from toxicological studies, a regulator exercises important influence over the design and conduct of such studies. For example, in the U.S., both the Environmental Protection Agency (EPA) and the FDA have been empowered to promulgate standards for various types of toxicological investigations and both have adopted requirements governing laboratory operations and practices. This is not strictly a top–down (regulatory to industry) operation. Communication between government regulators and industrial scientists flows in both directions. The testing standards promoted by the government are strongly influenced by the prevailing consensus of scientists within the discipline.

THE FOOD AND DRUG ADMINISTRATION

The FDA is within the U.S. Department of Health and Human Services and ensures the safety and wholesomeness of all foods, except meat, poultry and some egg products, sold in the U.S. It conducts unannounced inspections and sampling of foods it obtains from food-processing facilities and monitors for unsafe levels of pesticides in foods. FDA develops standards on composition, quality, nutrition, and safety of foods and food additives. The FDA can have products seized (with a court injunction) or suggest that a product be recalled. Within the FDA is the Center for Food Safety and Applied Nutrition (CFSAN), which is directly responsible for ensuring that foods are safe, wholesome, and accurately labeled.

For many years, the FDA played an advice-giving role to manufacturers in prescribing the type and design of tests to be performed. The FDA cataloged this information in their reference entitled *Toxicological Principles for the Safety Assessment of Direct Food Additives and Color Additives Used in Food*, known as the *RedBook*. The first *Redbook* appeared in 1982 and the sequential *Redbook II* is available in part online.

CENTERS FOR DISEASE CONTROL AND PREVENTION

The Centers for Disease Control and Prevention (CDC) is a branch of the U.S. Department of Health and Human Services and supports surveillance, research, prevention efforts, and training in the area of infectious diseases through the National Center for Infectious Diseases. Within the center, the Foodborne and Diarrheal Diseases Branch is responsible for surveillance, outbreak investigation, control, and prevention of foodborne diseases. This branch often works closely with state and local health agencies, serving as a consulting resource. The CDC has laboratories that provide diagnostic resources, evaluate methods for rapid detection, and aid in the identification of toxins and virulent substances. Also, the Biostatistics and Information Management Branch of the CDC is a good resource on processing of surveillance data.

U.S. DEPARTMENT OF AGRICULTURE

The Foods Safety and Inspection Service (FSIS), Agricultural Marketing Service (AMS), and Animal and Plant Health Inspection Service (APHIS) are three branches within the USDA charged with responsibilities for food safety. FSIS is responsible for inspecting meat and poultry products intended for sale within the U.S. or internationally. Although industry has assumed responsibility for ensuring wholesome and safe food, mandatory inspections are facilitated by FSIS to verify, review records and operations, check accuracy of labeled products, and take samples. Also, FSIS plays a crucial role in monitoring for microbial contamination and for residues of drugs, pesticides, and other chemicals in meat and poultry products.

The APHIS is charged with safeguarding animal and plant from exotic invasive pests and diseases. This branch of the USDA helps monitor and manage agricultural pests and diseases within the U.S. and provide the country with safe and affordable food. Another auxiliary role of the APHIS is to ensure the humane care and treatment of animals. Inspectors from the APHIS work at all ports of entry for foods to prevent the introduction of exogenous pests and diseases. Lastly, the APHIS is involved in permitting field testing of new plant varieties, including those produced by genetic engineering.

The AMS is responsible for egg product inspection, both for domestic and foreign distribution. In addition to keeping bad eggs from being sold into the wholesale market, this agency has been very active in developing public awareness strategies for consumers about the problems of salmonella in fresh eggs.

In addition to regulatory branches, the USDA has a large research program dealing with many aspects of agriculture, including food safety and nutrition. The Agricultural Research Service (ARS) conducts research in support of the department's regulatory activities and several of its centers, throughout the U.S., are devoted to human nutrition research.

U.S. Environmental Protection Agency

Manufacturing, labeling, and use of pesticides as designated under FIFRA are regulated by the U.S. EPA. The EPA's Office of Pesticides and Toxic Substances is responsible for licensing pesticides and ensuring that when such substances are used according to label directions, they are reasonably safe and do not pose significant risk to human health or to the environment. In addition to reviewing scientific data on pesticides before registration, the EPA sets limits for the amount of pesticide residues that can remain in or on foods used in the U.S. The agency also has authority to cancel registered use of a pesticide if required to ensure health.

Design and conduct of studies on pesticides and toxic substance are under the control of EPA because of its premarket approval authority. The Toxic Substances Control Act gave the EPA authority to mandate testing. Animal studies of pesticides must comply with the EPA's own GLP regulations, which were inspired by the same investigations that prompted the FDA to establish standards for testing laboratories.

Occupational Safety and Health Administration

The Occupational Safety and Health Administration (OSHA) requires employers to provide their workers with safe working conditions and gives OSHA the authority to mandate occupational safety and health standards. Workers in the food industry, including farm field workers, are covered by such standards. The basis of the 1970 Occupational Safety and Health Act is that no employee should suffer material impairment of health or physical capacity. The meaning of these contradictory phrases was for many years a source of controversy. Pivotal to the debate is OSHA's obligation to weigh the economic costs of its standards vs. health benefits.

The National Marine Fisheries Service

The National Marine Fisheries Service (NMFS) is part of the U.S. Department of Commerce. It conducts inspections on a voluntary fee-for-service on vessel and plant sanitation, product evaluation, the laboratory analyses and review of product labels. Inspection may involve grading and certification of fish for the U.S. or export. The NMFS has an HACCP-based inspection program that targets safety, wholesomeness, and concerns about species substitution (economic fraud).

Local and State Agencies

Local and state regulatory bodies often work in cooperation with federal agencies in setting and monitoring state standards for food products. Many states have their own meat and poultry inspection programs. Local restaurants, food industry, and food services are under local regulatory agencies for food safety and sanitary controls. Within the state exist departments of health and departments of agriculture, which work with the authority of state laws. If the state chooses, these agencies may inspect processing and distribution of foods within the state.

International Agencies

The Codex Alimentarius Commission was created in 1963 by the Food and Agricultural Organization (FAO) and World Health Organization (WHO) to develop food standards, guidelines, and related texts such as codes of practice under the Joint FAO/WHO Food Standards Program. The main objectives of this program are protecting the health of consumers, ensuring fair trade practices in the food trade, and promoting coordination of all food standards work undertaken by international governmental and nongovernmental organizations.

The Codex Alimentarius, or the food code, has become the global reference point for consumers, food producers and processors, national food control agencies, and the international food trade. The code has had an enormous impact on the thinking of food producers and processors as well as on the awareness of the end users, the consumers. Its influence extends to every continent, and its contribution to the protection of public health and fair practices in the food trade is immeasurable. The Codex Alimentarius system presents a unique opportunity for all countries to join the international community in formulating and harmonizing food standards and ensuring their global implementation. It also allows them to participate in the development of codes governing hygienic processing practices and recommendations relating to compliance with those standards.

The Codex Alimentarius is relevant to international food trade. With the ever-increasing global market, in particular, the advantages of having universally uniform food standards to protect consumers are self-evident. It is not surprising, therefore, that the Agreement on the Application of Sanitary and Phytosanitary Measures (SPS) and the Agreement on Technical Barriers to Trade (TBT) both encourage the international harmonization of food standards. A product of the Uruguay Round of multinational trade negotiations, the SPS agreement cites Codex standards, guidelines, and recommendations as the preferred international measures for facilitating international trade in food. As such, Codex standards have become the benchmarks against which national food measures and regulations are evaluated within the legal parameters of the Uruguay Round agreements.

Since the first steps were taken in 1961 to establish a Codex Alimentarius, the Codex Alimentarius Commission has drawn world attention to the field of food quality and safety. During the past three decades or more, all-important aspects of food pertaining to the protection of consumer health and fair practices in the food trade have come under the commission's scrutiny. In the best traditions of the FAO and the WHO, as part of its persistent endeavors to develop the Codex Alimentarius, the commission has encouraged food-related scientific and technological research as well as discussion. In doing so, it has lifted the world community's awareness of food safety and related issues to unprecedented heights and has consequently become the most important international reference point for developments associated with food standards.

U.S. FOOD LAWS

The original 1906 Food and Drugs Act contained two prohibitions only, which remain as part of the current law. The first forbids the marketing of a food containing any added poisonous or deleterious substance that may render it injurious to health. The second forbids the marketing of food containing nonadded toxicants that make them ordinarily injurious to health. The FDA had the burden of proving that a food was adulterated, and there was no required premarket approval. The act has been amended several times to improve the FDA's ability to ensure the safety of foods. The most important amendment was the 1958 Food Additives Amendment, for which additives had to be demonstrated as safe before marketing. However, the amendment excluded substances generally recognized as safe (GRAS) by scientific experts. There was, and still is, a distinction made between cancerous and all other toxic agents. For all other noncarcinogenic substances, regulators embraced standard safety assessment formulae, using the concept of acceptable daily intakes (ADIs) or thresholds below which no toxicity can be observed. However, this approach was not considered appropriate for carcinogens, as the premise is that cancer-causing substances cannot be assumed to have safe concentrations. Thus, the famous Delaney Clause was enacted as part of the Food Additives Amendment in 1958, which excludes the use of any food additive shown to induce cancer in humans or in experimental animals. GRAS items were not subject to the Delaney Clause because they are not technically food additives.

Pesticide residues, animal drug residues, and food contact materials (packaging material) are under distinct regulatory standards. Pesticide residues are under the 1954 amendment to the Food, Drug, and Cosmetic Act, which allows residues if they meet a tolerance established by the agency. This now falls under the jurisdiction of the EPA. Pesticide residues that satisfy the tolerance standards are exempt from the food additive provisions of the Food, Drug and Cosmetic Act, including the Delaney Clause. However, if the concentration of the pesticide in a processed food exceeds the tolerance standard and is considered a carcinogen, then it is prohibited from use by the Delaney Clause. Essentially, an animal drug residue must be shown to be safe for humans under the same standards that apply to food additives. A food contact substance requires approval as a food additive.

The FIFRA indicates that no pesticide may be marketed unless it has been registered by the EPA. The EPA has for several decades been engaged in a comprehensive review of previously registered pesticides and reregistration of those that meet current standards for marketing. The Toxic Substance Control Act (TSCA) of 1976 covers all chemical substances manufactured or processed in or imported into the U.S. The act gave the EPA the powers to restrict, ban the manufacture, processing distribution, use, or disposal of a chemical substance based on unreasonable risk of injury to health or environment.

STUDY QUESTIONS AND EXERCISES

1. Name the U.S. regulatory agencies concerned about food safety and discuss their respective jurisdictions and responsibilities.
2. Outline and draft a set of SOPs for measuring a toxicant metabolite (biomarker) in blood plasma.
3. Describe some factors in an animal long-term drug study that if not controlled may seriously jeopardize the study and lead to scrutiny by the FDA.
4. Describe the pros and cons of the Delaney clause regarding how scientists and consumers view carcinogens.
5. Describe the roles of SD, quality assurance, and SOPs in GLP-compliant toxicity tests.

Food Safety Assessment: Compliance with Regulations

TABLE 5.1
U.S. Food Laws

Law	Year	Action
Federal Meat Inspection	1906	
Pure Food and Drug Act	1906	Prohibits interstate commerce of misbranded and adulterated foods
Federal Food, Drug, and Cosmetic Act	1938	Expands the 1906 law and placed FDA in charge of food additives
Federal Insecticide, Fungicide, and Rodenticide Act	1947	Covers whether the pesticide is added to or is concentrated in a processed food.
The Pesticide Chemical Amendment	1954	Covers chemical fertilizers, herbicides, and pesticides used in or on raw agricultural commodities
Federal Poultry Product Inspection Act	1957	
The FIFRA Reauthorization	1988	Required complete reregistration of more than 600 pesticides
Delaney Clause	1967	No additive will be deemed to be safe if it is found to induce cancer when ingested by humans or animals
Color Additives Amendment	1960	Defines color additives and classifies them as certifiable or exempt from certification
Fair Packaging and Labeling Act	1966	Establishes mandatory food standards that require labeling of foods.
Wholesome Meat Act	1967	
Good Manufacturing Practices	1967	Regulation for manufacturing practices
The Food Additive Amendment	1988	Responsibility of determining whether a food additive was safe or was shifted from the government to the manufacturers
The Organic Foods Product	1990	Establishes a national set of standards easing intrastate commerce
Nutritional Labeling and Education Act	1990	Mandates nutrition labeling on all FDA-regulated processed foods and promotes voluntary labeling of fresh meat and produce
Dietary Supplement Health and Education Act	1994	Defines supplements, sets criteria for regulating labeling and claims, and establishes government agencies to watch regulation of supplements
Pathogen Reduction Act	1996	Requires that all plants which produce meat products install a plan to eliminate the points in a process, where if control is lost, contamination could occur

RECOMMENDED READINGS

Centers for Disease Control and Prevention, http://www.cdc.gov.
Environmental Protection Agency, Hazardous waste management system: General, 40 C.F.R. Part 260, 1993.
Food and Drug Administration, http://www.fda.gov.
Food and Drug Administration, Good laboratory practice for non clinical laboratory studies, 21 C.F.R. Part 58, 1994.
Middlekauff, R.D., Regulating the safety of food, *Food Technol.*, 43, 296, 1989.
Scientific Status Summary, Office of Scientific Public Affairs, Institute of Food Technologists, The risk/benefits concepts as applied to food, *Food Technol.*, 42, 119, 1988.
United States Department of Agiculture, http://www.usda.gov.
USDA FSIS, http://www.usda.gov/fsis.
Vanderveen, J.E. Nutritional equivalency from a regulatory perspective, *Food Technol.*, 41, 131, 1987.
World Health Organization Food Safety Program, http://www.who.int/fsf.

6 Risk

RISK–BENEFIT

The consumer is constantly blitzed by the media about some toxic substance. For food, there are claims that it is overprocessed, oversalted, oversugared, and oversaturated. The media has also claimed that the food is devitalized, filled with chemicals, drugs, and synthetic ingredients, and polluted by agriculture and industry. So, for many, it is hard not to succumb to the belief that a food safety crisis exists. Unfortunately, picking on chemicals makes for good press. In many media outlets, the definition of the term *chemical* has become almost analogous to *toxic substance* or *poison,* and conjures up images of cancer, birth defects, or tragic diseases. This chemophobia is based on the consumers' perception of what makes up the risk that chemicals are bad and more is worse (Figure 6.1). Consumers with a better understanding of science want to know how hazardous a substance is to their health during their lifetime. Exposure to a myriad of human-made (anthropogenic) chemicals and natural chemicals is an everyday event. How much or how little is too much? How hazardous is the exposure to one's health during a lifetime? These are questions that consumers often pose. Risk is associated with the chance of injury, damage, or loss. Risk can be physical, monetary, or even psychological — it can be anything that adversely affects people. There are no quantifiable limits of how big or how small a risk may be. Humans tolerate varying degrees of risks and may even ignore high-risk situations voluntarily. For example, the risk of death by motorcycling is 20,000 per 1,000,000 or death attributed to smoking 20 cigarettes/day is 5000 per 1,000,000. Each year, the sixth most frequent cause for accidental death in the U.S. is choking while eating, but it is rarely that the consumer would consider voluntary starvation over choking. Thus, there are acceptable risks that the consumer is willing to take voluntarily. However, there are other aspects of our lives, such as eating foods, which some believe should be risk free. *Safe* is another term that is grossly misused. Absolute safety would be the assurance that no injury or damage can occur from the use of a substance. For many consumers, this is a hard concept to grasp. However, one must concede that some risk exists with the use of any substance, chemical, or something found in food — no human undertaking is without some risk. Absolute safety is unattainable, but relative safety is defined as a practical certainty that injury or damage will not result from the use of a substance in a reasonably common manner and quantity. Some examples of relative food safety are given here. Eating peanut butter is relatively safe, yet peanut butter is responsible for approximately seven asphyxiations in young children each year. Drinking water is essential and safe; however, pure water not used in a reasonable and common manner and quantity

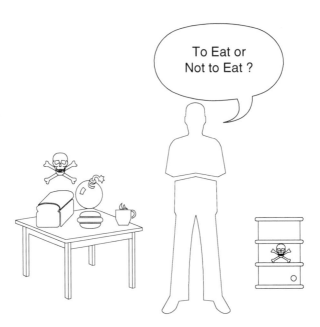

FIGURE 6.1 Chemophobia: consumers' perception of chemicals in our environment.

can result in renal shutdowns. Properly cooked fish is a safe and nutritious food source rich in certain unsaturated fatty acids that can be beneficial for health. However, this is not true for a person who suffers from severe fish allergies, for whom one bite of fish can be fatal, and in pregnant women eating fish with mercury and polychlorinated biphenyls (PCB) contamination may affect the fetus. Food safety must take into account the person who eats the food as well as the food itself. Foods considered safe for most people can be extremely toxic or even lethal to certain sensitive or allergic individuals even when used in a reasonable manner and quantity. Nuts are a good source of nutrition, but for those who suffer from allergies to nuts, eating them can be traumatic or even fatal.

Taking risks is part of life and humans are unique in the sense that they frequently ignore high risks taken by them voluntarily, but become terribly concerned about insignificant risks if they are imposed on them. There are risks associated with driving a car or flying a plane, but many choose these forms of transportation willingly.

Science cannot demonstrate that a risk does not exist. Research can determine the probable limits of possible risk, and if the limits are low enough or the benefits significant, or both, then the risk should be tolerable. For example, eating outweighs the concern about choking. Thus, food, eating, and every aspect of our lives involves some risk–benefit decision that may or may not be made consciously. The conflict that consumers can face is when any group imposes a risk on others, i.e., involuntary risk opposed to voluntary risk. When people attempt to avoid certain risks, they usually introduce other risks. Each time an individual rides in an automobile, there is risk, because of which a person may choose to stay home. However, falls at home result in more than 6000 deaths annually and home electrocution accounts for another 200 deaths each year. What is acceptable risk? When and to whom is the risk

Risk

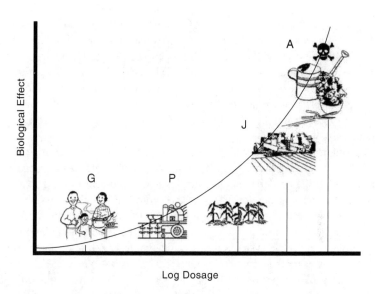

FIGURE 6.2 Exposure to any given chemical will vary with the population, depending on vicinity to the chemical and length of exposure.

acceptable? Such questions ultimately gravitate toward the ability of science to predict risk from existing toxicity and exposure databases. The role of risk assessment is to reveal the types of injury that may be associated with a toxic substance. Risk assessment is based on exposure level and frequency of exposure to the toxic substance and its inherent toxicity.

The risk associated with each substance may have to be handled differently, depending on the exposed populations. Figure 6.2 shows several populations that may be identified as having possible exposure to a range of concentrations of the toxic substance. Exposure populations include those that are the consequence of accidental and suicidal poisoning (A, e.g., a farm worker preparing pesticides for application), job-related exposure, or occupationally exposed workers (J, farm workers spraying fields with pesticides), passersby or bystanders such as workers nearby and dwellers in an adjacent farm (P), and the general public (G, grocery produce person and consumers). Poisonings tend to be over a narrow range, whereas occupational exposures are over a broader range. As expected, there is a tendency for overlap between the exposed populations. In an acute situation, if no adverse health effects are detected at high levels of exposure, it is a fair assumption that it is unlikely that anything adverse will be observed at a lower level of exposure. However, things may be quite different for the relationship of concentration to adverse effects in chronic exposure.

Occupational exposure, such as food handlers in a production line, may have intermittent exposures to a range of concentrations of a particular substance. Such exposures to a toxicant may result in toxic signs and symptoms that can be quantified. To protect workers, chemical substances' threshold limit values (TLVs), permissible exposure levels (PELs), short-term exposure limits (STELs), or time-weighted averages (TWAs) have been recommended. TLVs were designed to protect workers from exposures to solvents (American Conference of Governmental Industrial Hygienist, ACGIH, or OSHA, PELs) and are based on the best available information from industrial experience, animal tests, and studies with human volunteers. TWAs are values for a normal 8-h workday and 40-h work weeks. STELs are values for a short time period, i.e., 15 min. Thus, there is usually a very good database to work with to protect workers.

For the passerby or bystander, exposure is much more difficult to assess. The signs and symptoms may be ill defined or even bogus and the dosage range could be difficult to assess.

The problem of defining who is at risk becomes even greater for the general population. Ascertaining signs and symptoms of toxicity over background levels is difficult and is influenced by factors such as age, gender, health status, nutrition, and a host of other confounders. This is the difficulty in risk assessment and the crux of the entire risk assessment process. The assessor utilizes the best-available toxicology data for predicting risk to the health of the general population.

Risk assessment is the systematic scientific characterization of potential adverse health effects resulting from human exposures to hazardous agents. Risk assessment has the primary objectives of (1) balancing risks and benefits, e.g., in the use of drugs and pesticides; (2) setting target levels of risk, such as in food contaminants and acceptable water pollutants; (3) setting priorities for program activities, as might be done by regulatory agencies, manufactures, and certain environmental and consumer organizations; and (4) estimating residual risks and extent of risk reduction after steps are taken to reduce risk, i.e., determining the impact of mediation efforts.

It has been estimated that certain regulations, such as those advocated in part by the U.S. Environmental Protection Agency, can cost up to $7.6 million per life year saved, whereas the cost per life year saved in various medical intervention and injury-reduction measures is about $20,000 to $50,000. Thus, nine of the ten most expensive life-saving interventions are related to environmental control measures (Dr. Tammy Tengs, Harvard University).

The risk assessment process targets risk characterization or the level of potential risk to humans. The process involves hazard identification data, dose–response evaluation data, and human exposure evaluation data. Hazard identification is the qualitative evaluation of the adverse health effects of a substance in animals or humans. A potential hazard to human health may become discernible in several ways, such as a comment by a worker or a routine safety inspection. Subsequently, a risk assessor would search the literature for relevant data, studies, and case reports. Use of information regarding structure–activity relationships can be very useful, because key molecular structures can identify potential hazards. Many occupational carcinogens have structures belonging to the class of aromatic amines. When available, epidemiological data may provide very useful clues about human exposures. At this stage of the assessment, it is important to consider all the evidence. In the evaluation of animal studies, the risk assessor should be cognizant of sensitive species to the dosage range of concern. *In vitro* studies can be an important adjutant to animal studies, particular in giving valuable information regarding mechanisms of action. Once the initial hazard identification has been completed, the assessor can move toward developing relationships between the dose of the toxicant and various adverse health effects, i.e., a dose–response assessment.

Characterizing dose–response includes all the available information about LD_{50}, LC_{50}, ED_{10}, no observed adverse effect levels (NOAEL), margins of safety, therapeutic indexes, and models for extrapolation to very low doses. Data from animal studies are generally used because human exposure data are limited. The more times the same effect can be found in different animal model species, the better is the chance that the effect will be found in humans. However, the risk assessor is usually interested in low-level exposures for humans that are way below the experimental range of doses used in animal assays. Therefore, low-dose extrapolation and animal-to-human risk extrapolation methods are required. The premise for such extrapolations is that the intensity or frequency of the response is increased with the dose, which begins at zero and rises to measurable changes as the dose increases. After a dose–response assessment, the assessor can initiate exposure assessment.

Human exposure evaluation is the process of measuring the intensity, frequency, and duration of human exposure to the toxicant in the food or environment. The evaluation process describes the magnitude, duration, and route of exposure.

Risk management is the process by which policy actions to deal with the hazards identified in the risk assessment process are chosen. Attempts are made to control risk by eliminating or modifying the conditions that produce the risk. Often, people knowingly practice risk management in their daily lives. Making a home child-safe by putting medications out of their reach and covering electrical outlets to keep their little fingers from inserting metal objects are some examples. Farm workers donning protective clothing, gloves, and mask before working with pesticides and bicycle riders using a helmet to cover their heads are practicing risk management. Risk assessment asks, "How risky is this situation?" and risk management asks, "What shall we do about it?" At the level of government, risk management is practiced by passing regulations and rules for procedures to control risks, and imposing fines and penalties to those who ignore or abuse such procedures. The government gets involved with risks that affect the public or the consumer or other specific groups of people. Obviously, before the government can manage a risk, the risk must be identified and its importance to the population evaluated. This can be an enormous undertaking, requiring time, money, and extensive field and laboratory research.

To be most effective, risk management needs to go hand-in-hand with risk communication. Risk communication is the process of making risk assessment and risk management information comprehensible for lay people, i.e., lawyers, politicians, judges, business people and labor, environmentalists, and community people. When industries fail to communicate their activities to consumers in a timely manner and efficaciously, they may face public adversity and even opposition. Successful risk management can be achieved by those industries that explain their problems with true compassion and respect for their community neighbors and provide opportunity for a two-way flow of communication.

HAZARD IDENTIFICATION, DOSE–RESPONSE, AND EXPOSURE ASSESSMENT

Risk does not have quantifiable boundaries. Hazard is the relative probability that harm or injury will result when the substance is used in a normal manner. Hazard

TABLE 6.1
Major Issues That Animal Studies Should Address in Hazard Identification

Human surrogate suitability of the test species
Age, sex, and number of animals per study group
Types of observations and quantitative methods used
Pathological changes found
Species- and gender-related alterations in metabolic responses

identification involves qualitative evaluation of the adverse health effects of a substance in animals or humans. The evaluation involves searching the literature for relevant human and animal experiments, epidemiological reports, case studies, and sometimes anecdotal information about the substance. Data from relevant *in vitro* test models may be useful as clues for certain modes of toxicity. During the literature search, the assessor should concentrate on including results from studies with objective endpoints that can be predictive of human responses, particularly determination of a dose–effect relationship. Table 6.1 lists the major points that the assessor should look into in reviewing animal toxicity tests.

Animal experimentation is pivotal to the science of toxicology. Recognizing that species differ in their response to toxic substances is crucial for extrapolating results obtained using animals to judgements about human toxicity, and has been covered extensively in Chapter 3. It behooves the risk assessor to select the most sensitive surrogate species in the concentration range anticipated by the population exposed. It also is important to be confident that the toxicity seen for one species will be relevant to another species, particularly humans.

Dose–Response Assessment

The more number of times the same biological response can be evoked in different species, the more likely it is that, at some dose, the same response can be evoked in humans. Thus, one does not exclude results even if the dosage range found in an animal study for evoking a response is not within the encountered range of the substance experienced by humans. The literature may provide information that shows response in several species over a 1000-fold range of the concentration of the test substance. With a lack of reliable human data on exposure to the test substance, the risk assessor should initiate risk assessment by selecting results from the most susceptible species, based on low-dose extrapolation to some acceptable concentration.

Exposure Assessment

This is the process of measuring or estimating the concentration, frequency, and duration of a toxic substance in the human environment. For a foodborne substance, the risk assessor should estimate how much substance is present in a normal serving, whether cooking or processing affect its concentration in the food, and whether certain populations might be more susceptible than others to the adverse effects, i.e., elderly and young children vs. a healthy adult population. The process describes the magnitude, duration, and types of foods exposed and the number of likely subpopulations of human populations exposed.

An estimate is made of the number and magnitude of uncertainties in the measurements. There may be situations in which complete data is lacking or there are deficiencies in the available toxicity and exposure data. It also is useful to describe techniques that might be employed to reduce exposure to the toxic substance.

RISK CHARACTERIZATION

With information about the dose–response and exposure features of the substance, the risk can be characterized. Risk characterization is the process of estimating the probable incidence of an adverse health effect to humans who are under the circumstances of exposure. When every data is available, risk characterization should be based on human data. However, frequently human data is fragmented, incomplete, or even lacking. Thus, extrapolations are made from dose–response relationships established by controlled chronic animal studies. Whether the dose–response relationships are zero or nonzero thresholds, i.e., whether they are threshold or non-threshold, respectively, should be determined. Figure 6.3 provides graphical examples of such hypothetical options for extrapolated dose–response curves. The

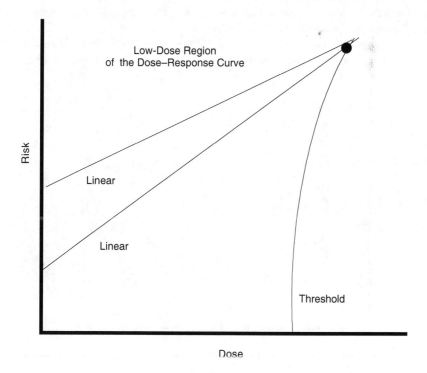

FIGURE 6.3 Graphical examples of hypothetical options for an extrapolated dose–response curve.

threshold represents a dose below which no response is observed in the low-dose region; alternatively, in the nonthreshold approach, numerous dose–response curves can be proposed in the low-dose region of the dose–response curve if a threshold assumption is not made.

THRESHOLD RELATIONSHIPS

For threshold responses, there will be a level below which adverse health effects are not likely to occur. Some examples include organ or tissue effects such as neurotoxicity, hepatotoxicity, nephrotoxicity, developmental effects, and germ-cell mutations or noncancer endpoints. Human exposure data are usually limited and animal bioassay data must be extrapolated. However, risk assessments usually require looking for dose–response at low human exposures, way below the experimentally observable range of response in animal bioassays. Extrapolation from animal data to the human risk situation represents a major aspect of dose–response assessment. Often, one has little idea of the exact shape of the lower end of the dose–response relationship, which is linear or curvilinear. This is because of difficulties in preselecting a range of doses in a chronic or subchronic toxicity testing that appropriately will result in a range of toxicological effects from overt toxicity through some intermediate toxicity expression to no toxicity, representing the highest, moderate, and lowest doses, respectively.

Figure 6.4 shows a theoretical dose–response relationship showing dose-related toxicity. A number of effect-related endpoints can be assigned at the lower end of the dose–response curve. The no observed effect level (NOEL) is that dose of the test agent at which exposed animals appear to be identical in all respects to control

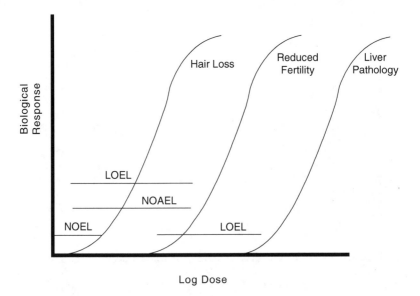

FIGURE 6.4 Dose–response relationships for adverse effects and endpoints for the lower end of the dose–response curves.

animals. The lowest observed effect level (LOEL) is that dose of a test agent at which the exposed animals may show some changes associated with the substance but the changes are not considered adverse effects. The no observed adverse effect level (NOAEL) is that dose at which there are no statistically or biologically significant increases in frequency or severity of effects between the exposed and the control groups. For each toxic substance, an adverse effect may be manifested by a separate threshold dose. Figure 6.4 illustrates progressively adverse responses: hair loss, reduced fertility, and liver pathology. The risk assessor would judge that hair loss is not an adverse effect and assign a NOEL. The lowest observed adverse effect level (LOAEL) is the dose of the substance at which there are statistically no biologically significant differences in the frequency or severity of adverse health effects between the exposed and the control groups. The lowest observed effect (LOEL) is shown with regards to the increased body weight and reduced fertility. At increased doses, fertility is reduced and NOAEL and LOAEL are assigned.

One or more of these values may be obtained and there might be some debate on which is best able to assess the toxic situation of the substance. In a practical sense, regulatory agencies will apply a series of safety factors to these endpoints in arriving at an acceptable concentration such as a reference dose (RfD), acceptable daily intakes (ADIs) promoted by the World Health Organization (WHO), or tolerable upper limit (UL), which has recently been identified for various dietary nutrients by the National Research Council. Typically, these are found by dividing the calculated NOAEL values by safety factors, i.e., uncertainty factors (UFs) or modifying factors (MFs), or both:

$$RfD = NOAEL/(UF \times MF)$$

$$ADI = NOAEL/(UF \times MF)$$

$$UL = NOAEL/(UF \times MF)$$

The purpose of the safety factors is to allow for human (intraspecies) or animal to human (interspecies) variation. UFs are often used to account for extrapolation of results of short-term animal studies to the real-world situation that involves chronic exposure. UFs can also account for the limited numbers of animals used or other limitations found in the experiments. The usual default value assigned to each uncertainty factor is 10. Modifying factors are used to further adjust the UFs in situations where data may be lacking regarding mechanisms of action or toxicokinetics, or if there are concerns about the relevance of the test animal's response to human risk. Anything not considered within the UFs can be adjusted for by modifying factors, either up or down. For example, to determine the UL in the dietary reference intakes (DRIs) for vitamin E, the UF was adjusted to 3 rather than 10 because the scientific thinking was that the research derived from the test animal, the rat, mimicked the human situation very well.

In practice, regulatory agencies prefer using NOEL over NOAEL and so on. For NOEL, the most suitable number derived from various study results may be divided by a factor of 100, accounting for 10-fold uncertainty for intraspecies variability and another 10-fold for interspecies differences:

$$NOEL/100$$

Applying such UFs considers the possibility that the human may be up to 10-fold more sensitive than the animal species used and allows for a 10-fold variability in sensitivity within the human population.

In a situation where only the NOAEL may be derived from the literature, the risk assessor may take a NOAEL/100 and include an additional safety factor of 5- to 10-fold to address the problem of lack of data:

$$NOAEL/500 \text{ or } NOAEL/1000$$

If there is only a LOAEL to work with, 1000 or 500 can be used as the safety factor:

$$LOAEL/1000 \text{ or } LOAEL/5000$$

Although the process of applying safety factors may appear to be subjective and even arbitrary, the system has been demonstrated to function reasonably well. Because of the paucity of definitive data, deriving an acceptable daily intake for humans cannot be taken directly from the results of animal studies without adjustment by an appropriate safety factor. One needs to account for many factors, such as multienvironmental exposures or the effects over an acute or chronic exposure or a lifetime. The number derived should be as conservative an estimate as possible.

Sometimes NOAEL values have been used in risk assessment to evaluate a margin of safety (MOS), which is the ratio of NOAEL determined in test animals (mg/kg/day) to the level to which a human might be exposed. For example, if a population is exposed through food ingestion of a toxicant at 0.5 mg/kg/day for a 60-kg man and the NOAEL found for neurotoxicity is 50 mg/kg/day, the MOS is 1000 for ingestion of the neurotoxicity. This large number, above 100, reassures the public that the risk is low. MOS values below 100 usually result in appropriate actions by regulatory agencies.

Nonthreshold Relationships

There are some types of toxic effect in which the perceived mechanism supports the notion that there may be no threshold for the biological effect. Theoretically, for a chemical carcinogen, a single molecule can be sufficient to interact with DNA and cause a permanent alteration of the genome of a single cell, which could become a cancer. The model is referred to as the one-hit type of exposure and gives a linear dose–response relationship with no dose threshold when extrapolated through zero, as shown in Figure 6.3. Much of the information and subsequent cancer modeling regarding this linear dose–response relationship is based on radiation research. Such models assume that for the toxicant, there are infinite number of target DNA, that the toxic response occurs only after a minimum number of the target DNA have been

TABLE 6.2
Models Used in the Determination of Low-Dose Response

Statistical or tolerance distribution: Probit, logit, Weibull
Mechanistic: One-hit, multihit, multistage
Time to tumor occurrence: Log normal, Weibull

modified, that the target DNA is critical, and that the probability of a hit in the low-dose range of the dose–response curve is proportional to the dose of the toxicant.

Public chemophobia has had a marked influence on the way regulatory agencies have handled their determination of permissible levels of toxic compounds. The 1958 Delaney Clause, described in Chapter 5, is an example of such a regulatory product, which excluded approval of a food additive found to induce cancer in humans and animals or the so-called zero tolerance (*de minimis*) approach to food additives and contaminants. However, the value of zero is completely contingent on the sensitivity of the methods used by the analytical chemist to detect the toxicant. What was available in 1958 in the analytical chemist's instrument arsenal has been far exceeded, going from part per million (ppm) to part per trillion (ppt) and beyond. Thus, in 1958, 1 DDT per million could be detected and currently DDT can be detected in everything, which presents a dilemma for the risk assessor, who has to consider zero tolerance and the increase in detection ability because of analytical advancement.

In essence, the concept of nonthreshold is contrary to observation. Very few things in the world have zero risk. Much of what has been or will be quoted about the risks associated with foods, drugs, or anything else in life is misunderstood by the public. Although everyone is exposed to trace amounts of numerous carcinogens, not everyone develops cancer in his/her lifetime. Observations suggest that in most cases the exposure to a carcinogen was too low for a response to be found, i.e., a practical threshold dose exists for the action of carcinogens.

The ultimate goal of risk assessment is to not underestimate human risk. A number of mathematical models have been developed to achieve this end, and some are listed in Table 6.2.

Thus, if a threshold assumption is not made, several dose–response curves can be proposed in the low-concentration region of the dose–response curve. The selection of the model is based on appropriate chronic animal studies. The statistical or tolerance distribution models are based on the assumption that each individual has a tolerance level for a toxicant and that level is a variable that follows a specific probability distribution.

RISK PUT INTO PERSPECTIVE

In 1987, Dr. Bruce Ames, a scientist from the University of California, Berkeley, ranked the low level of risk for many chemicals (human-made or naturally occurring) to which humans may be commonly exposed. Selected examples are listed in Table 6.3. The ranking was based on the chemical's carcinogenicity to rodents and the

TABLE 6.3
HERP Values for Selected Substances

Substance	HERP (%)
Ethylene dibromide (EDB)	0.0004
PCB	0.0002
Tap water	0.001
Saccharin	0.06
Comfrey herb tea	0.03
Basil	0.1
Wine	4.7

estimated extent of human exposure to the chemical. Human exposure/rodent potency (HERP) values or risk ranking for these chemicals were derived by Dr. Ames, and he concluded that carcinogenic hazards from current levels of pesticide residues, water pollution, or food additives are likely to be of minimal concern relative to the background of natural substances. For example, the HERP value for ethyl alcohol in wine is 10,000 times the possible hazard of ethylene dibromide (EDB). However, for wine, philosophically the risk is more acceptable because it is a naturally occurring toxic substance.

Although no uniform method or criterion for risk assessment exists among all the government agencies overseeing food safety, in general the FDA has interpreted the Delaney Clause according to the *de minimis* doctrine to permit the use of carcinogenic food additives with a cancer risk below 1 in 1 million. The National Academy of Sciences concluded that public health would be best served by subjecting all foods, raw or processed, to the same criteria regarding residues of carcinogenic compounds and to use the *de minimis* standard to define whether such compounds were decreed to be present at unacceptable levels. Thus, a substance would not be considered to violate the Delaney Clause if its presence results in less than a specified increase in risk, i.e., in an increase in a lifetime risk of cancer of less than 1 in 100,000 or 1 in 1,000,000.

STUDY QUESTIONS AND EXERCISES

1. What are the underlining principles for threshold and nonthreshold dose–response relationships?
2. Describe the process used for risk assessment of a new food additive.
3. How does the risk assessment of an environmental toxicant differ from risk assessment of an essential nutrient?
4. What components are considered for uncertainty factors (UFs) or modifying factors (MFs), or both, used in determining RfD or ADI?

RECOMMENDED READINGS

Gaylor, D.W. and Kodell, R.L., Linear interpolation algorithm for low dose risk assessment of toxic substances, *J. Environ. Pathol. Toxicol.* 4, 305-312, 1980.

Hallenbeck, W.H. and Cunningham, K.M., *Quantitative Risk Assessment for Environmental and Occupational Health*, Lewis Publishers, Chelsea, MI, 1987.

National Research Council, *Toxicity Testing, Strategies to Determine Needs and Priorities*, National Academy Press, Washington, D.C., 1983.

Tengs, T., Enormous variation in the cost-effectiveness of prevention: implications for public policy, *Curr. Iss. Publ. Hlth.* 2, 13-17, 1996.

Weisburger, E.K., Mechanistic consideration in chemical carcinogenesis, *Reg. Toxicol. Pharmacol.*, 12, 41-52, 1990.

7 Epidemiology in Food and Nutritional Toxicology

Extrapolation of data from animals to humans can be problematic because of differences between species. Human studies can be conducted by performing epidemiological studies. Epidemiology is the examination of the distribution and determinants of diseases or health-related circumstances, good or bad, in identified populations. Epidemiology's intent is to apply what is learned from such examination to the control of health-related problems. Epidemiological studies uncover relationships between exposure to substances and health effects. Epidemiological methods for study strategy, data collection, and data analysis are used for testing hypotheses linking health effects with the distribution of substances.

Epidemiological data play an important role in food and nutritional toxicology, such as in the assessing safety of food ingredients, the efficacy of phytochemicals, and incidence of foodborne illnesses. In foodborne illnesses, epidemiology is the tool used to estimate who will get sick from what food substance, how often, and under what conditions. With epidemiological data, one can assess the risks of foodborne hazards and establish priorities for which one may allocate resources. Such increased knowledge can become crucial to consumers, to policymakers for developing strategies to tackle food safety issues, as well as to evaluate the effectiveness of food safety programs.

Some examples of human epidemiological studies used in food and nutritional toxicology include linking aflatoxin B1 with liver cancer, food colors with allergic reactions, and prevention of lung cancer by carotenoids. Although links or correlations can be obtained by using epidemiological tools, the major disadvantage of epidemiological studies is the variety of things humans are exposed to, making it difficult to isolated effects of a specific substance on a population. Also, variability in population will affect the outcomes of epidemiological studies. Although epidemiological studies have limitations, they often can be used to corroborate the results of animal-based experiments.

There are two main types of epidemiology strategies: descriptive and analytical. Descriptive epidemiological strategies emphasize on the number and characterization of individuals, locales, and time. Descriptive epidemiology includes questions such as who became ill, what were the symptoms, when were the symptoms first seen, and how many people had the symptoms. Graphical plots of such information are

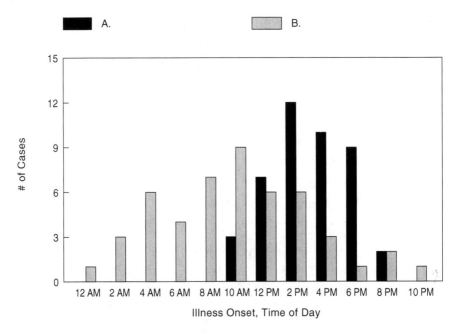

FIGURE 7.1 Epidemic curve.

referred to as epidemic curves, e.g., number of cases vs. onset time of illness. Figure 7.1 illustrates an epidemic curve having a span of onsets: A = 12 h and B = 24 h. Descriptive strategies are interested in existing distribution of variables; thus, they neither make inferences with regard to causality nor do they test hypotheses.

Epidemiological strategies that are designed to look at associations for causal relationships are analytical. Analytical strategies concentrate on ascertaining and estimating the effects of definite risk factors, e.g., comparing people who have been exposed or become ill to those who have not; looking for difference between the two groups, such as types of food consumed; and identifying factors that may have led to illness.

DESCRIPTIVE STRATEGIES

Descriptive epidemiology strategies can be considered as sentinel tools useful in developing hypotheses. The evaluation of data obtained from such studies can be useful in subsequent plans for conducting further and more elaborate analytical studies. Usually, descriptive strategies are less costly to conduct and of shorter duration compared with analytical strategies. Because no inferences can be made with regard to causality, descriptive strategies can be limited in their usefulness.

ECOLOGICAL STUDIES

Ecological studies concentrate on observations made with the group and not with the individual. Examples include farm workers or inhabitants of a city or country.

Nutritional data may be available only for the population under study, such as food balance sheets. The outcome variable under study in ecological studies is often mortality, e.g., mortality level due to cardiovascular diseases in different countries correlated with average saturated-fat consumption per capita in the countries. These studies involve observing disease frequency in large population-based groups and correlating such frequencies with exposure information. Thus, such studies are called correlation studies, relating exposure patterns of groups to disease incidence or mortality rates for whole populations. Different parameters such as nutritional status, occupation, geographic location, or economic status can be used to define the groups for study. For example, one might correlate low birth weights in infants in different Western countries with the frequency of maternal use of alcohol for such countries and find a correlation between low birth weights and the frequency of alcohol use. Similar designs may be used to examine a relation between a toxicant and a disease. Such studies are relatively inexpensive and quick to complete because they can usually utilize existing demographic governmental data and various registries containing information on health-related incidences, diseases, death certificates, etc. Traditionally, ecological studies are regarded as useful for generating a hypothesis. These studies do not make correlations between exposure and health outcomes among individuals and cannot be directly extrapolated to the individual. This is because the correlations are based on average exposure levels for the population groups and not all individuals within the group have the same exposure level. Overinterpretation of ecological studies can lead to an ecological fallacy. Therefore, the results of such studies are insufficient to demonstrate a relationship without other types of data to support them.

CASE REPORTS

These are anecdotal or clinical observations made that suggest a possible causal relationship between a change in a health parameter and exposure to a substance. There are probably unique experiences of a patient or a group of individuals with a similar diagnosis. Many medical observations of foodborne illnesses fit into this classification, and these are subsequently reported and published in medical literature. In retrospect, case reports have been used to substantiate an epidemic onset. Case reports can be useful in alerting health agencies as to the possible adverse health effects or benefits of an exposure. The more cases authenticated, i.e., case series, the greater is the value as evidence for generating a hypothesis. Case reports can provide the basis for an analytical strategy for examining the situation of concern.

ANALYTICAL STRATEGIES

Analytical strategies for epidemiology include cross-sectional, prospective, and retrospective studies. Such strategies are often initiated following a sequence of descriptive studies. They are more informative than descriptive strategies; however, they are expensive to run and time consuming to conduct. These types of epidemiology strategies have been used to obtain results that are used in safety evaluation of regulated products and provide the scientific base for governmental regulations of health claims on food and food labeling. Together, descriptive and analytical epidemiological strategies provide a perspective to health sciences that the mere use of experimental approaches in the laboratory does not, i.e., links to human exposure and disease. Whereas descriptive strategies generate hypotheses, analytical strategies test them.

CROSS-SECTIONAL STUDIES

In cross-sectional studies, the unit of study is the individual. Individuals are selected randomly, at one point in time, and information is gathered regarding exposures and health outcomes. In cross-sectional studies, data on exposure as well as biological effects are collected at the same time. Such studies are often used to describe the prevalence of certain diseases in a population. Prevalence is defined as the number of cases present in the population at a given point of time. Prevalence and incidence are related to each other. In a population where the number of new cases equals the number of cases that disappear, i.e., a steady-state population, prevalence (P) is equal to the product of incidence rate (I) and the duration (D) of the disease:

$$P = I \times D$$

Thus, the prevalence is determined by the duration of the disease if the incidence rates of two diseases are equal. In contrast, incidence is defined as the number of new cases that arise during a specific period of time. For example, the yearly cancer incidence is the number of persons who during a year were diagnosed to have cancer for the first time.

Cross-sectional studies are often referred to as surveys. For example, one might conduct a survey involving a random sample of individuals of a city to study the relationship of viral infection level with their dietary habits, lifestyle, age, and socioeconomic status. Such information may be obtained from a questionnaire and by examining databases from the local health agency. The correlations measured from such data can give an estimate of the proportion of people infected with the virus at a particular point in time, which is termed as prevalence.

The advantages of cross-sectional studies are that the design is simple, only a short duration of time is required to conduct them; usually no follow-up of individuals is required; and, compared to other analytical strategies, they are relatively inexpensive. The shortcomings of cross-sectional studies are that they reveal nothing about the temporal sequence of exposure and disease: only one time point used, and essentially based on current exposure as a representative for past exposure. As such, these studies do not investigate causal relationships for exposures that change over time.

PROSPECTIVE STUDIES

Prospective studies are often referred to as cohort or follow-up studies. Cohort refers to people exposed and those not exposed to suspected risk factors, i.e., the entire contacted group of people. In contrast to the cross-sectional studies, a study popu-

Epidemiology in Food and Nutritional Toxicology

lation of exposed and nonexposed individuals (groups) is selected and both groups are followed to determine the incidence. Prospective studies along with retrospective studies (discussed later) are longitudinal studies because they follow a certain property over the course of time and the investigator takes data points at various times. Because exposure is discerned before disease, prospective studies are considered the gold standard of epidemiological research.

The groups can be defined on time, such as the summer college class of freshmen, or defined on specific requirements (e.g., fire fighters or workers, menopausal women, retired men aged 50 to 55). Thus, people are enrolled into a cohort and baseline data are collected on factors of interest to the study, such as their lifestyle and exposure to the substance. The range of people enlisted in prospective studies can be from 100 to 100,000, and as time passes, some individuals will develop the disease of interest.

Prospective studies involve a large population or a prolonged period of time (years), or both. Prospective studies are expensive. One might need to contact 15,000 people and wait 5 years before 12 individuals contract the disease of interest.

In prospective studies, the incidence rates of the disease under study can be measured directly, which is a major advantage in epidemiology research. Therefore, absolute and relative risks can be directly measured. In prospective studies, it is possible to enquire into the association of a particular exposure with more than one disease and establish a temporal relationship between such exposure and the other diseases. Besides the expense involved, other disadvantages include difficulty in conducting large and long studies, potential bias if every member of the cohort is not kept track of, and insufficiency of the projected length of the study for the latency period of the disease. In addition, in contrast to case-control studies (discussed in the next section) perspective studies can be very inefficient for studying rare diseases.

An intervention study is a type of prospective study that can be very conclusive as well as very expensive. In intervention studies, the epidemiologist intervenes with the study population, e.g., smokers given a pill containing vitamin E, vitamin C, and beta-carotene to test the effect of supplemental antioxidants on the incidence of lung cancer. Thus, the investigator exerts a degree of control over the risk factors of interest, i.e., intakes of antioxidants.

Retrospective Studies

In retrospective studies, or case-control studies, data are obtained regarding past exposure to possible etiological factors from selected cases with a specific disease, and appropriate controls without the disease. The two populations are matched by considering all other variables (age, socioeconomic status, medical history, conditions of the work place or other environment, etc.). One contacts people who exhibit a certain trait and those without it (the controls) and then attempts to determine the risk factor from their past history. The history of exposure to a substance or other factors, such as occupation, is obtained for each person. The rates of exposure of these groups can be compared, and if differences are found, potential causal factors for the specific health effects can be studied. Usually, 50 to 1000 people each for cases and controls are enrolled in this type of study. Compared with prospective studies, retrospective studies are much less expensive and require less time to conduct, mostly because they need a smaller population size.

Retrospective studies are useful to study rare diseases, such as most cancers, because of the lower number of individuals needed and because the studies start by collecting individuals with the disease of interest. Because such studies select only cases of the disease of interest, there is no bias in ascertaining the endpoint. Retrospective studies are the preferred method to study diseases that have some unique and specific cause, e.g., infectious agents.

The disadvantages of case-control studies are the logistics, such as selecting controls and obtaining measurements of pass exposures without introducing bias. Thus, bias can occur during detection and selection of cases and during assessment of exposures. Care must be taken to ensure that controls are identical to exposed people with only the exception of the factor of interest. Retrospective studies have played an important role in safety evaluations at FDA, such as the use of artificial sweeteners and the National Bladder Cancer Study, and in evaluating the etiology for outbreaks of foodborne disease.

META-ANALYSIS

Meta-analysis involves combining or pooling data from different epidemiology studies, usually those involving analytical strategies. Meta-analysis can sometimes overcome the lack of statistical power found in the original studies. In the original epidemiology studies, exposed and nonexposed populations are the subjects of the studies; in meta-analysis, the results of the original studies function as the subjects of the studies. Weights can be assigned to the results of the individual studies, based on their reliability or the sample size. Meta-analysis can help learn how variables affect study results. Variables include exposure concentration, study design, methods of statistical analysis, geographical location of studies, and even less obvious factors such as date of publication or the original study. One methodological pitfall is the potential for publication bias. Editors of journals prefer to publish results indicating positive associations, even if they are only weak and perhaps inadequate from a methodological point of view. Thus, only papers showing positive effects are published and the outcome is a distorted picture of the real human health risk, skewed from the negative effects, because such effects are not published. Fortunately, journal editors are recognizing the need to publish negative findings; however, researchers still need to be encouraged to submit such findings for publication.

MOLECULAR EPIDEMIOLOGY

Molecular epidemiology seeks to link biological events with epidemiological research. It involves application of molecular tools, such as biological markers (biomarkers), to population-based studies in the attempt to better understand the development of disease, such as mechanisms of disease and metabolic pathways affected. In addition, molecular epidemiology can provide information regarding useful markers for detection or prognostic purposes, treatment, and prevention of disease. The search for biomarkers is a key determinant in molecular epidemiological research because of their ability to predict the incidence or outcome of a particular disease. Biomarkers can be any substance or functional process that can be measured in the organism or products and fluids thereof (blood, plasma, blood cells, feces, urine, milk, bile, saliva, gases from expiratory air, sweat, hair, etc.). Biomarkers reflect some phase between exposure and effect. They can be biochemical, metabolic, molecular, genetic, or immunological substances or events in biological systems. Biomarkers must be specific in assessing the human exposure to a substance. The molecular epidemiological approach can provide a better measure of exposures, both past and current. Ultimately, the combination of molecular biology and epidemiology will help reduce misclassification of the disease and provide insights on genetic susceptibility, i.e., given the same exposure, why only some fractions of individuals develop disease.

Before using a biomarker in large-scale epidemiological studies, the biological measure must be well described. This involves basic research on the disease by using several animal models, *in vitro* and *in vivo* approaches, and in humans. So-called transitional studies are done to bridge laboratory research with epidemiology, using small population-based studies. Such studies deal with issues such as processing of biological samples, accuracy and precision of methodology, and the effect of potential confounding factors. The objectives of transitional studies are to determine the optimal conditions required for collecting, processing, and storing biological samples and whether a particular biomarker assay is specific, reliable, and accurate. Subsequently, the biomarker may be applied in larger and extensive epidemiology studies.

Confounding is the effect of a third variable that influences the exposure–disease relationship under study and is very important in epidemiology. The confounder variable is associated with the exposure being studied and is an independent risk factor for the health outcome under analysis. A cohort study on the relation between alcohol intake and risk of lung cancer might find a relative risk. However, people who consume alcohol often smoke (a confounding variable). Smoking is a known risk factor for lung cancer. Confounding variables usually have a stronger effect than the exposure under study. To find the correct relative risk of alcohol on lung cancer, either the study population has to be restricted to nonsmokers or else smokers and nonsmokers have to be separated. Therefore, a corrected estimate of the relative risk can be obtained by calculating a weighted average of the stratum-specific relative risks for smokers and nonsmokers, which usually involves statistical procedures to adjust for confounding, such as, logistic regression. Sometimes an unknown or perhaps not measured confounder is present. Because such confounders cannot be adjusted for by statistical analyses, a biased study results. Thus, in addition to confounding factors, epidemiology studies must watch out for bias and interaction effects. Interactions, also referred to as affect modifications, include the phenomena of additive, antagonistic, or synergistic effects. Bias effects tend to skew results from the true value. Bias can be divided into selection bias and information bias. Selection bias occurs when the effect measured is corrupted because of the selection of study subjects, e.g., if subjects are systematically excluded from or included in the case or control group. Case-control studies are especially sensitive to selection bias, e.g., in cases being recruited from hospitalized persons with controls recruited from the same hospital, because hospitalized persons are likely to differ from the general population.

Information bias is defined as errors in the information obtained or misclassification errors. Such bias may lead to underestimation or overestimation of the effect.

Three types of molecular epidemiological studies are employed to examine discrete details of the exposure–disease continuum. Exposure dose studies use biomarkers in epidemiological studies to assess the effect of doses of exposure on disease outcomes. Physiological studies look at the association of physiological alterations in diseases. Gene–environment interactions are studies that define the contribution of inherited genetic background in the development of disease.

Exposure–Dose Studies

The critical issue in such studies is the half-life of the substance being measured. The range of a half-life of biomarkers (e.g., the heavy metal cadmium) in either blood or urine can vary from minutes to years. In addition, tissue difference can be found for the same substance. The half-life of lead in blood is about 1 month but between 10 and 50 years in bone tissue. Therefore, blood may be a useful specimen to assess recent exposure of lead but bone may be a good biomarker for assessing past exposures.

In general, the stability of many biomarkers is limited and reflects recent exposures. Thus, finding suitable biomarkers to study chronic disease can be difficult. Recent research has emphasized the use of protein or DNA-adducts, or both, as biomarkers; however, such measures usually reflect only recent exposures because most adducts are short-lived molecules.

Physiological Studies

Usually, research shows an association between blood levels of an endogenous chemical or a metabolite, or a hormone, and its involvement with a process, e.g., some specific kidney tumor formation. A cohort study may be carried out in which blood samples of each individual can be collected and stored at baseline evaluation. After years of follow-up, some of those individuals could develop the specific kidney tumor. Blood samples from those individuals could be revived and analyzed for the hormone, and an association between the specific tumor and blood levels of the hormone may be established. It is likely that the relationships reflect some inherited differences between individuals before the tumor formation and that the factors (hormone and tumor formation) are important determinants of the specific kidney tumor.

Therefore, biological measures can be used in molecular epidemiology studies to identify causes of a disease. Such studies can be beneficial by providing insights into mechanisms of the disease. In addition, they provide ways to diagnose and even prevent the disease.

Gene–Environment Interactions

A complex combination of genetics and exposure appears to control which individuals develop or do not develop a disease. A genetically susceptible subgroup of a population may be at risk from exposure to a particular substance; conversely, the risk of carrying a particular genotype may be evident in an exposed population. Polymorphism is when a germline variation is present in the population at a frequency ≥1%. DNA variations may be due to deletions, insertions, and base substitutions. These variations can have dire consequences on genetic transcription and translation, and thereby have a functional consequence. Thus, common inherited variations in genes can increase the risk of developing disease, and thus functional polymorphisms are relevant in the etiology of the disease.

Case-control studies are the usual design for susceptibility gene analysis. For example, a number of studies have focused on the analysis of drug-toxicant metabolism genes involved in phase I and phase II reactions of various carcinogens and their respective cancers. Polymorphisms for several phase I and phase II enzymes have been related to the risk of cancer. Arylamines are carcinogenic compounds from tobacco smoke, and functional polymorphisms have been found for the genes that code for the enzymes that produce the carcinogenic metabolites. In one case of the gene, a variant allele produces a protein that activates arylamines to form a more reactive compound. Case-control studies demonstrate a statistical significance for the interaction between the gene and exposure to smoke and tumor formation.

FOODBORNE DISEASES AND EPIDEMIOLOGY

When two or more persons experience similar illness after eating the same food, it constitutes an outbreak. This is opposed to a single occurrence of a foodborne illness, or an incident. If the incident has follow-up evidence, microbiological, clinical, or epidemiological data, a case is formed. Such evidence may establish the etiology (cause) of the disease. However, if the illness is an isolated event, the disease is labeled as a sporadic case.

Outbreak investigations usually begin by local health agencies, sometime assisted or joined by state and federal governmental agencies. In the U.S., final reports are filed to the Centers for Disease Control and Prevention (CDC). Investigations usually include interviews with affected people, inspections of food preparation practices, and, when possible, analysis of clinical and food samples. Lack of resources often hinders local agencies, leading to incomplete or inaccurate investigations filed with CDC. About 60% of reported foodborne disease outbreaks are filed at CDC with unknown etiology.

A rise of epidemiological studies in the past decade has contributed to our insight about food and nutritional toxicology, particularly regarding links between nutritional imbalances and chronic diseases. Such studies will likely play pivotal roles in understanding the significance of various phytochemicals and xenobiotics in human health.

STUDY QUESTIONS AND EXERCISES

1. How are incidences of foodborne illnesses derived?
2. Describe the types of epidemiological studies and the factors that dictate the use of one type over another.

3. Define some potential biomarkers for cancer, heart disease, birth defects, and macular degeneration.
4. Describe how you would develop an epidemiological study to look at the relationship between adverse health outcomes and arsenic in the drinking water of a specific population.

RECOMMENDED READINGS

Doll, R. and Peto, R., The causes of cancer, *J. Natl. Canc. Inst.* 66, 1195-1308, 1981.
Hennekens, C.H. and Buring, J.E., Epidemiology in medicine, Little, Brown, Boston, MA, 1987.
Knapp, R.G., and Miller M.C., III, *Clinical Epidemiology and Biostatistics,* Harwal Publishing, Malvern, PA, 1992
Gordis, L., *Epidemiology,* W, B. Saunders, Philadelphia, 1996.
Schulte, P.A. and Perera, F.P., *Molecular Epidemiology,* Academic Press, San Diego, CA, 1993.
Stern, M., Norbert, P.E., Koper, P., and Taylor, J.A., Molecular epidemiology, in *Introduction to Biochemical Toxicology,* 3rd ed., Hodgson, E. and Smart, R.C., Eds., John Wiley & Sons, New York, 2001.

8 GI Tract Physiology and Biochemistry

ANATOMY AND DIGESTIVE FUNCTIONS

Like nutrients, foodborne toxicants enter the body by way of the gastrointestinal (GI) tract or alimentary tract, particularly through the wall of the small intestine. The GI tract is a tube extending from the mouth to the anus. This hollow tube is several times longer than the height of a person, and is ca. 30 ft. The GI system includes the gut, with salivary glands, pancreas, liver, and gall bladder. The primary function of the GI tract is to break down complex food components into substances appropriate for absorption into the body. Also, it provides a means for waste removal from the digestive and metabolic operations. Lastly, the wall of the GI tract represents a barrier between the body and the outside world, i.e., the last frontier. The cell lining the GI tract not only controls the form in which nutrients enter the body but also has the ability to keep substances that are of no value or are potentially dangerous out of the body. To perform its functions, the GI tract system engages in digestive, motility, secretory, and absorptive operations (Table 8.1).

The GI tract consists of the oral cavity, pharynx, esophagus, stomach, small intestine, and large intestine (Figure 8.1). Special organs of the GI tract include the teeth, tongue, salivary glands, liver, gall bladder, and pancreas. Food and ingested material move through the open area of the muscular tube called lumen, which technically is the outside of the body, separated from the interior of the body by a lining known as the mucosa. The lining of the GI tract has additional layers, some of which are made of smooth muscle, which move contents through the lumen by rhythmic contractions. Sections of the GI tract are separated by circular muscles, called sphincters, which control the passage of food. Figure 8.2 illustrates parts of the stomach (fundus, body, atrum) and the esophageal (cardiac) sphincter and the pyloric sphincter.

Food enters the mouth, where chewing mixes it with saliva to moisten and lubricate the material. Amylase is released in the mouth to degrade polysaccharides into absorbable sugars, and, combined with the mastication, also destroys some of the bacteria. The lipid-digesting enzyme lingual lipase is released into the mouth, serving a similar function. About 1 to 2 qt of saliva is produced each day. A small bolus of food can be thrust to the back of the mouth, where simultaneously the epiglottis slips over the top of the trachea, thus preventing food from entering the respiratory tract. In the late stages of rheumatoid arthritis, elderly patients are prone to develop weakness in these muscles and become susceptible to respiratory infec-

TABLE 8.1
Functions of the Gastrointestinal Tract

Function	Detail
Digestion	Process of breaking down food into components
Absorption	Nutrient transport into the body
Elimination	Waste removal
Barrier	Last frontier between the body and the outside world

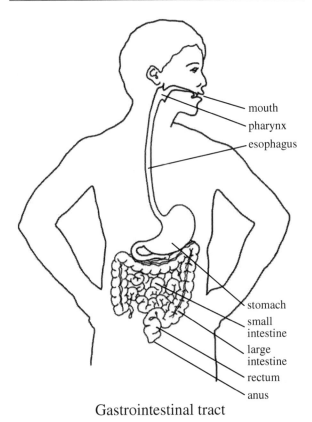

Gastrointestinal tract

FIGURE 8.1 Sections of the GI tract.

tions, pneumonia, and require surgical invention for nutrition support. Food passes through the esophagus by contractions and gravity. The cardiac sphincter at the bottom of the esophagus allows food to enter the stomach and at the same time prevents digestive juices and food from being moved back. The stomach functions as a reservoir, storing ca. 1 to 2 l of chyme until the lower tract is ready for the food. With the introduction of food in the stomach, the hormone gastrin is released, which stimulates the release of hydrochloric acid and pepsinogen, a proteolytic enzyme, by the stomach wall. However, very little absorption occurs in the stomach,

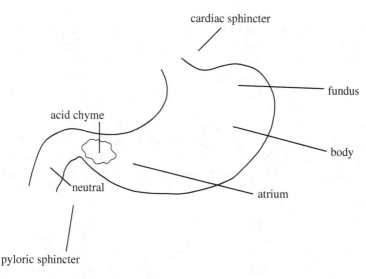

FIGURE 8.2 Stomach, esophagus, and sphincters.

the exceptions being water, alcohol, and some toxicants. Figure 8.3 shows that the walls of the stomach are characterized by the presence of several exocrine and endocrine glands. Oxyntic glands are exocrine glands that secrete HCl, pepsinogen, intrinsic factor, and mucus. Chief cells are zymogenic cells that produce the enzymes of the gastric section. The low pH of about 2.0 for the stomach is a critical defense and protects the body from many pathogens by the partial denaturation of proteins. *Salmonella* is particularly sensitive to acid, and the elderly, who often consume antacids or because of surgery, can have low stomach acid and be at risk.

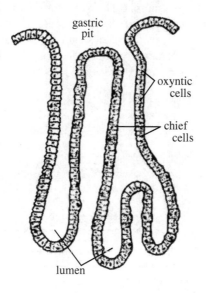

FIGURE 8.3 Cells and glands of the stomach.

It takes approximately 4 to 6 h to churn the chyme in the stomach, which involves the processes of preparing the nutrients in food for absorption, i.e., peristalsis, mixing with digestive secretions. The approximately 10-ft-long small intestine is the major section of the GI tract where absorption occurs. The mucosal surface of the small intestine is highly specialized for the absorptive process. A completely liquefied chyme leaves the stomach and enters the duodenum. The duodenum and stomach are separated by the pyloric sphincter, a muscular outlet that functions to regulate the amount of liquid chyme into the small intestine. The relatively short duodenum, approximately 8 in., is one of three segments of the small intestine, followed by the jejunum and ending with the longest segment, the ileum. The duodenum receives secretions from the pancreas, which include particular enzymes for fat, carbohydrate, and protein digestion, and bile, which helps emulsify fats for easier digestion and absorption. Bile, made in the liver and stored in the gall bladder, is composed of six primary ingredients: bile salts, cholesterol, lecithin, bile pigments, various minerals, and end products of organic and xenobiotic metabolism. Enterohepatic circulation or first-pass effects, in which toxicants may be excreted by the liver (activated or deactivated) into the bile and thus pass into the intestine, has been discussed previously. If the properties of such a toxicant are favorable for intestinal absorption, a cycle may result in which biliary secretion and intestinal reabsorption continue until metabolic degradation to urinary excretion eventually eliminates the toxicant from the body.

Absorption of substances occurs throughout the length of the small intestine. The histology of the GI tract wall is similar throughout the length of the tract. Figure 8.4 illustrates that the walls have several distinct layers. The layer closest to the lumen is the mucosa. The outermost region of the mucosa, the muscularis mucosae, is composed of smooth muscle. Adjacent to the muscularis mucosae is the submucosa, which is followed by circular smooth muscles, which in turn is followed by a layer of longitudinal smooth muscle. The outermost layer of the small intestine is the serosa. Buried within the different layers of muscles of the GI tract are blood vessels, which transport nutrients, hormones, and oxygen to and from the wall. In addition, the muscles contain nerve plexuses, which provide control to wall activity, and connective tissue and supporting ligaments.

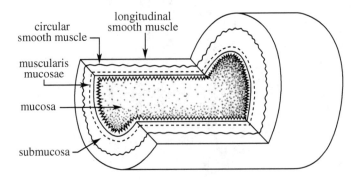

FIGURE 8.4 Layers of the intestinal tract.

The inner surface of the small intestine has finger-like projections. These circular folds are ca.10 mm in height and on the surface of these folds are small 0.5- to 2-mm-high projections called villi. Villi are tightly packed and dense and each villus is covered with even smaller 1-mm-high projections called microvilli. The combined effect of circular folds, villi, and microvilli multiplies the inner surface area of the small intestine by 300 times the size it would be if the small intestines were only a smooth-walled lumen.

The surface of each villus is made of a layer of specialized cells one cell in thickness. A few of the cells produce mucus, hormones, and other chemicals from the immune system, but most are absorptive cells. The mucus protects the inner intestinal wall and is part of the barrier discussed earlier. The hormones and chemicals of the immune system represent other components of the intestinal barrier and protect against infectious microorganisms and toxins in foods. Figure 8.5 shows the

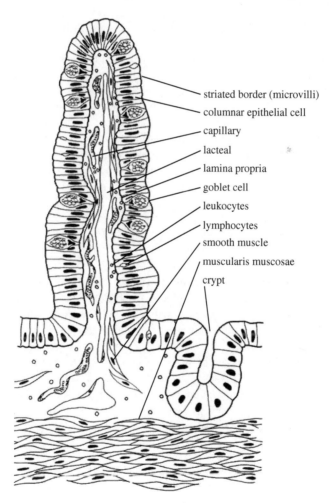

FIGURE 8.5 Composition of the villus.

composition of a villus. Projecting from the villi are the microvilli, which contain many enzymes and receptors. Absorption occurs by the columnar epithelial cells near the villus tip. Mature absorptive cells of the villus differentiate from precursor cells in the crypts. The tips have a short half-life of a few days and are sloughed off. In addition, there are goblet cells, which that produce mucin, and endocrine cells, which produce various gastrointestinal hormones. Mucins are glycoproteins that contain numerous negatively charged oligosaccharide chains, which can help protect the wall from microbial intrusion. The lamina propria contains phagocytic cells such as macrophages and lymphocytes that protect against invasion, and lacteal, which is part of the lymphatic system and directly empties into the blood circulation.

The intestinal barrier is composed of four components: tight epithelial junctions between cells; goblet cells, which secrete mucin; immune response and antibody production; and inflammatory cells.

GUT ABSORPTION AND ENTEROCYTE METABOLISM

Absorption of substances can occur throughout the alimentary tract. Direct absorption occurs from the oral cavity; however, the absorption area is quite small compared with that of the intestine and the high lipid-to-water coefficient accounts for the prevalent mechanism of substances diffusing from the mouth into the body. Direct absorption from the oral cavity obviates the passage of the compound through the liver (no first-pass effect) and enters the circulation directly. Usually one needs to keep the substance in long contact with the mouth because of limited absorption. This can be achieved by placing the substance under the tongue (sublingual), permitting the compound to go into solution with salivary secretions. Nitroglycerin is an example, which if swallowed can be hepatotoxic.

In the stomach, pH favors absorption of weak acids but not weak bases, which tend to be protonated. Normally, the stomach is not a site of appreciable absorption. Strong acids are poorly absorbed because such compounds are almost completely ionized.

In the small intestine all mechanisms described in the following subsections are operative, whereas in the large intestine little absorption occurs because of the bulk of solids. However, rectal absorption is useful clinically for drugs because this route has no digestive enzymes and there is no direct delivery to the liver.

There are no specific systems or pathways for the sole purpose of absorbing toxicants. Toxicants are absorbed by the same processes responsible for the absorption of essential substances, foodstuffs, and oxygen. As shown in Figure 8.6, nutrients are absorbed from the lumen in several ways: passive diffusion, facilitated diffusion, active transport, and endocytosis.

Passive Diffusion

Passive diffusion is the free movement of substances through the cell membrane. Substances move down their concentration gradient, from the side of the membrane where they are most concentrated to the side where they are less concentrated. Osmosis, a special case of passive diffusion, is the passive diffusion of water across

GI Tract Physiology and Biochemistry

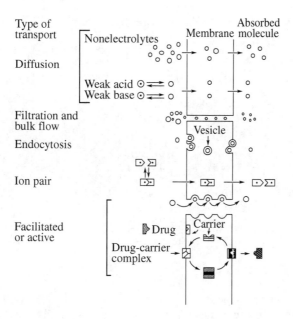

FIGURE 8.6 Nutrient absorption.

a semipermeable membrane. Osmosis is the major process by which water enters the body. Many nutrients, including water, move by passive diffusion from the GI tract lumen into the absorptive cells and eventually from the cells into blood or lymph.

Carrier Mediated

Many nutrients require a specific carrier protein in order to be absorbed into cells by a carrier-mediated process. The specific carrier protein binds to a nutrient or the mucosal side of an absorptive cell membrane and is transported into the cell, from where it can move across the cell and into the blood or lymph. Facilitated diffusion is a carrier-mediated process in which a protein acts as a shuttle to transport nutrients across the membrane. The process relies on an appropriate concentration gradient in order for the nutrient to flow out of the GI tract and no energy is expended. In contrast, active transport involves a carrier acting like a pump, actively transporting nutrients into the absorptive cells, even if the movement of nutrients is to a higher concentration gradient. Movement of a substance up a gradient requires the expenditure of energy, and such transport systems are coupled to energy-releasing reactions, such as the hydrolysis of adenosine triphosphate (ATP) to adenosine diphosphate (ADP) and inorganic phosphate (Pi).

Endocytosis and Exocytosis

Endocytosis and exocytosis are processes by which materials are engulfed into or extruded out of the cell, respectively. In endocytosis, a portion of the cell membrane invaginates to form a membrane-bound vesicle, which eventually pinches off from

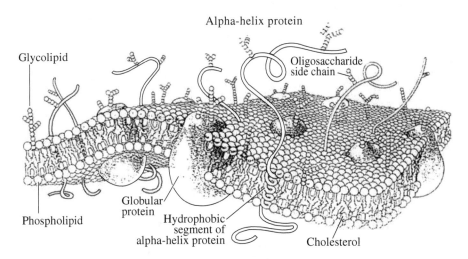

FIGURE 8.7 Membrane structure.

the membrane and enters the cell. Within the cell the vesicle fuses with the lysosome, a cellular organelle that contains various digestive enzymes. The reverse of endocytosis is exocytosis, in which secretory products of cells are passed to the exterior.

MOVEMENT OF SUBSTANCES ACROSS CELLULAR MEMBRANES

The plasma membrane of cells is the first barrier to toxicants. Figure 8.7 illustrates a recent model of membrane structure. This mosaic structure is composed of a discontinuous, bimolecular lipid layer containing various glycoproteins or lipoproteins embedded in the lipid matrix. Ionic and polar groups protrude out of the membrane, as do channels or pores. In addition, the structural matrix can contain enzymes and receptor proteins. The plasma membrane surrounding all types of cells is remarkably similar, whether they are stratified epithelia of the skin, thin cell layers of the lungs or GI tract, or the capillary endothelium. Plasma membranes are about 7 to 9 nm thick and contain a phospholipid bilayer with polar head groups on the outer and inner surfaces. The fatty acids fill the inner spaces and proteins cross it, which allows formation of aqueous pores. The GI tract is considered exterior to the body, and thus poisons in the GI tract usually do not produce systemic injury until they are absorbed, unless such noxious agents are caustic or cause irritation to the gut lining.

Overall, absorption can occur along the entire GI tract, including the mouth and rectum. If a toxicant is an organic acid or base, the substance tends to be absorbed by simple diffusion in that part of the GI tract in which it exists in the most lipid-soluble form.

Lipid-to-Water Partition Coefficient

The ability of a substance to diffuse across membranes is expressed in terms of the lipid-to-water coefficient, which can be defined as the ratio of the concentration of the substance in two immiscible phases: a nonpolar liquid or organic solvent and an aqueous buffer, usually at pH 7.5. The lipid-to-water partition coefficient decreases as the polarity of a substance increases. An increase in polarity can occur by either increasing the substance's degree of ionization or by adding groups such as carboxyl, hydroxyl, or amino groups. Alternatively, reducing a substance's polarity results in an increase in the lipid-to-water partition coefficient. Polarity can be reduced by suppressing ionization or by adding of lipophilic components such as phenyl or *t*-butyl groups.

Ionization and Dissociation Constants

Organic substances or toxicants are usually weak acids or bases. Organic electrolytes do not dissociate completely (do not form ions as dissolved salts do). Only a certain proportion of an organic electrolyte ionizes at a given pH. The degree of ionization by an organic electrolyte influences the substance's lipid-to-water partition coefficient and hence its ability to diffuse across the membrane. Equation 8.1 and Equation 8.2 give the dissociation of a weak acid and weak base:

$$RH \leftrightarrow H^+ + R^- \text{ (Acid)} \tag{8.1}$$

$$B + H^+ \leftrightarrow BH^+ \text{ (Base)} \tag{8.2}$$

Equation 8.1 and Equation 8.2 can be rewritten to derive a dissociation constant K_a:

$$K_a = \frac{[R^-][H^+]}{[RH]} \text{ (Acid)} \tag{8.3}$$

$$K_a = \frac{[H^+][B]}{[BH^+]} \text{ (Base)} \tag{8.4}$$

Taking the logs of Equation 8.3 and Equation 8.4 and substituting pK and pH for the negative log of K_a and [H$^+$], respectively, one arrives at the Henderson–Hasselbalch equations for the degree of ionization of a weak acid or weak base:

$$pH = pK_a + \frac{\log[R^-]}{[RH]} \text{ (Acid)} \tag{8.5}$$

$$pH = pK_a + \frac{\log[B]}{[BH^+]} \text{ (Base)} \tag{8.6}$$

The Henderson–Hasselbalch equations can be used to determine the fraction of a substance that is in the unionized or lipid-soluble form and estimate the rate of absorption from the intestinal or stomach lumen or from the intestinal or stomach

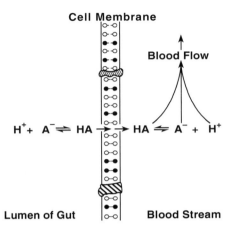

FIGURE 8.8 Unionized vs. ionized solutes in the gut wall.

cells into the blood stream or alternatively from the blood stream into various tissues, such as the brain, and is schematically illustrated in Figure 8.8.

On rearranging the Henderson–Hasselbach equations:

$$pK_a = pH + \frac{\log[RH]}{[R^-]} \quad \text{or} \quad pH + \frac{\log[\text{unionized}]}{[\text{ionized}]} \quad \text{(Acid)} \tag{8.7}$$

$$pK_a = pH + \frac{\log[BH^+]}{[B]} \quad \text{or} \quad pH + \frac{\log[\text{ionized}]}{[\text{unionized}]} \quad \text{(Base)} \tag{8.8}$$

Consider how a weakly electrolytic substance distributes across the gastric mucosa between plasma (pH 7.0) and gastric fluid (pH 2.0). For the plasma, a weak acid with $pK_a = 4 = 7 + \log$ [unionized]/[ionized] = –3. Thus, the ratio of [unionized]/[ionized] = 10^{-3}. When [unionized] = 1, [ionized] = 1000. For the stomach, a weak acid with $pK_a = 4 = 2 + \log$ [unionized]/[ionized] = 2. When [unionized] = 1, [ionized] = 0.01. For the intestine, a weak acid with $pK_a = 6 = -2 + \log$[unionized]/[ionized] = 10^{-2}. When [unionized] = 1, [ionized] = 100.

TRANSPORT INTO THE CIRCULATION

DELIVERY OF TOXICANT FROM THE SYSTEMIC CIRCULATION TO TISSUES

After a substance enters the plasma, it is available for distribution or translocation throughout the body. In general, distribution can occur rapidly. The rate of distribution for a particular substance to a specific organ is determined by the blood flow through the organ and the ease with which the substance crosses the capillary bed and penetrates cells, referred to as capillary permeability and blood flow–tissue mass ratios, respectively. Blood flow–tissue mass ratio is analogous to perfusion rate. The transfer of a substance from capillary to interstitial spaces is faster than the diffusion

GI Tract Physiology and Biochemistry

TABLE 8.2
Blood Perfusion Rates in Various Organs

Tissue	Percent Cardiac Output	Perfusion Rate (ml/min/100 g Tissue)
Kidney	20	350
Brain	12	55
Lung	100	400
Liver	24	85
Muscle	23	5
Skin	6	5
Adipose Tissue	10	3

that occurs across cell membranes unless protein binding is involved. The substance may also travel by bulk force through pores in the capillary bed. Thus, movement of substances through capillary bed pores is a function of molecular size rather than lipid solubility. Penetration depends on diffusion and transport processes. Substances can accumulate in various parts of the body because of protein binding or high solubility in lipid depots, or both. The site of substance accumulation could be a site related to its toxic action or it may just be a site acting as storage and represent a protective mechanism to keep the substance away from more sensitive sites.

Table 8.2 lists blood perfusion rates of various human organs, expressed as either percent cardiac output or volume per minute. The delivery of a toxicant and its eventual equilibration with tissue space are largely determined by the extent of organ flow. Usually, composition of the capillary bed is not a major factor except for the (CNS), where tight intercellular junctions between endothelial cells prevent passage of water-soluble substances.

Once a substance has entered the blood, the rate at which it subsequently penetrates tissues and other body fluids depends on the following factors: capillary permeability, blood flow–tissue mass ratios, extent of plasma protein and tissue binding, regional differences in pH, transport mechanism available, and permeability characteristics of specific tissue membranes. The last factor can be a unique situation, e.g., the tight junctions of the CNS.

STORAGE SITES

Plasma Proteins

Substances found in blood or the vascular compartment bind reversibly with plasma proteins such as albumin, globulins, glycoproteins, lipoproteins, and more specifically transferrin and ceruloplasmin. Figure 8.9 shows a typical electrophoretic pattern of plasma proteins and depicts where various substances are likely to bind. Albumin can bind many substances and has a propensity for acidic compounds. More alkaline compounds are likely to bind with lipoproteins and glycoproteins. The binding is due to various protein–ligand interactions and hydrophobic forces, and can be reinforced by hydrogen bonds and van der Waals forces.

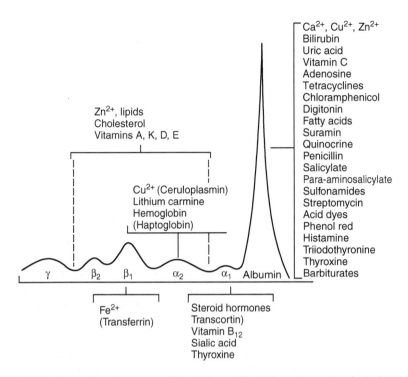

FIGURE 8.9 Electrophoretic pattern of blood plasma illustrating where a chemical might bind.

Protein-binding results in substances that cannot cross capillary walls. Thus, such substances are unavailable for metabolism and excretion. However, the reaction of a substance with protein is reversible, and there can be situations wherein substances with higher affinity for nonspecific binding sites displace a compound with the weaker affinity.

Substances usually bind to lipoproteins by dissolving in the lipid portion of the lipoprotein core. Because of the lipid content, the order of dissolution of lipid-soluble substances is as follows: very-low-density lipoproteins (VLDLs) > low-density lipoproteins (LDLs) > high-density lipoproteins (HDLs).

LIVER AND KIDNEY

Both the liver and kidney have a very high ability to bind chemicals, which is related to the importance of these organs in the elimination of toxicants (see discussion later). Some liver proteins have high affinity for substances such as organic acid. Metallothionein is a protein found in the liver and kidney, which exhibits a high binding capacity for cadmium and zinc.

BONE

Even though bone is a relatively inert tissue, it can accumulate a number of substances, e.g., lead, fluoride, or strontium. Such substances may be incorporated and stored in the bone matrix. Ninety percent of the body's lead eventually makes it way into the skeleton. Incorporation of a toxicant into bone occurs between the interface of the extracellular fluid and the surface of the bone. The surface of the bone is made of hydroxyapatite crystals. The crystal structures of hydroxyapatite create a large surface area for contact of the extracellular fluid. Some toxicants displace other compounds of similar size and charge, such as F^- for OH^- or strontium for calcium. Sometimes, such an exchange and the deposition of a toxicant into bone can be detrimental to bone health, e.g., fluoride deposition resulting in skeletal fluorosis. Other times, toxicant deposited in bone may eventually be released from the bone and such mobilization can cause toxic side effects.

Lipid Depots

Lipophilic substances concentrate in fat. Because the blood flow through lipid depots is low, distribution to fat is slow. Chlordane, DDT, and polychlorinated biphenyls accumulate in fat depots. Fat depots can constitute 20 to 50% of the body weight, depending on whether the individual is the lean, athletic type or obese. Compounds with high lipid–water partition coefficients may be stored in body fat. Storage of toxicants in fat should lower the concentration of the toxicant amount in circulation and lessen the exposure to target sites or receptors. Thus, an obese person should be more protected than a lean individual. However, short-term starvation can result in the release of toxicants from fat depots. Studies in laboratory animals exposed to organochlorine insecticides have shown that starvation produces signs of intoxication.

Physiologic Barriers to Toxicants

The blood–brain barrier, placental barrier, and blood-to-testis barrier are physiological barriers to toxicants. Capillary borders exist between the plasma and brain cells. This boundary is much less permeable than the boundary between plasma and other tissues to water-soluble compounds. The boundary is a single row of brain capillary endothelial cells that are joined by continuous, tight intercellular junctions. Thus, water-soluble compounds must pass through cells rather than between them, which can only occur if the compounds exhibit high lipid–water partition coefficients, enabling them to penetrate the cell membrane. Some areas of the brain are more permeable to toxicants than others. This may be a function of increased blood supply to those areas or a more permeable barrier to substances, or perhaps both. Cortex, lateral nuclei of the hypothalamus, the pineal body, and the posterior lobe of the hypophysis are more permeable than other areas of the brain. The toxicant enters into brain cells by the same principle that governs entrance into other cells. The amount of free toxicant opposed to that which is protein bound and lipid soluble is a key factor governing entrance of a toxicant into the brain. A few foreign compounds gain entrance to brain cells by carrier-mediated processes. Methyl mercury combines with cysteine to form an entity similar to methionine, which can be accepted by large neutral amino acid carriers of the capillary endothelial cells.

At birth, the blood–brain barrier is not fully developed. Thus, infants are more susceptible than adults to some chemicals.

Tissues of the placenta are derived from both fetal and maternal tissues and are perfused by both fetal and maternal blood. The blood vessels are separated by a number of tissue layers, which collectively constitute the placental barrier. Pore sizes begin at ca. 25 μm and are reduced to 2 μm, and leads to molecular size playing a role in the crossing of compounds across the barrier, i.e., less than 600 MW. The pH of fetal blood is 7.3 whereas that of maternal blood is 7.44. These differences give rise to unequal concentrations in mother and fetus.

It is known that the testis has a barrier because of the absence of staining in testicular tissue following intravenous injections of dyes. The barrier assists in the regulation of steroid passage through the testis.

FLUID BALANCE AND DIARRHEA

Diarrhea is an unpleasant physiological effect of toxicant ingestion. It is important to understand the factors and mechanisms responsible for the effect in order to better understand the toxic response and how treatment can be devised. Diarrhea is the frequent evacuation of watery feces. The term is derived from Late Latin *diarrhoea* and Greek *diarrhoia*, from *diarrhein*, which means *to flow through*. Food poisoning, laxatives, and alcohol ingestion can cause acute diarrhea, but it is usually caused by an acute infection with bacteria such as *Salmonella*, *Staphylococcus aureus*, and *Escherichia coli*. Acute diarrhea is usually self-limiting in infants and the major concern to influence the prognosis is prevention of dehydration. Travelers' diarrhea is very common and affects up to half of those traveling to developing areas of the world.

A lack of coordination of the inner circular and outer longitudinal muscular layers of the intestinal wall usually results in an accumulation of excess contents in the lumen, and consequent distension is the physiological response. This distension may cause pain and usually results in hyperactive contractions of the normal segment next to the distended area. Such contractions may be strenuous enough to produce severe, cramping pain. The most common cause of disturbed motility in the small intestine is food that contains an unsuitable component.

There are at least four mechanisms responsible for the increase in fecal water content during diarrhea (Table 8.3). The normal GI fluid balance in an adult consists of an intake of ca. 14 l of fluid per day, which is reduced to 1 l on entering the colon. There is a constant flux of water and sodium across the mucosa, which may total as much as 50 l/d in each direction. However, the flux in the distal small intestine

TABLE 8.3
Mechanisms That Promote Diarrhea

- Defective solute absorption
- Increased solute secretion
- Intestinal structural abnormalities
- Changes in intestinal motility

favors overall absorption. Between the colon and cecum, the volume of water in the normal stool becomes only 100 ml/d. The colon has a large capacity to absorb water, up to three times more than other parts of the gut; thus, diarrhea results in a substantial volume of water to exceed such reserve capacity.

Water and various ions are transported in both directions across the intestinal mucosa. Water and sodium passively move from the blood to the lumen in the duodenum. The jejunum absorbs against an electrochemical gradient sodium, chloride, and bicarbonate ions. The ileum actively absorbs sodium and chloride and secretes bicarbonate. Disturbing the balance may result in the abnormal secretion of ions and water, i.e., secretory diarrhea.

Decreases in solute absorption can result from overeating, deficiencies in gut enzymes or bile flow, or ingestion of poorly absorbed ions such as laxatives. Bacterial enterotoxins can interfere with intestinal electrolyte transport and stimulate secretion because of enterotoxin damage to mucosa walls, which results in the lack of solute absorption and the unabsorbed solutes result in an osmotic effect. Such situations lead to increased stool volume and interference with the absorption of nutrients. Also, mucosal damage can lead to the release of cells and cell debris into the lumen, increasing the hyperosmolarity of the lumen content. Motility usually is not solely responsible for diarrhea but can be a factor in each of the other mechanisms. If cellular membrane damage occurs, it can result in a reduction of surface area and can aggravate diarrhea. Increased volume of fluid can stimulate intestinal motility. Besides dehydration, diarrhea can lead to malabsorption problems, more frequently involving the small intestine, and inflammation, often localized in the large intestine. Pathogenesis of diarrhea in the small intestine includes decreased absorption of fluids and electrolytes, incomplete absorption of nutrients, and increased secretion of fluid and electrolytes, whereas the pathogenesis of the large intestine usually includes decreased absorption of fluids and electrolytes.

The characteristics of diarrheal stools vary with the mechanisms. Stools tend to be watery in a compromised electrolyte balance, i.e., rice-water stools due to a high ratio of water to solids. Stools are black when there is mucosal injury and blood is released into the feces. When fat absorption is compromised, the stools are foul-smelling, emulsion-like particles.

TREATMENT

Identifying and treating the disease is crucial because diarrhea is a symptom. Recovery of fluid and electrolyte balance is the next priority, followed by nutritional concerns.

Obviously, dehydration, or lacking sufficient fluids to maintain function properly, is a key concern with diarrhea. Both the elderly and children are at particular risk and warrant prompt action to avoid serious health problems. Severe diarrhea is debilitating and can be fatal, especially in infants. Large amounts of sodium, potassium, and water are washed out of the colon and the small intestine in the stools, causing dehydration, hypovolemia, and eventually shock and cardiovascular collapse. Lost fluids and electrolytes should be replaced by increasing the oral intake of fluids, particularly those high in sodium and potassium (bouillon and fruit juice). Fluid replacement may include a diet of broth, tea, and toast, but avoid solutions containing sugar, excess caffeine, and sweeteners derived from carbohydrates, e.g., sorbitol.

Gradual introduction of more foods can occur once stool formation is more pronounced. Adding the dietary fiber pectin and other foods high in potassium to the diet may be useful to replace electrolytes. Scraped raw apples or an unsweetened applesauce given every 2 to 4 h, as tolerated, is useful. A solution of glucose and electrolytes in water has been most effective for infants and small children. (Pediatricians recommend 2% concentration of glucose and 45 to 90 mEq/l of sodium and 20 mEq/l of potassium.)

When the diarrhea ceases and the patient begins to tolerate food, the amounts given should be gradually provided, starting with refined foods followed by protein foods and fatty foods. Also, it is useful to avoid lactose early in the recovery phase because gastroenteritis usually results in decreased activity of the enzyme lactase.

During chronic situations of diarrhea, nutritional deficiencies can be a cause for concern and there is a need to replace vitamins, minerals, and protein besides electrolytes and fluids. For example, GI bleed subsequent to diarrhea may be severe enough to cause anemia, and loss of potassium may alter bowel motility followed by anorexia. After the diarrhea, more fiber can be recommended to assist in larger stool formation and to restore bowel motility to normal.

STUDY QUESTIONS AND EXERCISES

1. Where is hydrochloric acid secreted in the GI tract and how is self-digestion by HCl prevented?
2. Describe the types of processes for the absorption of nutrients and give examples of food toxicants that are absorbed by similar mechanisms, e.g., lead or aflatoxins.
3. Why should soft drinks or alcoholic drinks not be given to a patient suffering from diarrhea?
4. Describe how the GI tract is protected against foodborne toxicants.

RECOMMENDED READINGS

Carpenter, C.C.J., The pathophysiology of secretory diarrheas, *Med. Clin. N. Am.*, 66, 597-609, 1982.
Caspray, W.F., Physiology and pathophysiology of intestinal absorption, *Am. J. Clin. Nutr.*, 55, 299S, 1992.
Ganon, W.F., *Review of Medical Physiology*, Appleton-Lange, Norwalk, CT, 1995.
Schneeman, B., Nutrition and gastrointestinal function, *Nutr. Today*, 20, January/February 1993.
Kelsay, J., Effects of fiber, phytic acid and oxalic acid in the diet on mineral bioavailability, *Am. J. Gastrol.*, 82, 983, 1987.
Spellett, G., Nutritional management of common gastrointestinal problems, *Nurse Pract. For.*, 5, 24, 1997.

9 Metabolism and Excretion of Toxicants

The amount of free plasma toxicant is a function of the toxicant's absorption, distribution, and elimination (Figure 9.1). In Chapter 8, a variety of factors that govern the absorption of toxicants in the gastrointestinal (GI) tract were discussed. This chapter focuses on factors that influence distribution and elimination of toxicants.

METABOLISM OF TOXICANTS

CONVERSION WITH INTENT TO EXCRETE

Toxicants and other foreign compounds (xenobiotics) undergo metabolic transformation in the body. In many situations, the rate of metabolism is the primary determinant of the substance for both duration and intensity of action. Compounds that are deactivated by metabolism tend to be more active and linger in the body when the metabolic rate is slow compared with compounds that are rapidly metabolized. Any substance if not eliminated could eventually reach a toxic level. A feature characteristic of most toxicants is that the subsequent metabolic products are more polar than the original compound. Thus, metabolism of toxicants decreases biological activity and increases polarity or reduces lipid solubility. The implication of increased toxicant polarity is that such compounds are more likely to be excreted by renal or biliary processes. On the other hand, compounds with high lipid–water partition coefficients pass effortlessly across membranes and diffuse back freely from the tubular urine through the renal tubular cells into the plasma, and such compounds thus tend to have a low renal clearance and a long endurance in the body. But if a toxicant is metabolized to a more water-soluble compound or one with a lower partition coefficient, the compound's tubular reabsorption is greatly reduced. The terms *metabolism* and *biotransformation* are often used synonymously, particularly when applied to xenobiotic compounds such as drugs. Sometimes the connotation associated with metabolism is to describe the total fate of a compound, including absorption, distribution, biotransformation, and elimination. But more often, metabolism is used to mean biotransformation, because metabolites are the products of xenobiotic biotransformation. Metabolism has evolutionary significance because if humans had not evolved with such capabilities, compounds such as pentobarbital would be pharmacologically active for hundreds of years. Toxicant-metabolizing systems have developed as adaptations to terrestrial life. It is likely

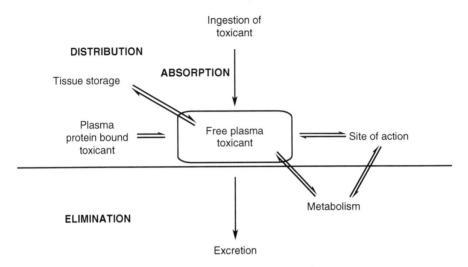

FIGURE 9.1 *In vivo* distribution of a toxicant.

that toxicants have been metabolized by living systems since the first cells were formed in the primordial slime. Marine organisms often lack the major toxicant-metabolizing systems found in mammals; however, they excrete lipid-soluble compounds directly into the surrounding water across the gill membranes. Conversion of a methyl group to a carboxyl group could reduce the biological half-life of a compound from many hours to a few minutes. Enzymatic biotransformation of xenobiotics facilitates the elimination of such compounds from the body. Without such enzymes, lipophilic xenobiotics would stay in the body for a prolonged duration following exposure. These compounds would accumulate in the body with repeated exposures, reaching toxic levels. Animals, especially herbivores, which consume a wide variety and amount of plant material laden with unusual secondary products, need to be able to biotransfer xenobiotics.

Some compounds that undergo metabolism become more toxic, e.g., carbon tetrachloride or benzo(α)pyrene. Decreased lipid solubility of a toxicant does not necessarily mean increased water solubility, e.g., acetylsulfathiazole transformed from sulfathiazole. The reduced water solubility of acetylsulfathiazole results in a compound with serious toxicity, which results from precipitation in renal tubules.

Overall, two scenarios can be mediated by biotransformation reactions: (1) xenobiotics (toxic) converted to intermediates (toxic or nontoxic) converted to products (nontoxic), or (2) xenobiotics (nontoxic) converted to intermediates (toxic) converted to products (nontoxic). The main site of toxicant metabolism is the liver, but other tissues may play an active part too. Table 9.1 summarizes the relative tissue distribution of toxicant metabolism. The hepatopancreas and the fat bodies are major organs involved in biotransformation in lobsters and insects, respectively.

Thus, the liver is the richest source of enzymes for metabolizing toxicants, but there is ample evidence that enzyme systems are ubiquitous, which can be rationalized on the basis of the importance of such enzymes in detoxifying various compounds. Intestinal microflora plays an important role in the biotransformation of

TABLE 9.1
Organs, Tissues, and Cells Involved in Toxicant Metabolism and Their Percent Distribution

Organ/Tissue/Cell	Percent Distribution
Liver	50–90
Kidney	8
Intestine (Gut flora)	6
Adrenals	2
Lung	20–30
Gonads	5
Placenta	5
Skin	1

xenobiotics because of the impact of evolution on the survival of the species. Ruminants may be able to cope with relatively high intakes of fungal toxins, e.g., aflatoxin, because of their breakdown by the rumen bacteria.

Within the liver and other organs, the microsomes or endoplasmic reticulum and the cytosol or soluble fractions of the cytoplasm are the principal sites of xenobiotic metabolism. The lipid-rich endoplasmic reticulum is a strong attractant for lipophilic xenobiotics. To a lesser extent, metabolism occurs in the mitochondria, nuclei, and other subcellular organelles.

Although some extrahepatic sites contain relatively high levels of enzymes systems for xenobiotic metabolism, their size minimizes their overall contribution to the metabolism of such compounds. Tissue differences in their capacity to metabolize toxicants can have important toxicological consequences, such as in tissue-specific chemical injury.

BIOTRANSFORMATION ENZYMOLOGY

One of the unique facets of toxicant metabolism is that even though structures of these potentially toxic products, be they natural or synthetic, are so tremendously varied, the body seems to have evolved detoxifying processes that can cope with almost any of the many different compounds. Animals possess enzymes that can metabolize drugs, pesticides, secondary plant metabolites, and synthetic compounds as defense mechanisms, which are likely because of evolution in response to selective pressures for protection against many naturally occurring toxic products. There are two categories of animal enzyme systems: (1) those for the transformation of normal endogenous chemicals in tissue, such as nutrients and metabolic by-products of nutrients; and (2) those that alter structure of many foreign compounds and essentially have no established normal endogenous substrates. The first category of enzyme systems has been studied in detail for their general biochemistry. These are enzymes of intermediary metabolism and are characterized by high turnover numbers and enormous rate enhancements over uncatalyzed reactions. Also, these reactions demand a precise chemical fit between substrate and enzyme (lock and key model),

TABLE 9.2
Catalytic Specificity and Efficiency of Enzymes

Intermediary Metabolism	Xenobiotic Metabolism
High efficiency (high turnover)	Broad substrate specificity
High substrate specificity	Low catalytic efficiency

and the fit dictates stringent substrate specificity. Typically, enzyme systems involved with intermediary metabolism have low K_M values or are tightly bound and high K_{cat} values or high efficiency and rapid turnover. Examples include cholinesterase and the hydrolysis of acetylcholine, and monoamine oxidase acting on epinephrine, tyramine, and short-chain amines.

The genetic capacity and thus the metabolic ability of an organism limits its ability to produce numerous distinct enzymes to detoxify all the foreign compounds that it may come in contact with. Thus, enzymes systems involved in xenobiotic metabolism exhibit broad substrate specificity and low catalytic efficiency. Such enzyme systems represent a metabolic compromise. To offset specificity or the cost of reduced precision of substrate binding to enzymes, these enzymes can metabolize diverse substrates. Table 9.2 lists the differences in these enzyme systems.

The ultimate goal of xenobiotic metabolism is to increase the hydrophilic property of the compound. Such metabolism is delineated in Figure 9.2, showing the integration of phase I and phase II biotransformation reactions. When an organism deals with a toxicant or an inactive compound that might be converted to a toxicant, biotransformation usually proceeds by a two-phase process. The aim of the enzymatic reactions responsible for biotransformation is to form hydrophilic products that are less toxic and can be excreted by the body.

Phase I or Type I Reactions

These biotransformation reactions involve oxidation, reduction, and hydrolysis of foreign compounds. Table 9.3 to Table 9.5 give a detailed description of phase I reactions.

In addition, the hydration of epoxides and dehydrohalogenations can be considered as phase I reactions. Many foreign compounds that enter the body are lipophilic, because of which they can easily penetrate lipid membranes and be transported by lipoproteins in body fluids. Therefore, the essence of such reactions is to introduce or expose a functional group that decreases the lipid solubility of the compound. They promote insertion, addition, or exposure of functional groups on the structure of the lipophilic compound to form electrophilic compounds (Figure 9.1). Such action gives the compound a polar group, making it a suitable substrate for phase II reactions. Phase II reactions alter compounds by combining them with endogenous substrates to produce a water-soluble conjugated products that can readily be excreted.

The predominant biotransformation enzyme systems in phase I reactions are cytochrome P450 and mixed-function amine oxidases. Other phase I enzymes

Metabolism and Excretion of Toxicants

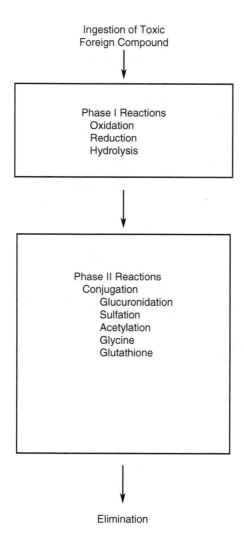

FIGURE 9.2 Metabolism of a toxicant.

TABLE 9.3
Oxidative Reactions

Reaction	Substrate Effect
Hydroxylation	Direct insertion of a hydroxyl functional group
Oxidative dealkylation	Cleavage of alkyl groups and aromatic groups from amines or ethers
Oxidative deamination	Loss of amino groups
N-Oxidation	Oxidation of the nitrogen
Oxidation of aliphatic alcohols	

TABLE 9.4
Reductive Reactions

Azo reduction
Nitro reduction
Keto reduction

TABLE 9.5
Characteristics of Hydrolytic Reactions

Compounds possessing ester linkages (amides and esters)
Formation of alcohol and acids

include flavin-containing monooxygenase (FMO), prostaglandin synthetase (PGS; carries out cooxidation), molybdenum hydroxylases, alcohol dehydrogenase, aldehyde dehydrogenase, esterases and amidases, epoxide hydrolase, DDT-dehydrochorinase, and glutathione reductase. Cytochrome P450 and the flavin-containing monooxygenase are located in the microsome.

Microsomal Enzymes

Cytochrome P450 (CYP) Enzymes
Cytochrome P450 enzymes of microsomal enzyme systems are embedded in phospholipid, which is important because the phospholipid facilitates interaction between the enzymes NADPH-cytochrome P450 reductase and cytochrome P450 (Figure 9.3). Cytochrome P450 derives its name from the fact that reduced cytochrome P450 (Fe^{2+}) forms a ligand with carbon monoxide (CO), which can be observed at a spectral absorption of 450 nm. It has been determined that cytochrome P450 is more than one enzyme and the location of the gene on a particular chromosome has been determined for cytochrome P450 isoenzymes. A system of nomenclature based on such findings has been used since 1987. Since the most recent update, P450 human genes are designated as CYP. Each designation is followed by an arabic numeral designating the individual gene, followed by a letter designating the subfamily, and finally an arabic numeral designating the individual gene.

Cytochrome P450 microsomal monooxygenase reactions are similar, but the enzyme classes differ in their substrates and products. Hence, these activities are classified on the basis of chemical reactions. Classes can overlap and the same substrate may undergo more than one oxidative reaction.

- *Aliphatic and aromatic hydroxylations (Figure 9.4)*. Alkyl side chains of aromatic compounds are easily oxidized to alcohols. Epoxides of aromatic rings are intermediates in aromatic hydroxylations. Oxides of polycyclic hydrocarbons (arene oxides) are known to be involved in carcinogenesis. The proximate carcinogens derived from the metabolic activation of benzo(α)pyrene are isomers of benzo(α) 7,8-diol-9,10-epoxide.

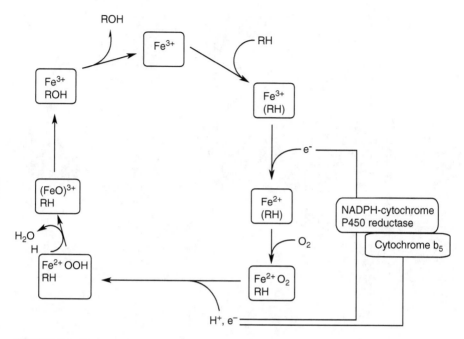

FIGURE 9.3 The cytochrome P450 enzyme system.

- *Dealkylation.* The reaction can involve O-, N-, and S-dealkylation. An example of O-dealkylation is the demethylation of *p*-nitroanisole. Many drugs and insecticides undergo N-dealkylation (Figure 9.5).
- *N-oxidation.* These reactions can result in hydroxylamine formation, oxime formation, and N-oxide formation (Figure 9.6). Several amines can undergo N-oxidation to form hydroxylamine. The classical example is aniline. Imines and primary amines can undergo N-hydroxylation. N-oxide formation is mostly a function of flavin-containing monooxygenase.
- *Oxidation (S and P).* Both microsomal monooxygenases and flavin-containing monooxygenase act on thioethers to oxidize them to sulfoxides and trisubstituted phosphines to phosphine oxides (Figure 9.7). Sulfoxides are further metabolized to sulfones, a common reaction for insecticides and drugs, chlorinated hydrocarbons and chlorpromazine, respectively.
- *Desulfuration and ester cleavage.* These reactions can convert the P–S double bond to P–O double bond. When cholinesterases are converted, powerful cholinesterase inhibitors are produced, e.g., paraoxon from parathion (Figure 9.7).

Flavin-Containing Monooxygenase

These microsomal enzymes are involved in the oxidation of several inorganic compounds and organic compounds containing nitrogen, sulfur, or phosphorus. The catalytic cycle of FMO is shown in Figure 9.8, and it requires NADPH and oxygen

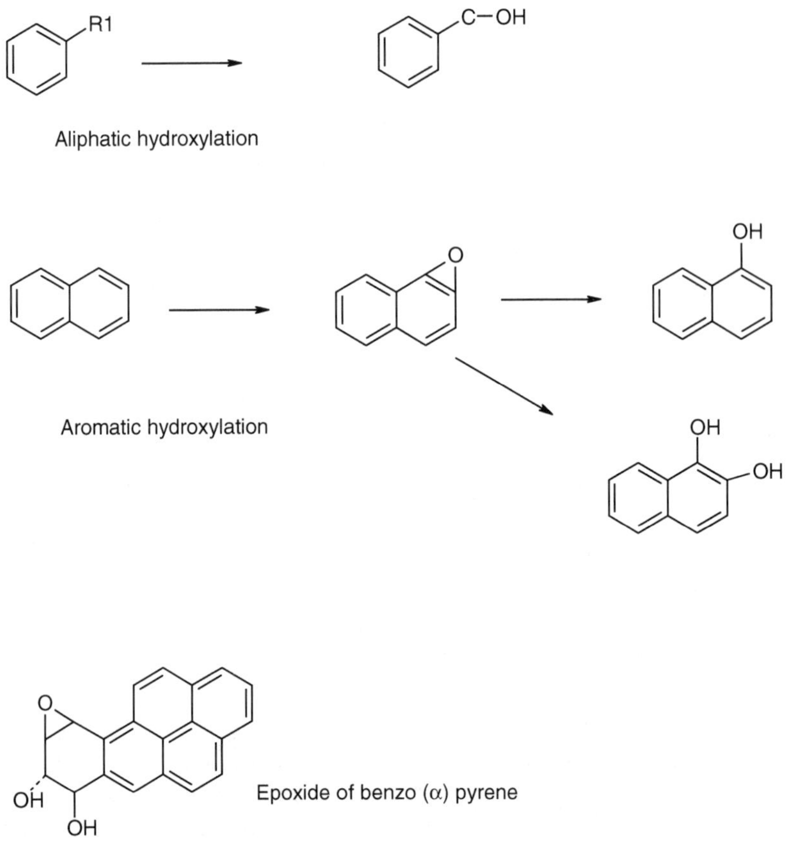

FIGURE 9.4 Aliphatic and aromatic hydrdoxylations.

as cytochrome P450 does. Many of the reactions catalyzed by FMOs can be catalyzed by cytochrome P450 too. Several techniques can determine whether compounds are metabolized by FMOs or by cytochrome P450. FMO is inactivated in the absence of NADPH by subjecting the microsomes to 50°C for 1 min, with no effect on cytochrome P450. Cytochrome P450 can be inactivated with nonionic detergents, which have no effect on FMO. Antibodies for cytochrome P450 can identify the particular P450 enzyme that catalyzes the reaction. Substrates oxidized by the FMO include inorganic compounds (HS^-, I^-, IO^-, I_2, and CNS^-); organic nitrogen compounds (acyclic and cyclic amines, N-alkyl and N, N-dialkylarylamines, hydrazine, primary amines); organic sulfur compounds (thiols and disulfides, cyclic and acyclic sulfides, mercaptopurines, pyrimidines, imidazoles, dithio acids and dithiocarbamides, thiocarbamides and thioamides); organic phosphorus compounds (phosphines, phosphonates); and selenides and selenocarbamides.

Nonmicrosomal Enzymes

These oxidoreductases are located in either the mitochondrial fraction or the cytosolic fraction (soluble supernatant) of the tissue homogenate.

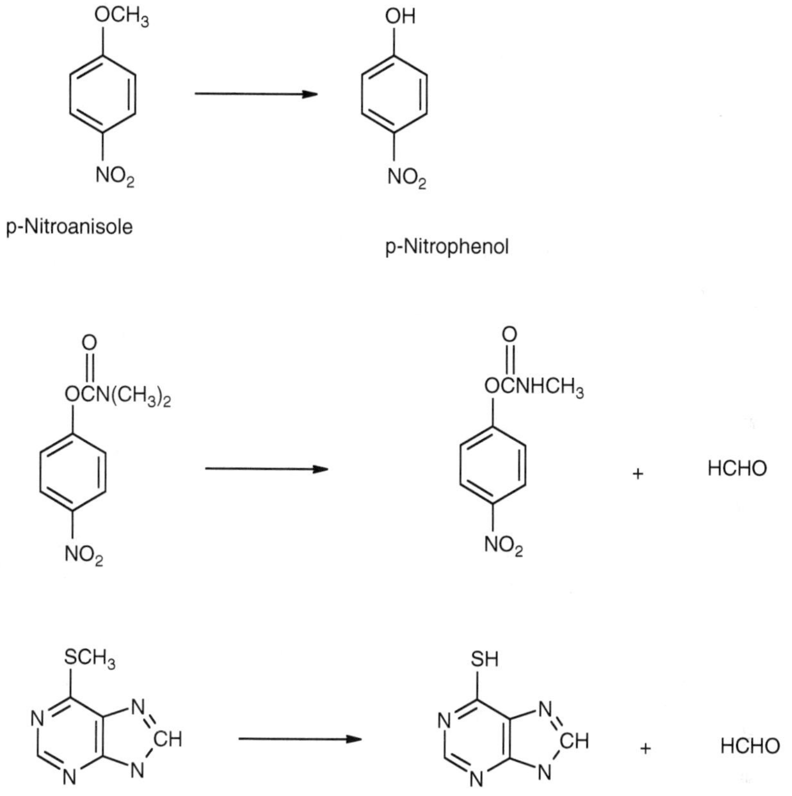

FIGURE 9.5 N-dealkylation.

Alcohol dehydrogenase catalyzes the conversion of alcohols to aldehydes or ketones:

$$RCH_2OH + NAD^+ \leftrightarrow RCHO + NADH + H^+$$

The aldehydes require a further metabolism to acids because such compounds are usually toxic and because of their high lipid solubility are not easily excreted. Metabolism is faster with primary alcohols than with secondary alcohols, followed by tertiary alcohols (which are not readily oxidized). Other dehydrogenases play important roles in steroid, lipid, and carbohydrate metabolism, but their substrate specificity is narrow and they thus do not play important roles in the metabolism of foreign compounds.

Aldehyde dehydrogenases can handle a wide variety of substrates, such as oxidation of aliphatic and aromatic aldehydes to acids. The acids can either be excreted or go through phase II reactions to become more polar.

Amine oxidases are involved in the oxidation of endogenous biogenic amines. Monoamine oxidases (MAOs) are important in the control of serotonin and other catecholamines. Amine oxidases are also involved in the oxidative deamination of

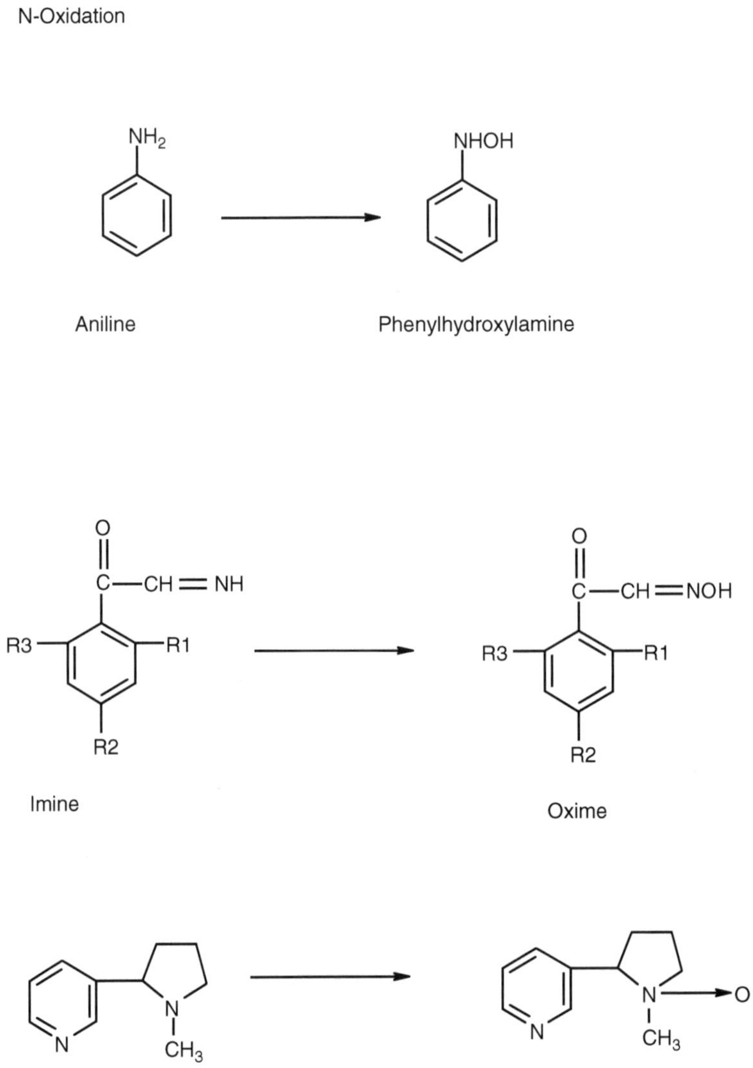

N-Oxidation

FIGURE 9.6 N-oxide formation.

foreign compounds. Monoamine and diamine oxidases are mitochondrial flavoprotein enzymes. MAOs deaminate primary, secondary, and tertiary aliphatic amines.

Molybdenum hydroxylases (aldehyde oxidase and xanthine oxidase) are molybdenum-containing enzymes important in carbon oxidation of foreign compounds, particularly aldehydes and N-heterocycles.

Reduction Reactions

Several functional groups are susceptible to reduction, i.e., nitro, diazo, carbonyls, disulfides, sulfoxides and alkenes. Various aromatic amines can be reduced by

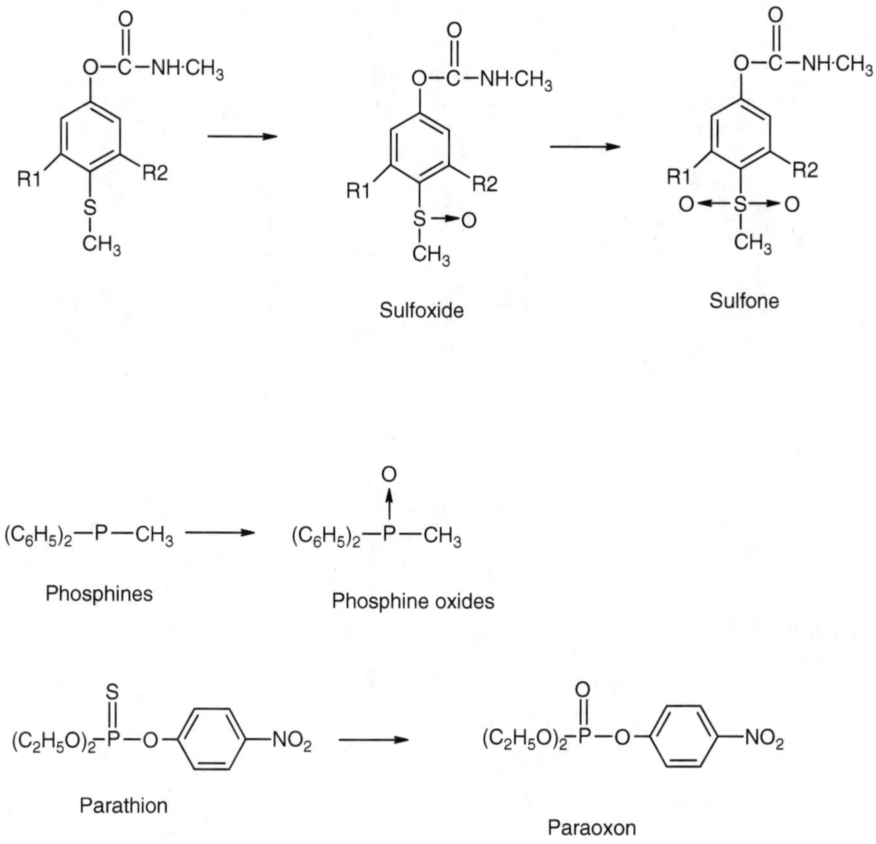

FIGURE 9.7 Oxidation (S and P).

nitroreductase systems of both bacteria and mammals. The reaction utilizes NADPH and NADH and anaerobic conditions. The reduction process proceeds through nitroso and hydroxylamine intermediates.

Azo reduction occurs through azoreductases, whose requirements are similar to those for nitroreductases, i.e., anaerobic conditions and NADPH. Mammals have a poor ability to reduce azo compounds and it is a function of specific tissues. Thus, most of the azo reduction is by intestinal bacteria, which can be eliminated by antibiotic pretreatment.

Hydrolysis

Esters, amides, and various substituted phosphates with ester bonds are susceptible to hydrolysis. In contrast to the other phase I reactions, hydrolysis occurs without utilization of energy. There are many hydrolases in the plasma and various tissues (both cytosolic and microsomal). Products of such reactions include various acids and alcohols, which can be directly excreted or undergo conjugation by phase II reactions.

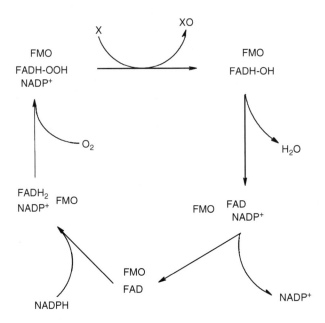

FIGURE 9.8 Flavin-containing monooxygenase (FMO).

TABLE 9.6
Conjugation Reactions

Reaction	Cellular Location
Glucuronide	Microsomes
Sulfate	Cytosol
Glutathione	Cytosol, microsomes
Acylation	Mitochondria, cytosol
Methylation	Cytosol
Amino acid	Mitochondria, cytosol

Phase II or Type II Reactions

These biotransformation reactions (listed in Table 9.6) can involve various cofactors that react with functional groups either present in the parent compound or introduced during phase I reactions (Figure 9.2). Tissue enzymes conjugate various chemical groups, such as acetyl, glucuronic acid, sulfate, glycine, ornithine, and glutathione, to the reactive groups of a toxicant. Phase II biotransformation results in further xenobiotic hydrophilicity and greater ability for excretion. Phase II biotransformation of compounds may or may not be preceded by phase I biotransformation.

Glucuronidation

Most glucuronidation reactions occur in the liver, intestinal mucosa, and kidney. Glucuronides are the most common conjugates of toxicants, and most products are

Metabolism and Excretion of Toxicants

excreted in the bile. Very low levels of glucuronidation occur in other tissues and organs. Four general compound classes make up a variety of compounds that can serve as substrates for glucuronidation: O-, N-, S-, and C-glycosides. UDP-glucuronosyl transferases (UGTs) are the enzymes involved in glucuronidation reactions. UGTs are part of a multigene superfamily.

Age, nutrition, gender, species, strain, and genetic difference affect glucuronidation. The levels are low to undetectable in fetal tissues and increase with age. Low levels of the conjugating system in newborns are responsible for increases in bilirubin levels and the development of neonatal jaundice.

Sulfation

The metabolism of foreign compounds and many endogenous compounds depends on sulfate conjugation. Endogenous compounds include the biosynthesis of thyroid and steroid hormones, certain proteins, and peptides. Primary, secondary, and tertiary alcohols, phenols, and arylamines can form sulfate esters via sulfation. Sulfate esters are completely ionized and water soluble and quickly excreted by the organism. Although most compounds undergoing sulfation are converted to less toxic products, a few form reactive intermediates that have been implicated in carcinogenesis.

Phenols, alcohols, and N-substituted hydroxylamines are the common compounds that undergo sulfation. Most sulfate conjugates are excreted in the urine and some in the bile. The superfamily of sulfotransferase enzymes is either membrane bound or cytosolic.

Methylation

Methyl groups are transferred from one of two methyl donor substrates, S-adenosylmethione (SAM) or N^5-methyltetrahydrofolic acid. Methylation occurs with a variety of methyl-acceptor substrates, including proteins, nucleic acids, and phospholipids. Interestingly, methyl conjugates are generally less water soluble than the parent compound. However, methylation is generally considered a detoxification reaction.

N-methylation reactions involve primary, secondary, and tertiary amines as substrates. The source of the methyl group that is transferred is SAM, forming secondary, tertiary, or quaternary N-methylamines and S-adenosyl-L-homocysteine (SAH).

The enzyme catechol-O-methyltransferase (COMT) is widely distributed throughout the plant and animal kingdom and is involved in O-methylation. COMT catalyzes the transfer of a methyl group from SAM to a phenolic group of a catechol. Several catechol-like substrates, such as pyrogallol, flavonoids, pyrones, and pyridenes, act as irreversible inhibitors of COMT.

An example of S-methylation is the transfer of methyl groups from SAM to thio-containing foreign compounds and drugs. In general, aromatic thiols are better substrates than aliphatic thiols. Both soluble and microsomal forms of thiol methyltransferases have been identified.

Acylation

Amide conjugates are formed from the acylation of foreign carboxylic acids and amines. There are two types of acylation reactions. The first involves an activated conjugating intermediate, acetyl CoA, and the foreign compound, acetylation. The second reaction involves the activation of the foreign compound to form an acyl CoA derivative, which can react with an amino acid to form an amino acid conjugate:

$$CH_3C(O)SCoA + RNH_2 \rightarrow RNHCOCH_3 + CoASH$$
$$\text{Acetyl-CoA} \qquad \text{amine} \qquad \text{Acetyl conjugate} \qquad \text{CoA}$$

$$RC(O)SCoA + NH_2CHCOOH \rightarrow RC(O)NHCH_2COOH + CoASH$$
$$\text{Acyl-CoA} \qquad \text{Glycine} \qquad \text{Amino acid conjugate} \qquad \text{CoA}$$

Conjugation of carboxylic acid compounds with amino acid requires the activation of the compound to a CoA derivative, and the acyl CoA reacts with an amino acid to produce the acylated amino acid conjugate and CoA. Amino acid conjugation occurs with glycine, glutamine, arginine, and taurine in mammals; other amino acids may be used by other species.

Glutathione-S-Transferases (GSTs)

This is a family of isoenzymes involved in the conjugation of reduced glutathione with electrophilic compounds. GSTs are widely distributed throughout the animal and plant kingdoms. Both soluble and membrane-bound GSTs are found in most tissues. GSTs are involved in the conjugation of epoxides, haloalkanes, nitroalkanes, alkenes, organophosphates, and methyl sulfoxide compounds.

OXIDATIVE STRESS

Oxidative stress and generation of reactive oxygen species (ROS) (see Table 9.7) seem to be involved in a wide variety of diseases and in many chemical-induced cellular injuries. Thus, preventing oxidative tissue damage is a subject of considerable investigation. Oxidative stress is the situation wherein prooxidants dominate over antioxidants. Prooxidants are compounds that oxidize (remove electrons from) other cellular compounds or molecules. The oxidized molecules can be DNA, resulting in mutations, or an enzyme, resulting in loss of enzymatic activity. Oxidative stress can be detrimental by reacting with critical lipid components such as polyunsaturated fatty acids (PUFAs) that comprise membranes and lipoprotein particles. ROS affect the unsaturated fatty acids, altering membrane structure and function. Because any type of macromolecule can be affected, the process of oxidative stress can result in deleterious consequences, the extent of which is determined by the tissue and type of prooxidant.

Many compounds that are prooxidants are by-products of normal oxidative metabolism. Cellular mitochondria, for example, are responsible for most of the cell's oxygen consumption, producing water as an end product. However, a small fraction of the oxygen (ca. 4%) is reduced normally to ROS. Some chemicals, toxicants, and infectious agents can disrupt the normal mitochondrial function and increase the percentage of oxygen converted to ROS. ROS increase as a consequence of normal aging processes, because mitochondria lose their efficiency due to age-dependent changes in them. Other enzymes involved in oxidation reactions also contribute to the production of ROS, such as the cytochrome P450 system, which in turn can be influenced by toxicants such as ethanol. In addition, differences in age, health, and environmental exposures can create additional load for ROS.

TABLE 9.7
Reactive Oxygen Species (ROS)

O_2^-	Superoxide anion
H_2O_2	Hydrogen peroxide
·OH	Hydroxyl radical
ROO·	Peroxyl radical
NO·	Nitric oxide
ONOO$^-$	Peroxynitrite
$^1O_2$	Singlet oxygen
O_3	Ozone

ROS are various forms of oxygen that are much more reactive and damaging to biological systems than molecular oxygen. Molecular oxygen, although a radical, is not very reactive with biological molecules. The two orbital electrons in molecular oxygen have the same spin states.

Processes that produce a one-electron reduction of oxygen produce a more reactive radical, the superoxide anion. The superoxide anion can be formed from oxygen by an enzyme in white blood cells and other enzymes or certain toxic agents. ROS can be eliminated by the enzymes superoxide dismutases, which convert two molecules of superoxide to one molecule each of hydrogen peroxide and oxygen (Figure 9.9). Hydrogen peroxide is another ROS that can be formed by some two-electron transfer reactions. As illustrated in Figure 9.9, hydrogen peroxide is detoxified by glutathione peroxidase and catalase. Superoxide and hydrogen peroxide can react together to form the more toxic ROS, the hydroxyl radical, in the Haber–Weiss reaction (Figure 9.10). This reaction occurs when iron (Fe^{2+}) and copper (Cu^+) ions are present. Superoxide anions can be generated by several other cellular processes, such as microsomal or mitochondrial electron transport systems and xanthine dehy-

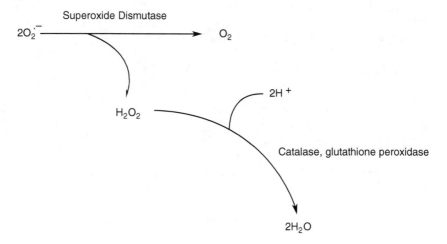

FIGURE 9.9 The superoxide dismutase system.

$$H_2O_2 + O_2^{\cdot -} \longrightarrow O_2 + OH^{\cdot} + OH^{-} \quad \text{Haber–Weiss reaction}$$

$$O^{\cdot -} + H_2O_2 \xrightarrow{Fe^{+2} \text{ or } Cu^+} O_2 + OH^{\cdot} + OH^{\cdot} \quad \text{Iron/copper-catalyzed Haber–Weiss reactions}$$

FIGURE 9.10 The Haber–Weiss reaction.

drogenase/oxidase. Phagocytic cells generate superoxide anions through NADPH oxidase, which reduces oxygen with NADPH to produce large amounts of superoxide anions. Such products are used by the cell to effectively destroy bacteria. Peroxyl radicals are produced when lipids undergo oxidative stress. Peroxyl radicals are also associated with prostaglandin synthesis and are the product of one-electron transfer from a carbon-centered radical to oxygen (Figure 9.11A). Although peroxyl radicals are not very reactive, they can migrate a considerable distance and react with thiols to generate thiyl radicals (see Figure 9.11B). Nitric oxide (NO·) is a ubiquitous critical oxidative biological signal molecule occurring in a variety of diverse physiological processes, such as smooth muscle relaxation, neurotransmission, and the immune response. Nitric oxide is generated by a reaction involving the enzyme nitric oxide synthase, which uses arginine as its substrate (Figure 9.12). Nitric oxide synthase occurs in macrophages and neutrophils, and along with superoxide anions and peroxynitrite, is prominent in the oxidative burst occurring during inflammation. As shown in the figure, peroxynitrile is formed by the interaction of nitric oxide with superoxide.

$$R-\overset{|}{\underset{|}{C}}\cdot \; + \; O_2 \longrightarrow R-\overset{|}{\underset{|}{COO}}\cdot \qquad A$$

Peroxyl radical

$$R-S^- \; + \; ROO\cdot \longrightarrow R-S\cdot \; + \; ROO^- \qquad B$$

Thiolate anion → Thiyl radical

FIGURE 9.11 Peroxyl radicals and thiyl radicals.

$$\text{Arginine} + O_2 + \text{NADPH} \xrightarrow{\text{Nitric oxide synthase}} \text{Citrulline} + NO + NADP$$

$$NO\cdot + O_2^{\cdot -} + H^+ \longrightarrow ONOOH$$

FIGURE 9.12 Nitric oxide generation.

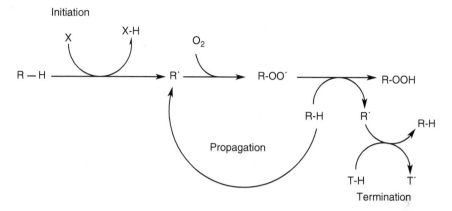

FIGURE 9.13 Lipid peroxidation.

Lipid components, such as plasma membrane and lipoproteins, are vulnerable to oxidative injury, particular if the content of PUFAs is high. Lipid peroxidation is defined as the process of oxidative deterioration of PUFAs, and is analogous to what occurs during the autoxidation of stored fats, or rancidity. Figure 9.13 shows a generally accepted simplified scheme for the mechanism of lipid peroxidation initiated by free radicals. Hydrogen from an unsaturated fatty acid molecule is first abstracted (initiation phase) by a free-radical initiator. Some of the most powerful catalysts that initiate lipid peroxidation, such as hemeproteins and coordinated iron, are in close molecular proximity to these unsaturated lipids *in vivo*. After hydrogen abstraction, oxygen attacks the subsequently formed carbon radical (R·), resulting in a fatty acid peroxyl radical (ROO·). Propagation is the consequence of peroxyl radicals reacting with another molecule of unsaturated fatty acid to produce a semistable unsaturated hydroperoxide (ROOH), which can then also regenerate a molecule of free radical. A free-radical lipid peroxidation reaction might be propagated through the PUFAs of the phospholipid in a membrane or lipoproteins. In membranes and other lipid structures, the propagation of each chain reaction leaves a fatty acid hydroperoxide product, which leads to further branching reactions. Propagation continues until the formed free radicals are quenched by a free-radical chain breaker such as vitamin E (termination).

If the process of lipid peroxidation is uncontrolled, membranes and lipid structures that contain high contents of PUFAs and are exposed to oxidants would be expected to result in their loss and the formation of their metabolites. This would be followed by a loss of intracellular membrane integrity, a change in membrane permeability, and the eventual loss of membrane function. For example, damage to a lysosomal structure would ultimately result in the destruction and inactivation of proteins, enzymes, nucleic acids, and other constituents of normal cell function.

Ozone and singlet oxygen are other ROS. Ozone is derived from photochemical processes in the atmosphere. It is not a free radical but is a much more powerful oxidizing agent than ground-state oxygen. The toxicity of ozone is likely due to direct oxidation. In the case of singlet oxygen, this radical can be generated in tissues by the oxidation of other partially reduced oxygen species, resulting in an oxygen with paired electrons in the reactive orbital.

Cellular Reductants and Antioxidants

Thiol groups are very important because they are often found at the active sites of various enzymes or other important proteins. Cysteine can be oxidized to cystine, cysteic acid, and other products. Also, glutathione, or γ-glutamyl-cysteyl glycine, plays an important role in maintaining many tissues. Two molecules of glutathione can be oxidized to a disulfide. Living cells have copious amounts of reduced glutathione but only trifle amounts of the oxidized form without reduced glutathione. This is important to prevent enzymes from inactivation, which occurs if functional sulfhydryl groups are oxidized. Research has shown that exposure to oxidants, such as ozone, results in large decreases in tissue glutathione content.

As a biological lipid-soluble antioxidant, vitamin E performs a crucial function in scavenging free radicals. Reversal of vitamin E deficiency by administering a variety of other antioxidants is evidence for this role. Also, vitamin E–deficient animals are very sensitive to oxidant-induced lung damage. Vitamin E refers to a family of compounds that includes tocopherols and tocotrienols. These compounds inhibit lipid peroxidation by scavenging lipid peoxyl radicals much faster than the rate at which these radicals can react with adjacent fatty acid side-chains or with membrane proteins. Tocopherols can both quench and react with singlet oxygen and protect membranes from this oxidant. Tocopherol reacts slowly with superoxide anions and its reaction with hydroxyl radicals is diffusion-controlled. Tocopherol also reacts with peroxyl radicals to give nonradical products. One molecule of tocopherol is capable of terminating two peroxidation chains. The products of such termination can include tocopheryl radical and tocopherylquinone. Tocopherylquinone is excreted in the urine. Physiological mechanisms may exist for reducing the radical form back to tocopherol. A synergy between vitamin E and vitamin C was suggested in 1968 by Professor Al Tappel, now retired from the University of California, Davis, and pulse radiolysis studies confirmed that ascorbate can reduce the tocopherol radical back to tocopherol (Figure 9.14). The ascorbate is simultaneously converted to ascorbyl radical, which in turn can be reduced to ascorbate by glutathione and other endogenous reductants, i.e., ascorbate and tocopherol cycling.

Just as vitamin E serves as a lipid-soluble antioxidant, ascorbic acid (vitamin C) serves as a key aqueous-soluble antioxidant. In addition to studies showing that

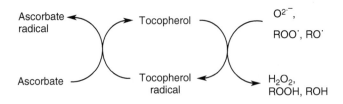

FIGURE 9.14 Vitamin E and vitamin C cycles.

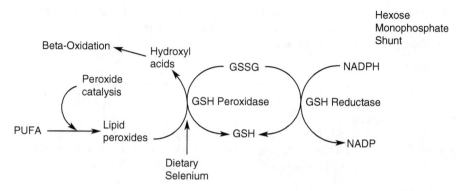

FIGURE 9.15 The glutathione peroxidase system.

the two vitamins are synergistic in the way they protect against lipid peroxidation, vitamin C has been shown to improve drug metabolism, reduce serum cholesterol, play a vital role in collagen metabolism, and is required in dopamine-β-hydroxylase. Ascorbate tends to reduce more-reactive species such as hydroxyl radicals, superoxide anions, and urate radicals.

Enzymatic Antioxidant Systems

Superoxide dismutase and catalase may prevent or minimize the oxidation of lipid hydroperoxides. In combination, these two enzymes have been referred to as the superoxide dismutase system. The glutathione peroxidase system also acts in concert to convert hydroperoxides to hydroxyl fatty acids. Enzymes include glutathione (GSH) peroxidase, GSH reductase, glucose-6-phosphate dehydrogenase, and enzymes of the pentose (hexose monophosphate) shunt pathway. Figure 9.15 illustrates the suggested pathway. GSH peroxidase is capable of hydrogen peroxide decomposition, similar to the action of catalase. GSH peroxidase is important because this enzyme can also reduce organic hydroperoxides as well as hydrogen peroxide. GSH peroxidase is a selenium-containing enzyme, which explains why selenium serves as a protective element against oxidative injury.

Targets of Oxidative Stress Products

Carbohydrates

Hydrogen atoms from carbon atoms of carbohydrate chains can be abstracted in reactions involving the hydroxyl radical, producing carbon-centered radicals. These reactions can lead to breaks in chains of crucial physiological molecules. For example, the production of ROS during the accumulation and activation of neutrophils during the inflammatory response can alter hyaluronic acid, causing a decrease in the synovial fluid surrounding joints. Hyaluronate degradation is caused by hydroxyl radical generation by the superoxide-anion-driven Fenton chemistry. Catalytic iron can be measured in fluids extracted from inflamed joints of rheumatoid arthritis patients. The catalytic iron could be liberated from necrotic cells by hydrogen-peroxide–mediated degradation of hemoglobin (microbleeding of the joint). In addition, the pentose-phosphate polymers of nucleic acids can be attacked by hydroxyl radicals, causing polymer alterations.

Lipids

Polyunsaturated lipids (PUFAs) are major constituents of cellular membranes and are important targets of ROS damage or lipid peroxidation. Lipid peroxidation is a ROS-initiated chain reaction that can be self-propagating in membranes. Subsequently, lipid peroxidation can have profound effects on membrane function. In addition, products of lipid peroxidation, such as unsaturated aldehydes, have been implicated in modification of other cellular constituents such as cellular protein.

Proteins

Metal-binding sites of proteins are especially susceptible to oxidative stress. Oxidative stress can result in irreversible modification of the amino acids involved in the metal binding, such as histidine. Also, reactive sulfhydryl groups on specific cysteine residues or reactive methionine can be oxidized to disulfides or methionine sulfoxide, respectively. In addition, the hydroxyl radical has been shown to fragment proteins in plasma. Thus, crucial proteins are liable to oxidative stress.

Nucleic Acids

Besides damage to pentose-phosphate polymers of nucleic acids, ROS can modify the base portion of the polymer. Such modification in bases can account for genetic defects produced by oxidative stress. 8-Hydroxyguanosine, a product of nucleic acid oxidation, has been used as a biomarker of DNA damage in humans. DNA damage has also been estimated by chain breaks and base modifications in cell cultures undergoing oxidative stress.

EXCRETION

Table 9.8 lists the principal routes for the elimination of a toxicant from the body, the most important route being urine. The major route through which foreign compounds that have been biotransformed into water-soluble products can be excreted is the urine. Biliary excretion into the feces is the second important route, followed by loss of volatile compounds through the lung. Either the parent foreign compound or its metabolite may be excreted into the feces through bile, and gaseous by-products

TABLE 9.8
Excretion Routes for Toxicants

Urinary
Biliary
Pulmonary
Mammary
Salivary glands
Cutaneous

of metabolism make their way out the body through the lungs. Alternatively, because toxicants may be distributed throughout the body, any body secretion may excrete chemicals, e.g., sweat, saliva, tears, and milk.

URINARY EXCRETION

Toxicants are removed from the body by the kidney by the same processes responsible for removing waste from intermediary metabolism. The kidney is the focal point for toxicant elimination, receiving a quarter of the cardiac output, of which 20% is filtered at the glomeruli. About 180 l of plasma water is filtered each day. Only those compounds that are not too large pass through the pores of the glomeruli; thus, significant protein binding of toxicants limits filtration through the glomeruli. Similar to products from intermediary metabolism, a toxicant filtered at the glomeruli may remain in the tubular lumen and be excreted in the urine, or, based on its physicochemical properties, it may be reabsorbed across the tubular cells on the nephron back into the bloodstream (see previous discussion on passive diffusion, lipid–water partition coefficient). Only free toxicant in the plasma water, and not protein-bound toxicant, can be filtered. Of the 180 l filtered, only 1.5 l is excreted as urine, the remainder being reabsorbed in the tubules. Toxicants with high lipid–water partition coefficients are readily reabsorbed and polar compounds and ions are unable to diffuse back and are excreted, unless a carrier transport system is available to the toxicant metabolite for reabsorption.

The proximal tubules, rich in mitochondria, carry on active energy-dependent reabsorption, i.e., for water, NaCl, glucose, and amino acids. The proximal tubules also are the site of active secretion of various toxicant metabolites from the plasma into the tubular urine. Further down in the distal tubules, acidification of the urine occurs. The renal proximal tubule can reabsorb small plasma proteins that are sometimes filtered at the glomerulus. If a toxicant binds to small plasma proteins and reaches the proximal tubule cells, it may exert toxicity. Such is the case with cadmium bound to metallothionein, a metal-binding protein, which causes kidney injury.

At birth, the kidneys are incompletely developed and therefore it takes longer for foreign compounds to be eliminated compared with adults. Penicillin clearance in infants is only ca. 20% of that found for older children. Sometimes, the underdeveloped kidney can be an advantage. Nephrotoxic compounds may occur in the adult but not in newborns, because active uptake of the toxicant by the kidney is not well developed in the newborn and the agent is not concentrated in the tubules.

When individuals suffer from renal shutdown, a kidney dialysis machine or "artificial kidney" must be used to treat uremia, where high levels of nitrogenous waste products accumulate in the patient's blood. Collapse of blood pressure and consequent renal failures are common consequences of poisoning (barbiturates, tranquilizers, narcotic analgesics, etc.). For rapid reduction of a high-plasma drug or toxicant level, an artificial kidney, also termed *extracorporeal dialysis*, may be employed. Blood of the patient is diverted to flow across cellophane membranes permeable to water and to low-molecular-weight solutes. On the other side of the membrane is an aqueous solution of the same ionic composition as plasma water.

The process of simple diffusion is used, resembling glomerular filtration. Frequent changes of the dialysate bath help eliminate the toxicant from the patient's plasma. The artificial kidney can achieve a urea clearance of 140 ml/min. A less costly and simpler alternative to extracorporeal dialysis is to wash out the peritoneal cavity with an isotonic solution, which removes metabolites of the toxicant.

To summarize, urinary excretion of a toxicant metabolite is a function of the degree of protein binding, the glomerular filtration rate of the metabolites, and the extent of active tubular secretion or reabsorption.

Biliary and Fecal Excretion

A toxicant may be excreted by liver cells into the bile and therefore into the intestine and be potentially eliminated through the feces. Fecal excretion of a substance is a complex process. If the properties of a toxicant favor intestinal absorption, the enterohepatic cycle may occur, in which biliary secretion and intestinal reabsorption alternate until metabolism and urinary excretion eventually result in elimination of the toxicant. On the other hand, biliary excretion is extremely important because of its relationship to the liver. The liver is in a focal position for removing toxic compounds from blood after absorption from the GI tract. The blood from the GI tract passes through the liver before going to the general circulation. The liver can extract compounds from blood, and before distribution to other parts of the body, it can metabolize the toxicant, and the metabolite can be excreted directly into the bile, depending on the physicochemical properties of the metabolite.

Toxicants bound to plasma proteins are fully available for active biliary excretion. Low-molecular-weight compounds are poorly excreted into the bile whereas compounds or their conjugates with molecular weights above 325 MW can be expected to be excreted in large quantities. Glutathione and glucuronide conjugates have a high probability of being excreted into the bile.

The hepatic excretory system is not fully developed in newborns. This is another reason why toxicants can be more harmful to newborns. The development of hepatic excretory function can be promoted in newborns by administering them with microsomal enzyme inducers.

In addition to removal of toxicants through biliary secretion, some toxicants can be eliminated in the feces because of the sloughing of intestinal epithelial cells, approximately every 3 days, described as mucosa block.

Pulmonary Gases

Gaseous substances and metabolites are eliminated mainly by the lungs. Highly volatile liquids, e.g., diethyl ether, are excreted almost exclusively by the lungs. Gases with low solubility in blood, such as ethylene, are rapidly excreted, and those with high solubility in blood, such as chloroform, are slowly eliminated. An increase in cardiac output will increase pulmonary blood flow and by simple diffusion increase pulmonary excretion. Most compounds are not metabolites, but usually intact toxicants, such as nitrous oxide. An exception is volatile dimethyl selenium compounds that the body makes when the selenium status is high.

Other Routes of Excretion

Milk

Many toxicants can be present in the mother's blood and are detectable in milk. Secretion of toxic substances into milk is important because the toxicant may be passed from the mother to her offspring while nursing. Also, compounds can be passed from cows to people through dairy products. The pH of milk is more acidic (pH = 6.5) than plasma, and basic compounds may concentrate in milk more than acidic compounds. Another important factor is that milk contains 3 to 4% lipids and lipid-soluble compounds accumulate in the fat portion. Compounds such as DDT and polyhalogenated hydrocarbons are known to occur in milk. Milk represents a major excretion path for these foreign compounds. In addition, metals that are chemically similar to calcium, such as lead, find their way into complexes that are excreted through milk.

Sweat and Saliva

Many of the physicochemical properties of substances that govern excretion into saliva apply to sweat. Excretion depends on diffusion of the nonionized, lipid-soluble form of an agent. Dermatitis may occur when the toxic material is excreted into the sweat. Toxicants in the saliva are eventually swallowed and absorbed through the GI tract.

PRINCIPLES OF TOXICOKINETICS

The study of the kinetics of chemicals in the whole organism was originally developed for drugs, and termed *pharmacokinetics*, which was derived from the Greek words *pharmako* (medicine, drug, or poison) and *kinetikos* (motion or movement). Thus, by definition, pharmacokinetics (PK) can apply to any foreign compound and not just drugs. However, those concerned about the use of semantically correct terms have referred to the study as chemobiokinetics or toxicokinetics (TK). TK, like PK, can be defined as the qualitative and quantitative study of the time course of absorption, distribution, biotransformation, and elimination of a substance in an intact organism, either plant or animal. By use of TK, one can study factors that influence the movement of substances throughout the body. Closely related terms are toxicodynamics (TD) or pharmacodynamics, which can be defined as the study of the action of substances and their effects on the organism. TK studies the effect of the body on the eventual distribution and fate of substances and TD studies the effect of the toxicant on the body. The toxicodynamic phase comprises the interaction between the molecules of the toxicant and the specific sites of action, i.e., the receptor. Some important mechanisms include interference with enzyme systems (e.g., uncoupling of biochemical reactions, removal of essential metals, and inhibition of oxygen transfer), blockages of oxygen transport (e.g., CO poisoning, formation of methemoglobin, hemolytic processes), and interference with DNA and RNA synthesis. PK studies can be an indispensable tool to evaluate the absorption, distribution, metabolism, and elimination of xenobiotics. Such information is useful in predicting the duration of the toxic action following exposure, the persistence of the substance and transformation products in target organs, and the disposition in storage sites with subsequent yields of body burdens of the substance.

TK data are useful for several reasons. It can be the means to calculate doses to achieve steady-state blood levels of a substance. With pharmacologically active substances, steady-state blood levels of a drug are related to therapeutic effect. With toxicological substances, steady-state blood levels may be related to the point at which the body can no longer effectively handle the substance without adverse effects. TK data are useful to predict accumulation of a substance in tissues, which might occur at storage or target sites of the toxicant. PK data can be useful to interpret toxicity tests, such as the relevance of specific organ tests, e.g., eye. In addition, TK data can be useful in interspecies extrapolation and in planning dose adjustments for altered physiological states (aging) or altered pathological states (liver disease).

DESIGN OF A TK STUDY

The first step involves the exposure of animals to a dose of the test substance. Following exposure to the test substance, serial samples are taken from the animal at selected times. The time course sampling is usually followed by the chemical analysis of serial samples of suitable biological fluids for the toxicant, parent or metabolite. Prospective fluids include blood, urine, milk, and amniotic fluid; in other situations, animal groups are serially killed for specific organ or tissue evaluation.

The important principle of the TK method is the description of complex phenomena that occur *in vivo* by means of mathematical equations derived from biological systems that may be conceived of as one or two components or compartments (noted by boxes, see Figure 9.16). One idea is that the body is a system of interlinked physiological compartments. These compartments are usually depicted as a series of parallel shunts connected by the systemic circulation. The compartment approach for TK is one of three approaches, the other two being the noncompartmental approach and the physiological TK modeling approach. Compartmental analysis is the traditional approach. It considers the rates of absorption, distribution, and elimination as first-order rate constants. The advantage of the compartmental analysis is the ability to simulate and predict plasma concentrations of the test substance. The disadvantage is the complexity of the mathematical equations involved with the analysis. For noncompartmental analysis, parameters of TK are easily obtained because they can be derived from the relationship involving the area under the plasma substance concentration–time curve and by using simple algebraic equations. However, noncompartmental analysis has limitations in predicting plasma concentration–time profiles. Physiological TK modeling focuses on the anatomical and physiological factors that influence substance uptake and disposition. Mass balance equations are written, describing the rate of change in the amount of substance in each organ system. Individual organ systems are studied for the partitioning of a substance between blood and organ and binding effects. This is a sophisticated model but has had limited use until recently.

Metabolism and Excretion of Toxicants

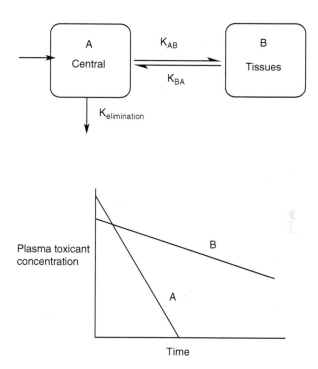

FIGURE 9.16 Kinetics: one or two compartments.

The three approaches to studying TK of compounds are not mutually exclusive. Fundamental parameters, such as clearance and volume of distribution, can be estimated by any of the methods.

ONE-COMPARTMENT TK

The one-compartment TK approach has had wide use in clinical situations, particularly for pharmaceuticals. The basic concept relies on a one-time bolus dose of a test substance, usually intravenous (IV). The amount of the test substance in the body immediately following injection is equal to the dose X_0. As the body's elimination processes, such as metabolism and excretion, begin, the amount of intact substance in the body declines in an exponential manner, as illustrated in Figure 9.17. The amount of the substance in the body for any particular time following IV bolus injection is given by the following equation:

$$X = X_0 e^{-kt}$$

where X is the amount of the test substance in the body at time t, X_0 is the IV dose equal to the initial amount of the test substance in the body, and k is the elimination rate constant. The determination of k from the equation can be simplified by transforming the amount of test substance to natural log values:

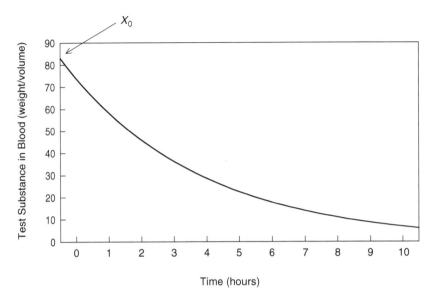

FIGURE 9.17 Relationship between time and bolus dose of a toxicant.

$$\ln X = \ln X_0 - kxt$$

This gives an equation with properties of a straight line where the slope of the line can be obtained by plotting log concentration vs. time = k.

$$\log X = \log X_0 - (k/2.303) \times t$$

$$k = 2.303/(t_2 - t_1) \times \log(X_1/X_2)$$

In the last equation, common log is more familiar than natural log, thus $\ln X = 2.303 \log X$ can be used and the elimination rate constant is obtained by multiplying the slope of the line by 2.303. $-k/2.303 = (\log X_2 - \log X_1)/(t_2 - t_1)$ and is shown in Figure 9.18. If $X = X_0/2$, when time $t = t_{1/2}$, it is the half time or half life. Log transformation results in $\log X_0/2 = \log X_0 - k/2.303 t_{1/2}$ or $0.693 = k t_{1/2}$. Figure 9.19 shows a plot of the concentration of the test substance in blood or plasma (as a log function) against time. The slope of the linear relationship is $-k/2.303$. Also, $\Delta y/\Delta x = -k/2.303$. Half life is a more frequently used expression for describing elimination and is defined as the rate at which a substance is removed from the body. The half life of a substance is the time taken for the amount of the substance in the body to decline to half of its original value.

Volume of Distribution

The amount of a test substance in the body is related to the concentration of the test substance in the blood by the volume of distribution (V_d). The concentration of a test substance can be measured in the blood, serum, or plasma; however, it is not

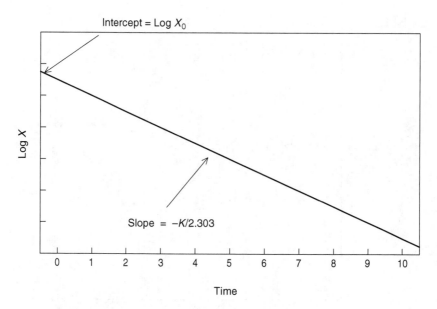

FIGURE 9.18 Relationship between time and log concentration of a toxicant.

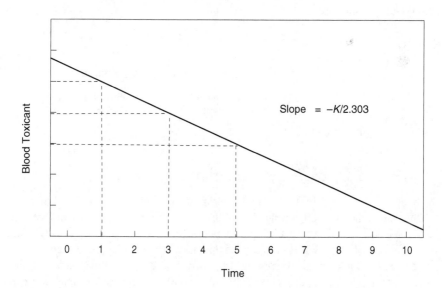

FIGURE 9.19 Plot of the concentration of a toxicant in blood vs. time.

possible to determine directly the amount of the test substance in the body. If D is the amount of the test substance in the body at any given time and C_0 is the corresponding concentration of the test substance in the blood at that time, then $V_d = D/C_0$, where D can have the units of mg/kg and X_0 can have the units of mg/ml, and V subsequently will have the units of ml/kg. The simplest way to estimate the V_d of a test substance is when C_0 is equal to X_0 or immediately after administering

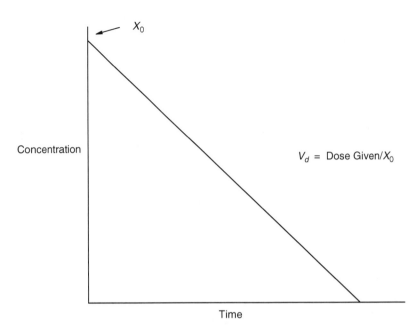

FIGURE 9.20 Estimation of the volume of distribution.

TABLE 9.9
Compounds Used to Measure Physiological Compartments

Compound	Compartment Volume (ml)	Physiological Compartment
Evans blue	3,500	Plasma
Inulin	14,000	Extracellular fluid
Deuterium oxide (D_2O)	38,500	Total body water

the bolus IV dose (Figure 9.20). Thus, dividing the dose by the concentration of the test substance in the blood at time X_0, which can be estimated by back-extrapolation, yields an estimate of V_d. Specific compounds can be used to measure body fluid compartments. Table 9.9 lists compounds that have little appreciable protein binding and can be used to estimate the respective plasma, extracellular fluid, and total body water physiological compartments. The body is really composed of many compartments in which fluid might be distributed. Thus, a substance can be distributed first into the plasma, followed by the highly perfused lean tissues, e.g., blood cells, heart, lungs, hepatoportal system, kidneys, various glands, and the central nervous system. Next, it is distributed to the poorly perfused lean tissues such as muscle and skin. Subsequently, a substance may distribute between the adipose and bone marrow. There is negligible perfusion in tissues such as bone, teeth, ligaments, tendons, cartilage, and hair.

Metabolism and Excretion of Toxicants

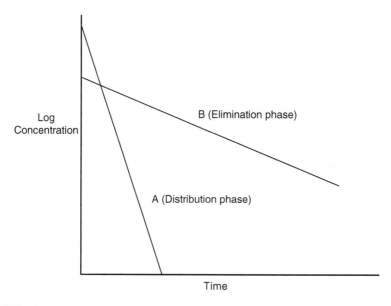

FIGURE 9.21 The two-compartmental model.

MULTICOMPARTMENT MODELS

The distribution of many substances can be explained by a one-compartment model; however, others cannot be explained or are best explained by two- or multicompartment models. A one-compartment decline of the substance concentration is governed only by a single first-order process, which is mostly due to the body's elimination processes. In a multicompartmental model, besides elimination, there are distribution processes involved with the movement of the substances between compartments. A two-compartmental model can be composed of a distribution phase and a postdistribution phase (Figure 9.21). The early time points contribute to the distribution phase, in which the concentration of the substance falls off quite rapidly with time. The early distribution phase is related to the rapid movement of the substance out of the blood and into tissues. In the postdistribution phase, the concentration of the substance declines more slowly. Physiologically, this represents the time when the concentration of the substance is in a pseudoequilibrium between the blood and tissues.

A and B are graphically represented by the lines in Figure 9.22. If all the points used to establish Line A are taken and added to the corresponding points in Line B, a plot of A and B is obtained.

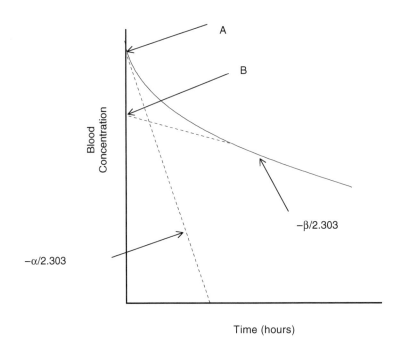

FIGURE 9.22 Graphical representation of the two-compartmental model.

STUDY QUESTIONS AND EXERCISES

1. Describe the major features of the following: cytochrome P450, glutathione, and glucuronic acid.
2. Give three examples each of phase I metabolic transformation and phase II transformation.
3. Describe the process of lipid peroxidation and discuss the major defense systems that protect against the by-products of lipid peroxidation.
4. Why is the plasma level of a toxicant an important piece of information for a toxicity study? How is the volume of distribution determined?

RECOMMENDED READINGS

Ariens, E.J., Simonis, A.M., and Offermeier, J., *Introduction to General Toxicology*, Academic Press, New York, 1976.

Ecobichon, D.J., *The Basis of Toxicity Testing*, CRC Press, Boca Raton, 1992.

Parkinson, A., Biotransformation of xenobiotics, in *Cassarett and Doull's Toxicology: The Basic Science of Toxicology*, 5th ed., Klaassen, C.D., Eds., McGraw-Hill, New York, 1996.

Reddy, A.K. and Omaye, S.T., Target organ toxicity: metabolic and biochemical responses following lung exposure, in *Inhalation Toxicology*, Salem, H., Ed., Marcel Dekker, New York, 1987, pp. 223-253.

Smith, D.A., Pharmacokinetics and pharmacodynamics in toxicology, *Xenobiotica* 27, 513, 1997.

10 Food Intolerance and Allergy

According to some surveys, 20 to 25% of people in the U.S. are allergic to certain foods. Self-reported information based on changes in dietary habits to accommodate a food problem is likely to be mostly erroneous. Often, patients who say they have a food allergy avoid a food and never seek medical advice. Diagnosis of food allergies is overworked, poorly defined, and misused. There are many misconceptions about food allergies, such as understanding of the causes of food allergies and their symptoms. A minority of practitioners who have overemphasized the magnitude of the role of food allergies in human illness have greatly contributed to this misconception. The American Academy of Allergy and Immunology has sharply criticized their concepts and questioned their practices.

Double-blind placebo-controlled studies indicate that food allergies occur in 2 to 2.5% of the population. It has been estimated that 1 to 3% of children under the age of 6 years have allergies to foods. The frequency of food allergies is highest in infancy and early childhood, but decreases with age. Childhood allergies to egg and cow's milk usually disappear, but allergies to nuts, legumes, fish, and shellfish tend to linger throughout life. Prevalence of childhood allergies is related to the gastrointestinal epithelial membrane barrier, which is immature during infancy. Thus, the barrier allows more proteins into the circulation, which can sensitize infants to ingested allergens. The mucosal barrier becomes less absorptive and more efficient for digestion as the child matures, and cow's milk and eggs become less offending.

Food allergies can be influenced by culture and eating habits. In Scandinavia, fish can be responsible for food allergies. In Japan, both fish and rice can cause food-induced allergies. In the U.S., the prevalent food that causes allergies is peanuts. Because of the internationalization of food supply, there is an increase in food allergies due to exotic foods, e.g., kiwi. Genetic influence is very strong for food-induced allergies. If one parent is allergic, then the risk of the same allergy occurring in offspring is increased by 50%. If both parents show food allergies, the chance of offspring having similar problems increases to 67 to 100%.

For a small population, the problem of allergies can be life threatening. Allergies cause more than 100 deaths/year in the U.S. Anaphylactic episodes due to food account for a third of all cases, with twice the incidence and three times the mortality compared with those by bee stings.

Allergy can be defined as a disease state caused by exposure to a particular chemical to which certain individuals have a heightened sensitivity (hypersensitiv-

TABLE 10.1
Food Sensitivities

Primary Food Sensitivity		Secondary Food Sensitivity
Immunological (Food Allergies)	Nonimmunological (Food Intolerance)	
IgE-mediated	Anaphylactoid reactions	Secondary to GI disorders
Non–IgE-mediated	Metabolic reactions	Secondary to drug treatment
	Idiosyncratic reactions	

ity), which has an immunological basis. Foods are not the only substances to which people can be allergic. Bee stings, insect bites, pollen, dander, mold spores, house dust, and drugs can also initiate allergies. For such allergens, the symptoms are identical to those found for food allergies, and many individuals suffer multiple sensitivities from food or other sources.

ALLERGY AND TYPES OF HYPERSENSITIVITY

Many people eat a variety of foods and show no ill effects; however, a few people exhibit adverse reactions to certain foods. Food sensitivities refer to the broad concept of individual adverse reactions to foods. Food sensitivities are reproducible, unpleasant reactions to specific food or food ingredients. There are many types of adverse reactions to foods, e.g., hives, headaches, asthma, and gastrointestinal complaints. Food sensitivities can be divided into primary and secondary sensitivities (Table 10.1).

PRIMARY FOOD SENSITIVITY

Primary food sensitivities can be divided into immunological and nonimmunological reactions. The basis of an abnormal immunological response after food consumption is a true food allergy or hypersensitivity. Primary sensitivities involving immunological reactions are further divided into IgE-mediated and non–IgE-mediated food allergies. Individuals who have IgE-mediated food allergy reactions to certain components (allergens) constitute only a small part of food sensitivities. The reactions are often noted as immediate hypersensitivity reactions, because the symptoms occur soon after ingesting the offending foods. Food allergens are defined as common food proteins which, in certain individuals, produce substances that induce allergic symptoms and can be life threatening. As in all people, the allergens are ingested, pass through the gut epithelium, and circulate in the blood; however, the immune system of some individuals reacts to these food allergens by manufacturing immunoglobulin E (IgE).

Foods contain many proteins, but only a few of them are allergens. Virtually all allergens are proteins, but not all proteins are food allergens. Allergens tend to be the most abundant protein found in a particular food. Overall, in most people, major muscle proteins in beef, pork, and chicken do not cause allergic reactions. Important

TABLE 10.2
Properties of Major Immunoglobulin (Ig) Classes

Ig Class	Half-Life (d)	Percent of Total Circulating Ig	Structure	Tissue in Which Found and Properties
IgG	7–21	80	Monomer	Blood and lymph, attaches to phagocytes, complement fixation
IgA	6	15	Monomer, dimer	Blood and lymph, secretory antibody
IgM	10	5–10	Pentamer	Blood and lymph, attaches to phagocytes
IgD	3	0.2	Monomer	Surface of B-cells
IgE	2	0.05	Monomer	Blood and lymph, attaches to mast cells and basophils, allergic response

allergens of the legumes are storage proteins, which make up the majority of the protein content of the seed, whereas the major allergenic protein from codfish is present in a small amount in the fish. Most allergenic foods contain multiple allergens; for example, egg white contains 20 proteins, of which 5 or 6 are allergenic. Most allergens are stable to digestion and processing, e.g., acid-resistant glycoproteins. Fruits and vegetables are the exceptions; however, there might be oral signs related to allergic reactions. Heat and processing tend to change the tertiary structure of food proteins, but this may be minimally important to their allergenicity.

IgE is one of five antibody systems that humans have to fight infection and resist disease, the other immunoglobulins being IgG, IgA, IgM, and IgD. Table 10.2 defines some properties of major immunoglobulin classes.

A particular role of IgE is in fighting parasitic infection. Usually, most humans have a low level of circulating IgE antibodies, but some individuals predisposed to developing allergies produce IgE antibodies that are specific for and recognize certain antigens.

The IgE and other immunoglobulins are produced by plasma cells derived from B cells, or B lymphocytes. IgEs have the ability to recognize food allergens. The B lymphocytes are mainly derived from lymphoid tissue of the bone marrow in higher animals and from the bursa of Fabricius in birds. The other major components of the immune system are the T lymphocytes, which are of thymic lymphoid tissue origin. The lymphoid tissues of the bone and thymus are referred to as primary lymphoid tissues. Secondary lymphoid tissues include the spleen, lymph nodes, tonsils, and adenoids. There are also some lymphoid aggregates at the three major portals of entry for environmental agents, the lung, gut, and skin: the bronchus-associated lymphoid tissue (BALT), gut-associated lymphoid tissue (GALT), and skin-associated lymphoid tissue (SALT). Thus, B cells are responsible for the synthesis of circulating humoral antibodies or immunoglobins, and T cells are involved in a variety of important cell-mediated processes, such as graft rejection, hypersensitivity reactions, and defense against malignant cells and many viruses.

IgE molecules are secreted out of the B cells and are distributed through the circulatory system, where they can find a mast cell. Mast cells are ubiquitous and

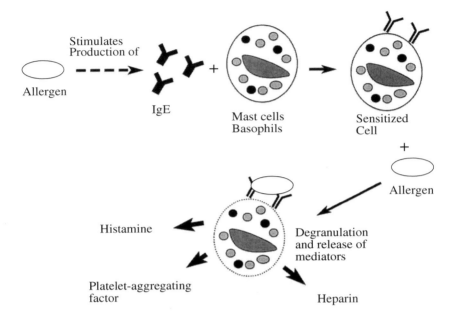

FIGURE 10.1 IgE-mediated allergic reaction.

in the blood stream are called basophils. Basophils and mast cells contain granules filled with active chemicals (mediators) that can be released during an allergic or inflammatory response. The mechanism of IgE-mediated allergic reaction, or immediate hypersensitivity (Type I; Figure 10.1), is composed of two major events. The first event or sensitization is when an allergen (antigen) is consumed. Other routes of exposure can be portals for sensitization, i.e., the respiratory tract or the skin. Serum concentration of IgE is low compared with that of other immunoglobulins, and its serum half-life is relatively short (Table 10.2). Once the allergen is consumed, the individual become sensitized. Sensitization results in production of allergen-specific IgE antibodies, which then bind to local tissue mast cells and on entering the circulation bind to circulating mast cells, basophils, and other tissue mast cells distal to the original site of entrance. The second event occurs after subsequent exposures or reexposure to the allergenic material, whereupon the allergen cross-links two IgE antibodies on the surface of the mast cell or basophil membrane via sites called F_c receptors. This cross-link results in a change in the membrane (degranulation) and stimulates the release of chemical mediators such as histamine, heparin, and platelet aggregating factor. These mediators promote vasodilation, inflammation, and bronchial constriction. Clinical manifestations vary from urticarial skin reactions (wheals and flares) to rhinitis and conjuctivitis to asthma and anaphylaxis.

The mechanism of IgE-mediated sensitivity is identical to that of allergic reactions to various environmental substances, such as pollen, pet dander, drugs, penicillin, and insect stings. The food allergen must be small enough to gain access through the body's barrier (GI membrane, skin, lungs) but large enough for the immune system to recognize. Some structural characteristics of allergens may be shared by similar foods and be biologically related, and sensitive people may consequently have IgEs that cross-react with the related foods.

Non-IgE-mediated primary food sensitivities are usually manifested by 6- to 24-h delayed hypersensitivity reactions following ingestion of food material. The allergic reactions develop slowly and peak at 48 h, subsiding 72 to 96 h later. Mounting evidence suggests that the allergic response involves the interaction between specific allergens from the food and sensitized, tissue-bound T cells, releasing inflammatory mediators. Celiac disease or celiac sprue is an example of a non-IgE-mediated immunological primary food sensitivity. Celiac disease sufferers are sensitive to glutens, particularly the gliadin fraction of wheat and related crops. Gliadin is a simple protein found in the gluten, consisting of 43% glutamine. Following ingestion of glutens, the absorptive epithelial cells in the small intestine become damaged by an inflammatory process. The intestinal damage results in a severe malabsorption syndrome, i.e., diarrhea, bloating, weight loss, anemia, fatigue, and muscle and bone pain. In children, celiac disease can cause failure to gain weight and growth retardation. Celiac disease is an inherited trait affecting people of European backgrounds and is very rare in Asians and Africans. Some believe that the affected population lacks an enzyme necessary to digest gliadin. Celiac disease is treated by avoiding gliadin foods, which restores the absorptive function and resolves the disease. Celiac disease sufferers can exhibit symptoms by ingesting even small amounts of gluten grains.

Nonimmunological Primary Food Sensitivities

These reactions have been referred to as food intolerances and involve nonimmunological mechanisms. Like true food allergies, food intolerances affect some people only, and usually they can tolerate small amounts of the offending food without adverse effects. Nonimmunological primary food sensitivities can be categorized as anaphylactoid reactions, metabolic food disorders, and idiosyncratic illnesses (Table 10.3).

Anaphylactoid reactions are adverse reactions caused by foods or food components that produce a spontaneous release of histamine and related mediators from tissue mast cells. Thus, except the IgE-mediated response, the reaction to foods or food components is identical to that for true food allergies. Substances found in the offending food may react with and destabilize the membrane of mast cells, releasing

TABLE 10.3
Nonimmunological Reactions

Anaphylactoid	Metabolic	Idiosyncratic
Strawberry	Lactose	Sulfite
Cheese	Favism	Tartrazine
Chocolate	Cabbage	MSG
	Licorice	BHT/BHA

histamine and other mediators. The mechanism is well established for certain drugs; however, no histamine-releasing substances have been isolated from such offending foods, e.g., strawberry allergy. Individuals affected by the ingestion of strawberries exhibit true food allergy symptoms, such as hives, but the symptoms are not IgE-mediated. One symptom mimics anaphylaxis.

Metabolic food disorders can be either due to inherited defects in the metabolism of a food or food component or due to genetically linked enhanced sensitivity to some food chemical. For example, individuals with lactose intolerance lack the enzyme lactase or β-galactosidase in the intestinal mucosa. As a result, such individuals cannot hydrolyze lactose or milk sugar into its monosaccharides, galactose and glucose. The undigested lactose cannot be absorbed, so it passes down the small intestine to the colon, where bacteria ferment it. Fermentation of lactose to carbon dioxide, water, and acetic acid results in gas, abdominal cramping, and diarrhea. Lactose intolerance is prevalent in some ethnic groups, such as Greeks, Arabs, Jews, African Americans, Hispanics, and Asians. In susceptible individuals, the activity of intestinal β-galactosidase is usually enough at birth to provide sufficient digestion of mothers' milk. With time, such individuals lose enzyme activity, and lactose intolerance can begin at any age. The condition can be very severe in the elderly.

Individuals who lack the red cell enzyme glucose-6-phosphate dehydrogenase (G6PDH) are susceptible to favism, a metabolic food disorder to ingested fava beans. Fava beans contain vicine and convicine, which are naturally occurring oxidants. These oxidants damage the red cell membranes of G6PDH-deficient individuals, resulting in erythrocyte hemolysis, causing individuals to suffer from hemolytic anemia. G6PDH is a critical red blood cell enzyme responsible for maintaining glutathione (GSH) and nicotinamide adenine dinucleotide phosphate (NADPH), which help prevent oxidative damage. G6PDH deficiency is common, affecting approximately 100 million people worldwide, with highest prevalence among populations of Jews, Greeks, and African Americans.

Individuals sensitive to cabbage exhibit goiter, because isothiocyanates present in cabbage interfere with the utilization of iodine. Some people are sensitive to licorice because the glycyrrhizic acid found in licorice mimics mineralocorticoids, resulting in hypertension and cardiac enlargement following sodium retention.

Idiosyncratic Reactions

Individuals who display idiosyncratic reactions to foods show a link between ingestion of such foods and their illness but without any defined mechanisms. The symptoms associated with idiosyncratic reactions can be from trivial to life threatening. For many cases, the role of specific food ingredients in causing idiosyncratic reactions remains to be determined. The cause-and-effect relationship can only be established through carefully controlled double-blind food challenges.

An example of a well-established idiosyncratic reaction is sulfite-induced asthma. Sulfites are widely used as food ingredients to control nonenzymatic and enzymatic browning and to prevent bacterial growth. Sulfites also are useful antioxidants and can condition dough and bleach certain foods. In some asthmatic populations, sulfite ingestion initiates an asthmatic reaction, which can be severe, and, on occasions, life threatening. The prevalence of sulfite sensitivity among asthmatics ranges from 1 to 10%. The most severe asthmatics seem to be the individuals who are most sulfite sensitive. Sulfite sensitivity is diagnosed by subjecting individuals to a sulfite challenge test, with the sulfite administered in a double-blind fashion.

Sulfite sensitivity may be due to a partial deficiency of sulfite oxidase in sulfite-sensitive asthmatics. Inhalation of sulfur dioxide vapors during the ingestion of foods and beverages may trigger an irritative reaction in the lungs of sensitive asthmatics. Some sulfite-sensitive asthmatics exhibit a positive skin test to sulfites, indicating a possible IgE-mediated mechanism.

Tartrazine sensitivity has been reported to cause asthma in some children, and such reports have been verified by double-blind studies. A high dose of monosodium glutamate (MSG) affects small populations. There have been a few isolated reports suggesting that butylated hydroxyanisole (BHA) and butylated hydroxytoluene (BHT) elicit sensitivity, but this has not yet been proven.

Secondary Food Sensitivity

Secondary food sensitivities are adverse reactions to food that occur as a consequence of other conditions. Examples include secondary sensitivities to gastrointestinal disorders or to drug treatment. Lactose intolerance is an adverse effect to lactose and occurs secondarily to a gastrointestinal disorder. Individuals who take antidepressant drugs have an increased sensitivity to tyramine. Secondary food sensitivities often disappear within a few weeks after recovery from the illness or discontinuation of drug therapy. A variety of gastrointestinal illnesses can enhance the chance of developing food allergies, such as bacterial or viral gastroenteritis, cystic fibrosis, Crohn's disease, and ulcerative colitis.

SYMPTOMS AND DIAGNOSIS

Usually, individuals prone to food allergies suffer only a few symptoms. Symptoms can vary among individuals, ranging from the common gastrointestinal symptoms to severe anaphylaxis. Table 10.4 summarizes the symptoms experienced during allergic reactions to foods. Rhinitis is runny nose, asthma is difficulty breathing, laryngeal edema is constriction of the throat, angioedema is swelling, urticaria is hives, and eczema/atopic dermatitis is skin rash. The potentially fatal form of food-

TABLE 10.4
Symptoms of IgE-Mediated Food Allergies

Respiratory	Cutaneous	Gastrointestinal	Systemic
Rhinitis	Angioedema	Abdominal cramps	Anaphylactic shock
Asthma	Urticaria	Diarrhea	
Laryngeal edema	Eczema/atopic dermatitis	Nausea	
		Vomiting	

allergic response, anaphylaxis, is rare, but may begin with mild symptoms (tongue swelling and itching, throat tightening, wheezing and cyanosis) and develop rapidly, resulting in cardiorespiratory arrest and shock. Death may occur rapidly if the individual cannot obtain medications.

In some individuals, exercise before or just after ingesting the offending food can induce symptoms of food allergies, including severe anaphylaxis. Certain foods, such as shellfish, wheat, and celery, produce symptoms provoked by exercise. The mechanism of action is unknown, but may involve enhanced mast cell responsiveness to physical stimuli.

The first step in the diagnosis of IgE-mediated food allergies is to establish an association between the ingestion of one or more offending foods and the elicitation of an adverse reaction. An allergist should be consulted, because self-diagnosis or parental diagnosis of children can be problematic, leading to erroneous findings. Careful history-taking, which includes a food diary by an experienced allergist, can often identify problem foods. This can be confirmed by using elimination diets of the suspected problem food, followed by challenges. The double-blind placebo-controlled food challenge (DBPCFC) is often used in clinical situations to document the existence of a food-associated adverse reaction. However, DBPCFC is not used in cases involving serious, life-threatening adverse reactions because of the risk to the patient. After the role of the specific offending food has been established, the involvement of the IgE mechanism can be documented through skin-prick tests by using extracts of the suspected foods. Alternatively, radioallergosorbent tests (RASTs) can be done to test for the presence of food-specific IgE antibodies in the blood of patients. A summary of steps in the diagnosis of IgE-mediated food allergies is shown in Table 10.5.

TREATMENT

Approaches for treating food allergies include (1) specific avoidance diet, (2) overall elimination diet, (3) pharmacological treatment, and (4) prophylactic treatment.

In a specific avoidance diet, the problem food or foods containing the offending substances are eliminated from the diet. Careful scrutiny of labels and considerable knowledge of food composition are important. Even with such knowledge, difficulties may be encountered because of the presence of allergenic residues that do not appear on a label and because labeling is inadequate in restaurant and eating establishments away from home. A patient must have considerable knowledge of possible hidden sources of the allergen in the diet. The potential problem with specific avoidance diets is that such diets could lead to nutritional deficiencies. Specific avoidance diets

TABLE 10.5
Steps in the Diagnosis of IgE-Mediated Food Allergies

Food diary
Double-blind placebo-controlled food challenge (DBPCFC)
Skin prick test (SPT) or radioallergosorbent test (RAST)

can be a successful treatment approach; however, it is important that such diets be based on solid data from patients' history and skin tests and food challenge tests. Unfortunately, very few medical foods are available for those with food allergies. Infants allergic to cow's milk can be given soybean and hydrolyzed casein products, but for the many other types of food allergies, very few substitutes are available.

The overall elimination diet is used in situations where a variety of possible allergenic foods have to be removed from the diet at one time. Such diets are used for patients with severe, chronic cases of an allergy, often due to multiple foods. Although this technique may resolve chronic symptoms of such individuals, the diets become unpalatable if used for long.

Pharmacological treatments include various antihistamines, which are used to treat the symptoms following an allergy episode, and epinephrine-filled syringes for life-threatening reactions. Physicians often advise individuals with a lifelong history of acute allergic reactions to carry antihistamines or epinephrine products to be rapidly administered. Prior treatment of some individuals with antihistamines allows some to tolerate offending foods, particularly patients allergic to cow's milk. Although immunotherapy has been useful in treating insect-sting and pollen allergies, no definitive evidence has been obtained for their use against food allergies.

Many studies have been done to address the usefulness of breast-feeding as a prophylactic treatment in preventing food allergies. The results have been mixed, with the edge given in favor of the benefits of breast-feeding. Many allergists are recommending exclusive breast-feeding for at least 6 months, particularly to infants with a family history of allergies. Some have recommended breast-feeding for even longer than 6 months because some studies have demonstrated that allergies to cow's milk can develop in infants exclusively breast-fed for 6 months. Others have suggested that if the infant's diet is well managed for the introduction of other foods early on, breast-feeding for beyond 6 months is not necessary. Little is known regarding the mechanism of prophylactic action of breast milk; however, the presence of secretory IgA antibodies in breast milk may play a role. Some infants even after being fed breast milk develop food allergies. It is likely that transmission of protein allergens occurs through breast milk or even via *in utero* sensitization. Both egg and soybean proteins have been identified in both human colostrum and mature breast milk.

STUDY QUESTIONS AND EXERCISES

1. Describe, in words and with an illustration, IgE-mediated sensitivities.
2. What are the major types of immunoglobulins? Describe their properties.
3. Describe food allergies, sensitivities, and intolerances. What are idiosyncratic reactions?

RECOMMENDED READINGS

Bruggink, T., Food allergy and food intolerance, in *Food Safety and Toxicity*, deVries, J., Ed., CRC Press, Boca Raton, FL, 1997, pp. 183-193.

Metcalfe, D.D., Food allergens, *Clin. Rev. Aller.*, 3, 331-349, 1985.
Selgrade, M.K., Germolec, D.R., Luebke, R.W., Smialowicz, R.J., Ward, M.D., and Sailstad, D.M., Immunotoxicity, in *Introduction to Biochemical Toxicology*, 3rd ed., Hodgson, E. and Smart, R.C., Eds., Wiley-Interscience, New York, 2001, pp. 561-598.
Sampson, H.A., Mechanisms in adverse reactions to food, *Allergy*, 50, 46-51, 1995.
Sampson, H.A., Food allergy: from biology toward therapy, *Hosp. Pract.*, pp. 67-83, May 14, 2000.
Taylor, S.L. and Hefle, S.L., Food allergies and other food sensitivities, *Food Techn.*, 55, 68-83, 2001.

Section II

Toxicants Found in Foods

11 Bacterial Toxins

Of the many different causes of foodborne diseases, bacteria are by far the most common. About half of all cases of diarrhea in the U.S. are of foodborne origin, and, according to the CDC, microbial diseases are on the rise. The reasons for the increase in foodborne illnesses are as follows. (1) There are better epidemiological capacities and better means to report cases, as well as better means to detect and identify foodborne illnesses. (2) Over the last few decades, people have made significant changes in their lifestyle and food consumption. They eat out more often, travel more, and choose exotic foods more often. Vegetables and fruits come from different countries, which sometimes have different sanitation standards and different strains of microbes. As a working society, we have gotten further away from food preparation and as such there is less emphasis on teaching about food preparation. At present, school curriculums rarely contain safety instructions for preparing food, i.e., home economics classes. People consume more meals in restaurants, where food passes through many hands, thereby increasing the chances of food contamination due to improper handling. Also, consumers' demand for natural or organic foods has resulted in more unpasteurized food production. (3) Food distribution is more global, which has increased the possibility of problems becoming more far-reaching. With larger operations, one mistake in food preparation can affect large numbers of people. Large production can increase the potential for cross-contamination. (4) Microorganisms are developing resistance to antibiotics. Overuse of antibiotics has increased the incidence and decreased the ability to treat microbial diseases.

We are also to blame because we fail to use sound food safety practices in our homes. Our food handling practices, such as lack of good cleaning techniques in the kitchen, careless hand-washing, and not observing food temperatures between 40° and 160°F (4° and 68°C, respectively), have put us at greater risk. Some still believe that foods should be cooled to room temperature before being refrigerated. This belief comes from the practice of placing hot food into iceboxes, causing the hot food to melt the ice, thereby spoiling all the food in the icebox.

Microbial-related foodborne diseases can be due to either infections or intoxications. Diseases involving the pathogen itself are infections, and those involving the pathogen's toxic products (toxin, toxic metabolites) as causal agents are intoxications. Intoxications also refers to foodborne illnesses resulting from other natural sources.

INTOXICATIONS

BACILLUS CEREUS

There are 34 species of *B. cereus*, which are aerobic endospores, but only two, *B. anthracis* and *B. cereus,* are recognized as pathogens. This group of bacteria is widely found and can colonize on a variety of habitats. In 1949, Hauge in Oslo, Norway, performed the classical investigation that implicated *B. cereus* in food poisoning. In three hospitals and a convalescent home, 600 people were affected. The source was traced to a vanilla sauce prepared the previous day and stored in a large container at room temperature. Hauge found by direct microscopic examination of the vanilla sauce a heavy infection of large Gram-positive rods. The first documented report of *B. cereus* diarrheal food poisoning was in 1969, involving 209 cases in North Carolina. Emetic syndromes from *B. cereus* have been linked to foods ranging from vegetables and salads to meat dishes and casseroles. There are frequent associations of *B. cereus* emetic effects with rice dishes, although the reason for the association is not known. Usually, the organism causes a self-limiting type of food poisoning. Occasionally, the organism can be fatal in immunocompromised individuals.

Bacillus refers to the genus consisting of rod-shaped, Gram-positive bacteria that aerobically form endospores. Endospores are a new kind of cell formation within the bacterial vegetative cell, differing from the parent cell in chemical structure, enzymatic content, and physiological function. This new kind of cell carries within it everything necessary to form another vegetative cell by germination. *Bacillus cereus* exists in water and soil and is motile, nonencapsulated, and β-hemolytic.

Bacillus anthracis is found in the soil, causing many animals to die of anthrax. The organism can be found in the gastrointestinal (GI) tract of an animal that survives the disease. Anthrax in humans is usually an occupational disease affecting veterinarians, butchers, ranchers, and meat industry workers usually by the cutaneous route through abrasions or scratches in the skin. The less common route is by inhalation, causing the so-called Woolsorters' disease. Fatalities are high (>80%), particularly by the inhalation route, unless treated with antibiotics. Another possible route of infection is through eating contaminated food, causing gastrointestinal anthrax. Eating meat from infected animals is the usual means of exposure, which is rare in the U.S. Fatalities can be between 25 and 60%. Anthrax cannot be passed through the air, so the infectious rate is low; however, the exception is cutaneous anthrax, wherein contact with drainage from an open sore can spread the bacteria.

Anthrax became infamous in the aftermath of September 11, 2001, as a suspected tool for bioterrorism. Several individuals contracted the deadly inhalation form, and many more came down with the cutaneous anthrax after being exposed to a powder material sent through mail. The U.S. Postal Service has been looking for ways to make the mail safer for its employees, including the use of irradiation.

Mode of Action

B. anthracis cells multiply locally, resulting in an acute inflammatory response. Polymorphonuclear leukocyte phagocytosis is inhibited by the capsule; thus, the organisms survive and multiply. Exotoxin is released locally and the organism branches out and invades adjacent tissues rapidly. This is followed by necrotic, black lesions; serosanguinous fluid; septicemia; and more tissue invasions. Woolsorters' disease is also characterized by toxemic and invasive symptoms. The organism rapidly germinates into vegetative cells in the respiratory system, releasing exotoxin and producing pulmonary necrosis, septicemia, and meningitis within 24 h. Gastrointestinal anthrax produces vomiting of blood, abdominal pain, nausea, and diarrhea. Treatment with antibiotics must be done in the earliest stages of infection to fight the bacteria. Cipro® (Bayer Pharmaceuticals) is the major antibiotic used to treat inhalation anthrax.

At least two enterotoxins are associated with *B. cereus* food poisoning, believed to be linked with the two symptoms described later. An enterotoxin is responsible for the diarrheal syndrome, and antibodies have been prepared against the toxin to detect the enterotoxin protein. The emetic toxin has been difficult to characterize because of the lack of a useful model system.

Clinical Symptoms

Anthrax is both a toxemic and invasive disease, showing symptoms as described previously. Inhalation anthrax results in malaise, fatigue, and sometimes a dry cough. Often the subject experiences improvement, but that is followed by a decline, with breathing trouble, sweating, and bluish discoloration of the skin. The subject experiences shock and death 24 to 36 h after the severe symptoms begin. For cutaneous skin anthrax, individuals experience low fever, skin lesions, and swelling. Often, the skin has lesions with black centers. Two distinct types of illnesses are associated with food poisoning from *B. cereus*. Within 4 to 16 h of incubation, there is the diarrheal illness, manifested as abdominal pain and diarrhea. Such symptoms usually subside within 12 to 24 h. There also is an emetic illness of shorter incubation, 1 to 5 h, producing nausea and vomiting.

CLOSTRIDIUM BOTULINUM

The botulism toxins are produced by *Clostridium botulinum*. These bacteria are Gram-positive, motile, Gram-rod-shaped, spore-forming anaerobes. *C. botulinum* is a group of bacteria, all the members of which are capable of producing neurotoxins. *C. botulinum* is commonly found in the soil and its spores can often be seen on fresh fruits and vegetables. The spore form is an important contaminant that can tolerate many environmental conditions. There are eight types of *C. botulinum*: A, B, C1, C2, D, E, F, and G. The letters indicate antigenically distinct types. Types A, B, E, and F are toxic to humans whereas Types B, C, and D are toxic to cattle and Types C and E toxic to birds. *C. botulinum* needs anaerobic conditions, thus practices such as packaging mushrooms with plastic film for extended periods should be avoided. Type A *C. botulinum* is the most lethal: ca. 25% of Type A outbreaks are lethal compared with about 8% for Type B outbreaks. Whereas irradiation can be a useful adjuvant in food safety, spores of Types A and B are resistant and low doses kill useful competing bacteria. *C. botulinum* is inhibited by acidic pH (<5) and low water activity. Water activity (a_w) is vapor pressure of the water in food divided by vapor pressure of pure water. Thus, a value of <0.95, or >30% sucrose, or >10% salt is useful in reducing bacterial growth (see later).

Botulus is the Latin term for sausage, which was the first food associated with cases of botulism. The categories of botulism are based on the way people acquire the toxin. In botulism arising from the category of food poisoning (food intoxication), individuals ingest the toxin with food. The second category is a rare wound botulism, in which *C. botulinum* forms the toxin in an infected tissue (infection). The third category is infant botulism, wherein toxin-forming bacteria colonize the lumen of the intestinal tract of infants (infection).

Cases of botulism-induced food poisoning are very rare in the U.S. Outbreaks occasionally occur from home-prepared products, particularly fruits and vegetables. Commercially canned foods can cause large outbreaks, but the industry has made progress to prevent such situations.

As regard infant botulism, honey produced in the U.S. is the only infant food in which *C. botulinum* spores have been consistently demonstrated. Soil on clothes can carry spores to infants, which can be inhaled. The inhaled spores have little effect on adults, who are normally resistant because their gut flora contains competitors of *C. botulinum*, but this is not the case for a child's gut. The ingested spores germinate in the intestine and produce the toxin, which is absorbed.

The spore form is the most important contaminant, because this form can tolerate many environmental conditions. Soil habitats give excellent opportunities for types A and B. Growth depends on anaerobic conditions. Contamination of raw food material usually occurs during growth and harvest.

Acidic pH is often used by the food industry, because spore germination is inhibited at pH 5. High salt (brining, >10%) and sucrose (>30%) are effective ways to reduce growth of organisms. Curing meats with nitrites chelates iron and prevents growth of organisms. Spores of types A and B are resistant to low radiation, and low radiation kills competing bacteria.

Mode of Action

Illness is attributed to foods prepared with inadequate heating. Purified cell extracts have low toxicities. It appears that when the intact protein is exposed to endogenous proteases, it becomes toxic. Toxin–protein complexes are often found with other food constituents, which protect the toxin from further GI tract deactivation. The neurotoxin is absorbed by the upper intestine and transported in the blood to peripheral nerves. The toxin binds at receptor sites, so that acetylcholine is not able to exert full response, producing paralysis. Receptor sites may be gangliosides at nerve endings. The toxin is inactivated in foods by heating to 80°C for at least 30 min.

Clinical Symptoms

Symptoms appear 12 to 72 h after ingestion. They include nausea, vomiting, headaches, tiredness, and muscular paralysis. Fatigue and muscular weakness are the first indications. These symptoms can be followed by eye effects such as droopy eyelids, sluggish response of pupils to light, and blurred vision. Individuals experience dryness of the mouth and difficulty in speech and swallowing. Symptoms last for 1 to 10 d, with high mortality. There is progressive paralysis of musculature enervated by cranial nerves. Respiratory paralysis and death result if the disease is not treated soon. Treatments consist of use of emetics, gastric washouts, and mechanical ventilation. There also is a horse serum antitoxin available which should be used. Recovery may take months.

Wound botulism is essentially the counterpart of tetanus and involves an infection at the site of injury. Infant botulism can affect babies one year or younger. The symptoms are different from food poisoning in that the child first experiences constipation, which precedes an obvious paralytic response. In the following hours or few days, breathing becomes difficult, and unless properly diagnosed, death occurs. Death is usually classified as sudden infant death syndrome. Usually, symptoms can be reversed by mechanical ventilation and treatment.

STAPHYLOCOCCI

The history of staphylococci and food poisoning goes back to 1914 when M.A. Barber reported his recollections of food poisoning from milk in the Philippines. Barber was able to trace the causative material to cream left at room temperature. Using himself as a guinea pig, he found that he could inoculate sterile milk with the bad milk and induce nausea and diarrhea within 2 h. In 1930, others found that it was a toxin that was causative and the term *enterotoxin* was used to illustrate the toxic effects on the intestine. Enterotoxins act on the viscera to produce nausea, cramps, diarrhea, and vomiting, usually lasting for several hours. For staphylococcal poisoning, the situation usually is not fatal, although some wish that it were.

Even though staphylococcal food poisoning occurs worldwide, it is seldom reported because of the relatively mild symptoms. Most staphylococcal food poisoning outbreaks involve small number of individuals, such as family groups, although a few larger outbreaks have occurred, such as one affecting 1300 people attending a picnic in Indiana.

There are 23 species of staphylococci, and *Staphylococcus aureus* is responsible for most of the outbreaks of food poisoning. Staphylococci are Gram-positive, nonmotile, facultative anaerobic cocci. The major characteristic of *S. aureus* is that it contains coagulase and thermonuclease (TNase). However, some intermediate species test positive for both coagulase and TNase and may be involved in food poisoning. Coagulases are soluble enzymes that coagulate plasma components, and TNases are heat-stable phosphodiesterases that can cleave either DNA or RNA to product $3'$ phosphomonucleosides. *S. aureus* is ubiquitous in nature, being a part of the normal flora of the skin, nose, throat, and GI tract of many humans and animals.

Causative agents for *Staphylococcus*-induced illnesses include a number of enterotoxins: A (SEA), B (SEB), C_1 (SEC_1), C_2 (SEC_2), C_3 (SEC_3), D (SED), and E (SEE). Enterotoxins produce their effects on the intestinal tract and can be identified by their reactions to specific antibodies. Enterotoxins are basic proteins, are resistant to proteolytic enzymes, and are heat stable up to 100°C for up to 30 min. The amount of enterotoxin required to produce illness is between 0.1 and 1 µg. The organism grows at a_w values as low as 0.83 and under either anaerobic or aerobic conditions. However, staphylococci do not grow well in the presence of other organisms. The common sources of outbreaks are from fermented sausages, salads, custards, and cream-filled bakery goods. Cheese and milk are less common sources. Because staphylococci can grow in a medium of salt up to 15%, any food can be a good medium.

Mode of Action

The causative agents in food poisoning are Enterotoxins A and D, which inhibit water absorption from the intestinal lumen and induce diarrhea. These enterotoxins also act on the emetic receptor sites, causing vomiting. Enterotoxin B damages the intestinal epithelium and produces colitis. Many *S. aureus* strains produce hyaluronidase, an enzyme that hydrolyzes the hyaluronic acid of connective tissues and facilitates the spread of the organisms in tissues. Staphylokinase (fibrinolysin) is another product of several *S. aureus* strains, which dissolves fibrin clots. *Staphylococcus aureus* contains lipases, which can disrupt cell membrane, and leucocidin, which can destroy leukocytes.

There are three modes of action: intestinal tract or the emetic reaction; circulatory system effects, low blood pressure, decrease in urine output, pulmonary edema, and pooling of blood in vascular beds resulting in shock and death; and others, such as allergic effects, particularly in clinical workers working with human specimens.

Clinical Symptoms

The damage to the host is due to ingestion of food containing preformed Enterotoxins A and D, which can act on emetic receptors and produce vomiting and inhibit water absorption from the intestine to produce diarrhea. An important observation is the absence of fever. Enterotoxin B can be induced in patients with normal bowels after taking oral broad-spectrum antibiotics. Such antibiotics can selectively permit overgrowth of antibiotic-resistant, enterotoxin-producing strains of *S. aureus*.

INFECTIONS

SALMONELLA

Most known species of *Salmonella* (Enterobacteriaceae family) are pathogenic to humans and are carried by a variety of animals. The virulence of *Salmonella* in human is dependent on the strain and individual susceptibility. Those in poor health are prone to illness. About 1% of the known *Salmonella* serotypes are associated with a single species, referred to as host adapted. For example, *Salmonella pullorum* and *S. gallinarum* are responsible for diarrhea and fowl typhoid, respectively, in poultry and are not usually found in other animals.

Salmonellosis is the disease associated with *Salmonella* and can include septicemia, typhoid fever, and enteric disease. However, the foodborne gastroenteritis form is often referred to as salmonellosis. It has been estimated that 50,000 cases of salmonellosis occur each year in the U.S., which may be grossly underreported.

Salmonellae can inhabit the GI tract of many animals, including poultry, rodents, birds, and others, where they can be harmless or cause disease. Over the past few years, the major source of human infection has been from commercial poultry and practices by that industry that involve overcrowding and sometimes poor hygiene. Improperly cooked poultry meat can serve as a source of foodborne infection. Eggs are now known to become infected in the ovaries of the hen; thus, consumption of raw eggs is very risky. Salmonellosis carriers are rare (ca. 1%), but in some cases wherein food handlers and babysitters have been suspected to be carriers, the people have been barred from working by local health authorities until their stool cultures have been shown negative.

Usually, the food poisoning can be traced back to the ingestion of improperly prepared previously contaminated food. Meat and dairy products are often sources, as are undercooked eggs, cheese, salads, and cold sandwiches. In the 1950s and 1960s, pet turtles were found to be a source of *Salmonella* infection, which could have been passed on to young children who touched the turtles and transferred the bacteria to their mouths. The infectious dose is ca. 10^5 organisms; however, in some cases, fewer than 100 organisms can cause infection. Salmonellae are killed easily by cooking temperatures of 60°C for 15 to 20 min or by chemical disinfectants and chlorine.

Salmonella species are Gram-negative, non-spore-forming bacilli, but *S. typhimurium* has a capsule. These organisms are facultatively anaerobic and grow on most types of medium. They can survive stomach acidity and enzymes, and can colonize the ileum and colon. The organisms invade the intestinal epithelium and are phagocytized by macrophages, in which they can intracellularly multiply. During their time in the macrophages, the bacteria are resistant to antibiotics. Thus, multiple treatments are required to prevent a relapse. As polymorphonuclear leukocytes respond to the invasion and destroy the organisms, endotoxin is released.

Clinical Symptoms

The incubation period is 8 to 48 h, producing nausea, vomiting, diarrhea, headache, chills, and fever. Individuals usually recover in about 2 d. People with immunocompromising diseases or other illnesses are more susceptible. In rare situations, enteric fever (hematogenous dissemination) or septicemia occurs, i.e., when the organisms are derived from the gut or transferred via blood. It such situations, the bacteria invade the GI tract and then the circulatory system via the lymphatic system, causing systemic disease. On occasions, complications from secondary pneumonia and osteomyelitis can occur. In these rare situations, mortality can be as high as 70% when there is no proper therapy. Treatment for enteric fever is by antibiotics, but for the more common food poisoning situations, antibiotics are not recommended because of the concern of encouraging the emergence of resistant strains.

Typhoid fever is the most serious form of *Salmonella* disease. Typhoid is endemic to many parts of the world, and about 500 cases occur each year in the U.S. Usually, cases in the U.S. can be traced to patients who have undertaken overseas travel. *S. typhi* is host adapted in humans (3%) and carriers can maintain the organism. The organism can be shed into water in the infected feces and sometimes transmitted by the hands of carriers (Typhoid Mary). Chloramphenicol is the drug of choice; however, ca. 15% of the isolates are resistant to the drug.

CAMPYLOBACTER JEJUNI

Campylobacter jejuni and *Salmonella* are the two most common foodborne pathogens. *C. jejuni* is a Gram-negative slender, curved, and motile rod. It is a microaerophilic organism, i.e., it has a requirement for reduced levels of oxygen. It is relatively fragile and sensitive to environmental stresses, such as 21% oxygen, drying, heating, disinfectants, and acidic conditions. *C. jejuni* requires 3–5% oxygen and 2–10% carbon dioxide for optimal growth and is an important enteric pathogen. Surveys have shown that *C. jejuni* is the leading cause of bacterial diarrheal illness in the U.S. and that it probably causes more disease than *Shigella* and *Salmonella* combined. *C. jejuni* is often isolated from healthy cattle, chicken, birds, and even flies, but is not usually carried by humans. But it is sometimes present in nonchlorinated water sources such as streams and ponds. *C. jejuni* causes the illness campylobacteriosis, which is also often known as campylobacter enteritis or gastroenteritis.

Clinical Symptoms

C. jejuni infection causes diarrhea, which may be watery or sticky and usually contains occult blood and fecal leukocytes. Other symptoms often present are fever, abdominal pain, nausea, headache, and muscle pain. The illness usually occurs 2 to 5 d after ingesting the contaminated food or water. Illness generally lasts 7 to 10 d, but relapses are common in ca. 25% of the cases. Most infections are self-limiting and are not treated with antibiotics. The infective dose of *C. jejuni* is usually small; about 400 to 500 bacteria may cause illness in some individuals, whereas greater numbers are required in others. The pathogenic mechanisms of *C. jejuni* are still not completely understood. In addition to being an invasive organism, it produces a heat-labile toxin that may cause diarrhea.

Complications are relatively rare, but infections have been associated with reactive arthritis, hemolytic uremic syndrome (HUS), and, following septicemia, infection of nearly any organ. The estimated case-to-fatality ratio for all *C. jejuni* infections is 0.1, meaning 1 death per 1000 cases. Fatalities are rare in healthy individuals and usually occur in cancer patients or in the otherwise debilitated. Only 20 cases of septic abortion induced by *C. jejuni* have been reported in the literature. Meningitis, recurrent colitis, acute cholecystitis, and Guillain–Barre syndrome are very rare complications.

Although anyone can have a *C. jejuni* infection, children less than 5 years old and young adults (15 to 29 years) are more frequently afflicted than people of other age groups. Reactive arthritis, a rare complication of these infections, is strongly associated with people who have the human lymphocyte antigen B27 (HLA-B27). Usually, outbreaks are small (fewer than 50 people), but in Bennington, VT, a large outbreak involving ca. 2000 people occurred while the town was temporarily using a nonchlorinated water source as a water supply. Several small outbreaks have been reported among children who were taken on a class trip to a dairy and given raw milk to drink. An outbreak was also associated with the consumption of raw clams. However, a survey showed that about 50% of the infections are associated with either eating inadequately cooked or recontaminated chicken meat or handling chickens. It is the leading bacterial cause of sporadic (nonclustered cases) diarrheal disease in the U.S.

CLOSTRIDIUM PERFRINGENS

This is a sporeforming, anaerobic organism that is widespread in the soil and a normal resident of human and animal intestinal tracts. *Clostridium perfringens* is distinct from other clostridia in being nonmotile, reducing nitrate to nitrite, and fermenting lactose in milk. The organism is common in the U.S. and Europe and can be found in cooked foods because of the heat-resistant endospores. The organism grows rapidly in warm foods and in the human intestine, where it produces an enterotoxin.

In most instances, the actual cause of poisoning by *C. perfringens* is temperature abuse of prepared foods. Small numbers of the organisms are often present after cooking and multiply to food-poisoning levels during cooling and storage of prepared foods. Meats, meat products, and gravy are the foods most frequently implicated.

C. perfringens poisoning is one of the most commonly reported foodborne illnesses in the U.S. Typically, dozens or even hundreds of people are affected. It is probable that many outbreaks go unreported, because the implicated foods or patient feces are not tested routinely for *C. perfringens* or its toxin. CDC estimates that about 10,000 cases actually occur annually in the U.S.

Clinical Symptoms

The common form of *C. perfringens* poisoning is characterized by intense abdominal cramps and diarrhea, which begin 8 to 22 h after consuming foods containing large numbers of *C. perfringens* bacteria capable of producing the food-poisoning toxin. The illness is usually over within 24 h, but less severe symptoms may persist in some individuals for 1 or 2 weeks. A few deaths have been reported as a result of dehydration and other complications.

Necrotic enteritis caused by *C. perfringens* is often fatal. This disease also begins as a result of ingesting large numbers of the causative bacteria in contaminated foods. Deaths from necrotic enteritis or pig-bel syndrome are caused by infection and necrosis of the intestines and from resulting septicemia. This disease is very rare in the U.S. The symptoms are caused by ingestion of large numbers (>10^8) of vegetative cells. Toxin production in the digestive tract is associated with sporulation.

ESCHERICHIA COLI

E. coli is part of the normal microflora of the intestinal tract of most warm-blooded animals. The organism is shed in the feces and most strains are harmless. They are lactose-fermenting, Gram-negative, non-spore-forming rods, most are motile with flagella, they produce gas from glucose, and some forms contain capsules. Most strains are harmless; however, a few are pathogenic to humans.

Since 1980, attention has been focused on *Escherichia coli* O157:H7 as the major provoker of Shiga-toxin *E. coli*–induced human diseases; however, current evidence suggests the need to expand understanding and be concerned about other *E. coli* serotypes too. There are four recognized classes of enterovirulent *E. coli* (EEC group) that cause gastroenteritis in humans: (1) enteropathogenic *E. coli* (EPEC) responsible for infantile diarrhea, often transmitted by contaminated and unchlorinated well water; (2) enteroinvasive *E. coli* (EIEC), responsible for the syndrome related to *Shigella* or a form of bacillary dysentery transmitted in water and food and by person-to-person contact; (3) enterotoxigenic *E. coli* (ETEC), the infamous travelers' diarrhea; and (4) enterohemorrhagic *E.coli* (EHEC), of recent notoriety as the toxin producing *E. coli* O157:H7.

Enteropathogenic *Escherichia coli* (EPEC)

EPEC sources and prevalence are controversial because foodborne outbreaks are sporadic. Frequent foods implicated in EPEC outbreaks are raw beef and chicken, and any food exposed to fecal contamination can be strongly suspect.

Infantile diarrhea is the disease usually associated with EPEC infections. EPEC outbreaks most often affect infants, especially those that are bottle-fed, in underdeveloped countries, suggesting that contaminated water is often used to rehydrate infant formula. Diarrhea in infants can be prolonged, leading to dehydration, electrolyte imbalance, and death. Mortality rates of 50% have been reported in Third World countries.

Clinical Symptoms

EPEC causes either a watery or bloody diarrhea. Watery diarrhea is associated with the attachment to, and physical alteration of, the integrity of the intestine. Bloody diarrhea is associated with attachment and an acute tissue-destructive process, perhaps caused by a toxin (verotoxin) similar to that seen in *Shigella* dysentery. EPEC is highly infectious to infants and the dose is likely very low; however, for diseases in adults, the dose is presumably similar to that for other colonizers ($>10^6$ total dose).

Enteroinvasive *Escherichia coli* (EIEC)

EIEC may produce an illness known as bacillary dysentery. It is not well established as to what foods may harbor EIEC, but any food contaminated with human feces from an ill person, either directly or from contaminated water, could cause disease in others. Some outbreaks have been associated with hamburger meat and unpasteurized milk.

Clinical Symptoms

Ingestion of EIEC results in the organisms invading the epithelial cells of the intestine, resulting in a mild form of dysentery, often mistaken for dysentery caused by *Shigella* species. The illness is characterized by the appearance of blood and mucus in the stools of infected people. The infectious dose of EIEC is thought to be as few as 10 organisms. Dysentery produced by EIEC usually occurs 12 to 72 h after ingesting contaminated food. Abdominal cramps, diarrhea, vomiting, fever, chills, and a generalized malaise are associated with the disease. Usually the dysentery is self-limiting with no known complications. However, a common sequel associated with infection, especially in pediatric cases, is the hemolytic uremic syndrome (HUS).

Enterotoxigenic *Escherichia coli* (ETEC)

Overall, this subgroup comprises a relatively small proportion of the species and has been etiologically associated globally with diarrheal illness of all age groups. The organism frequently causes diarrhea in visitors from industrialized countries and in infants in less-developed countries. The etiology of this cholera-like illness has been recognized for about 20 years. ETEC is not considered a serious foodborne disease hazard in industrialized countries because of their high sanitary standards and practices. In less-developed countries, contamination of water with human sewage may lead to contamination of foods. ETEC is infrequently isolated from dairy products such as semisoft cheeses, and infected food handlers may also contaminate foods.

A relatively large dose (10^8 to 10^{10} bacteria) of enterotoxigenic *E. coli* is probably necessary to colonize the small intestine, the site where these organisms proliferate and produce toxins that induce fluid secretion. With highly infective doses, diarrhea is usually induced within 24 h. Obviously, infants can be exposed to fewer organisms for infection to be established.

Clinical Symptoms

The most frequent clinical symptoms of infection include watery diarrhea, abdominal cramps, low-grade fever, nausea, and malaise. During the acute phase of infection, large numbers of enterotoxigenic cells are excreted in feces. These strains are differentiated from nontoxigenic *E. coli* present in the bowel by immunochemical, tissue culture, or gene probe tests designed to detect either the toxins or genes that encode these toxins. The clinical symptoms of the disease are usually self-limiting. It is important that infants or debilitated elderly individuals receive appropriate electrolyte replacement therapy.

Escherichia coli O157:H7 (Enterohemorrhagic *E. coli* or EHEC)

Similarities between the Shiga toxin produced in *Shigella* dysentery Type 1 and the toxin produced by *E. coli* O157:H7 prompted investigators to name the *E. coli* O157:H7 toxin as Shiga-like toxin or Shiga-toxin-producing *E. coli* (STEC). Coincidentally, the same toxin was named verotoxin by other investigators because such toxins could kill Vero cells in established tissue cultures from the kidneys of the African green monkey. The dire health and food safety concern is the association between STEC serotypes and HUS (5 to 10% of the patients) and kidney failure (another 5% of the patients). About 50% have long-term renal dysfunction, with mortality about 5%. Infection can progress to cause thrombotic thrombocytopenic purpurea (HUS with neurological complications) and can be fatal. Shiga toxins are thought to cross epithelial cell barriers of the gut and target microvascular endothelial cells of the intestine, kidney, and CNS. The mechanism of cell death may be because of the production of a functional inhibitor to Bcl-2, which plays a central role in apoptosis by suppressing cell death, i.e., by reprogramming cells to commit themselves to apoptotic pathways. People particularly susceptible include infants, young children, the elderly, and the sick. The infective dose is 50 to 100 organisms, but, in some cases, as few as 10 organisms are sufficient. Although the major exposure is usually from contaminated (fecal, soil) raw hamburgers, raw milk, and ruminant products, there is increasing concern about cross contamination to other food stuffs, e.g., bean sprouts or apple juice. *E. coli* O157 can survive in water at cold temperatures for long periods and can become acid tolerant. Flies and hand-to-hand contact, which might occur in day-care centers, may be modes of transmission.

Three gene sets found in *E. coli* O157:H7 are responsible for the destructive effects of this organism on the host. Genes that have the ability to produce Shiga-like toxins attach to cells lining the intestinal epithelial cells and possess a plasmid. Two Shiga toxins, Stx1 (VT-1) and Stx2 (VT-2), are encoded on a bacteriophage, which can be easily moved via the virus from organism to organism. The bacteriophage-encoded Shiga toxins may explain the use of antimicrobial agents to induce O157 to produce more toxin. Compounds such as 4-fluoroquinolones can induce bacteriophages. A feature significantly associated with the development of HUS in children has been the administration of antibiotics, suggestive of a situation of counterindication.

The attachment gene within *E. coli* can move between *E. coli*. Also, genes on the plasmid move to others by conjugation. Thus, there is danger of genes readily moving to other *E. coli* strains. In the U.S. and other countries, several investigators have found non-O157 serotypes with the ability to produce the toxins, and these have been associated with serious human diseases. However, because very few of the small number of laboratories researching to find Shiga toxins are geared for identifying non-O157 serotypes, the number of identified non-O157 serotypes may be quite conservative. In the U.S, non-O157 serotypes include O111, O26, O145, and O103.

It may not be enough for food producers and health practicians to be looking for O157 only. However, it may be too prudent to expect that it is cost effective to look for all STEC-forming organisms, because not all the positives are necessarily a health threat. Research that targets developing a better understanding about gene transfer and eventual impact on human health is needed.

The potential of more non-O157 serotypes expressing STEC is serious and represents a major threat to vulnerable populations. The consequences of exposure to STEC can be devastating and fatal. There is a need to increase effective diagnosis, provide better control of spread, and design treatment, as well as educate consumers, practitioners, and health care workers.

Undercooked or raw hamburger (ground beef) has been implicated in many of the documented outbreaks; however, *E. coli* O157:H7 outbreaks have implicated alfalfa sprouts, unpasteurized fruit juices, dry-cured salami, lettuce, game meat, and cheese curds.

Clinical Symptoms

The illness is characterized by severe cramping (abdominal pain) and diarrhea, which is initially watery but becomes grossly bloody. Occasionally vomiting occurs. Fever is either low grade or absent. The illness is usually self-limiting and lasts for an average of 8 d. Some individuals exhibit watery diarrhea only. In children, blood clots plug the convoluted tubules in the kidney. Patient may require dialysis treatment and the situation may be permanent. In some situations, children go into a coma and die. The acute disease caused by *E. coli* O157:H7 is hemorrhagic colitis. Hemorrhagic colitis infections are not too common, but this is probably not reflective of the true frequency. In the Pacific Northwest, *E. coli* O157:H7 is thought to be second only to *Salmonella* as a cause of bacterial diarrhea. Because of the unmistakable symptom of profuse, visible blood in severe cases, the victims probably seek medical attention, but less severe cases are probably more numerous.

LISTERIA MONOCYTOGENS

The organism is a Gram-positive, nonencapsulated short rod, and a facultative intracellular parasite. Its coccobacillary appearance, β-hemolytic characteristic on blood agar, and tendency to grow in short chains often results in an erroneous identification of streptococci. The organism is found in water, soil, sewage, and has been traced to improperly pasteurized food products. It also can be found in the GI tract, female genital tract, and throat of humans and animals. The organism can multiply and survive for years in the environment, but can be destroyed by antiseptic compounds and pasteurization.

Listeriosis is primarily a disease of animals, but serious diseases can be encountered in the human fetus, newborns, pregnant women, and sick individuals. Exogenous transmission can occur from the infected female genital tract *in utero* or at the time of delivery, producing disease of the fetus or newborn.

Clinical Symptoms

The organisms gain access to the circulation and are taken up by macrophages, in which they multiply and produce septicemia. Hemolysin released during multiplication causes lysis of macrophages. The organism can spread from cell to cell and can be carried to the meninges, producing meningitis. In addition, the organism can gain access to the liver and spleen, producing multiple abscesses and granulomas. In pregnant females, infection can result in abortion. Early treatment has a chance of success; however, treatment is often ineffective.

SHIGELLA

Shigella causes bacterial dysentery or shigellosis and is named after a Japanese physician, Kyoshi Shiga (1898). Shigellosis is far less common than salmonellosis and accounts for only 2% of the reported outbreaks of food poisoning. Transmission of shigellosis is usually by person-to-person contact by the fecal–oral route. Also, house flies and contaminated food and water can be modes of transmission, particularly because of improper personal hygiene or when cooked food is not held at a temperature sufficient to kill organisms. Shigellosis is a problem in developing countries where unsanitary conditions exist. It is also a problem where crowded living conditions occur, such as day-care schools. Foodborne sources include salads, especially those containing potatoes, chicken, tuna, or shrimp; raw oysters; watermelon; spaghetti; beans; apple cider; cream puffs; and hamburger.

Shigella is Gram-negative, rod shaped, and nonmotile. The organism had DNA homology with *E. coli*. There are four species: *dysenteriae, flexneri, boydii,* and *sonnei*. The organism is not very hardy and can be killed at 63°C in 5 min and can survive only within the pH range of 5 to 8.

The following adverse effects are associated with the toxin produced by *Shigella*: (1) nervous system, resulting in paralysis and neuron destruction; (2) GI system, resulting in fluid accumulation; (3) RNA, resulting in inhibition of protein synthesis; and (4) general effects, resulting in cell death.

Clinical Symptoms

Symptoms can vary from asymptomatic infection to mild diarrhea to dysentery (inflammation of large intestines with bloody stools). Severe situations may include bloody stools with mucus and pus, dehydration, fever, chills, toxemia, and vomiting. The onset is from 1 to 7 d and symptoms can persist from a few days to a couple of weeks. The major sites of infection are the ileum and colon. *Shigella* penetrates the epithelium and multiplies within the epithelial cells. The organism passes on to adjacent cells, producing necrosis and death of cell patches, leading to ulcers that exude blood. The organism is very infectious, and illness can occur with 10^2 to 10^4 cells. The Shiga toxin produced by the organism is a protein with enterotoxic, neurotoxic, and cytotoxic activities. In many situations, the illness is self-limiting and resolves in 1 to 2 weeks and antibiotics are not required. However, the illness can be quite devastating to the young, elderly, or immunocompromised individuals. Repeated bouts of bacterially induced diarrhea from *Shigella* have been suggested to cause chronic rheumatoid arthritis.

VIBRIO

The genus *Vibrio* consists of Gram-negative curved bacteria with a single turn, Gram-nonencapsulated rod, and motile with a single polar flagellum. The organism is a facultative anaerobe and can be divided into six subgroups based on somatic O-polysaccharide antigens. *Vibrio cholerae*, belonging to the family Virionaceae, is a species in the genus (two biotypes of serogroup 01). Cholera is the disease associated with the organism and the responsible toxicant is cholera toxin (choleragen). The organism can exist in saltwater for long periods of time and is found in plankton and shellfish. Transmission is by ingesting uncooked or undercooked seafood or by the fecal–oral route. The infective dose can be as low as 10^{11} organisms, and *V. cholerae* must be boiled for a least 10 min to inactivate the organism.

Clinical Symptoms

Between several hours and a few days, patients experience an explosive onset of watery diarrhea, vomiting, and abdominal pain. Fluid output can be voluminous, with up to 20 to 30 evacuations. The intestinal mucosa becomes shredded with damage, releasing plugs of mucus from intestinal cells resembling grains of rice

(rice-water stools). Mortality can be less than 1% if fluid replacement treatment is initiated; if untreated, 60% of the patients can become comatose and die.

The organism can rapidly multiply on the mucosal surface. The toxin choleragen produced by vibrios binds to ganglioside receptors of epithelial cells. Choleragen is made of five polypeptide B subunits circling a central polypeptide A subunit. The B subunit binds to ganglioside receptors and the A subunit enters through the cell membrane and activates the adenyl cyclase system to produce cAMP. Increased intracellular cAMP causes fluids and electrolytes to enter the intestinal lumen, i.e., hypersection of fluids and chloride and inhibition of sodium absorption and diarrhea. Other toxins with less-known roles are also released.

YERSINIA ENTEROCOLITICA

Y. enterocolitica is common in domestic animals. Human outbreaks (yersiniosis) have been attributed to contaminated milk, water, and various foods. Pig is the principal source of *Y. enterocolitica*. The organism is the etiological agent of diarrhea. It is Gram-negative and pleomorphic (sometimes ovoid and sometimes rod shaped). The organism is not motile at 37°C but becomes motile when grown at 30°C by producing a peritrichous flagella.

Yersiniae possess invasins, high-molecular-weight outer-membrane proteins that mediate adherence and cell entry. Invasins mediate uptake by epithelial cells of the mucosal lining of the GI tract. Also, yersiniae produce lipoprotein factors that inhibit phagocytosis. Many strains produce a heat-stable ennterotoxin that resembles the ST of *E. coli*.

Clinical Symptoms

Many characteristics are similar to those seen in acute appendicitis, including fever, abdominal pain, headache, vomiting, guarding, and peripheral neutrophilia. Frequently present is acute, watery diarrhea. Incubation period is 24–36 h and can last for 1–3 d.

STUDY QUESTIONS AND EXERCISES

1. Discuss the practices that likely are most effective in preventing an outbreak of salmonellosis.
2. Distinguish between the different serotypes of *E. coli* and discuss the diseases they cause.
3. Describe the pros and cons for the use of antibiotics in foodborne infections.
4. Define and give some examples of foodborne illnesses resulting from intoxications and infections.

RECOMMENDED READINGS

Acheson, D., Is testing for O157:H7 enough? *Food Qual.*, 35-37, January/February 2001.

Acheson, D.W.K. and Jaeger, J.L., Shiga toxin-producing *Escherichia coli*, *Clin. Microbiol. Newslett.*, 21, 183-188, 1999.

Bad Bug Book, http://vm.cfsan.fda.gov/~mow/intro.html.

Banatvala, N., Griffin, P.M., Greene, K.D., Barrett, T.J., Bibb, W.F., Green, J.H., Wells, J.G., and the Hemolytic Uremic Syndrome Study Collaborators, The United States nation prospective hemolytic uremic syndrome study: microbiologic, serologic, clinical, and epidemiologic findings, *J. Infect. Dis.*, 183, 1063-1070, 2001.

Boerlin, P., Evolution of virulence factors in Shiga-toxin-producing *Escherichia coli*, *Cell Mol. Life Sci.*, 56, 735-741, 1999.

Boerlin, P., McEwen, S.A., Boerlin-Petzold, F., Wilson, J.B., Johnson, R.P., and Gyles, C.L., Association between virulence factors of Shiga toxin-producing *Escherichia coli* and disease in humans, *J. Clin. Microbiol.*, 37, 497-503, 1999.

Greener, M., How *Escherichia coli* kills, *Mol. Med. Today*, 6, 411, 2000.

Hussein, S.H., Thran, B.H., and Hall, M.R., *Escherichia coli* O57:H7 as a foodborne pathogen: environmental, and nutritional factors affecting prevalence in ruminants and outbreaks in humans, *Environ. Nutr. Interact.*, 3, 277-311, 1999.

Law, D., Virulence factors of *Escherichia coli* O157 and Shiga toxin-producing *E. coli*, *J. Appl. Microbiol.*, 88, 729-745, 2000.

Sandvig, K. and van Deurs, B., Entry of ricin and Shiga toxin into cells: molecular mechanisms and medical perspectives, *EMBO J.*, 19, 5943-5950, 2000.

Talan, D. et al., Etiology of blood diarrhea among patients presenting to United States emergency departments: prevalence of *Escherichia coli* O157:H7 and other entero-pathogens, *Clin. Infect. Dis.*, 32, 573-580, 2001.

Zhang, W.-L., Bielaszewska, M., Liesegang, A., Tschäpe, H., Schmidt, H., Bitzan, M., and Karch1, H., Molecular characteristics and epidemiological significance of Shiga-toxin-producing *Escherichia coli* O26 strains, *J. Clin. Microbiol.*, 38, 2134-2140, 2000.

12 Animal Toxins and Plant Toxicants

Toxicants are produced by a variety of animals and plants and are widely distributed throughout each kingdom, from the unicellular to the multicellular. There is striking diversity of chemical structures for toxic compounds found in nature, making classification based on structure difficult.

The presence of toxicants in food may have come about because animals or plants evolved means of producing chemicals to protect themselves from predators, or insects, nematodes, microorganisms, or even humans.

The animal world has approximately 1200 species of venomous and poisonous creatures. Venomous animals refer to animals that are capable of creating a poison by a highly developed secretory gland or group of cells and delivering the poison during a bite or sting. The venom may have one or several functions, such as offense (capturing and digesting prey) or defense (protection against predators). Usually, venomous animals are not used by humans as a source of food, but when they are, care must be taken to avoid the poisonous glands containing toxicants. Poisonous animals are those whose tissues contain toxic materials. Such animals do not have a mechanism or structure for the delivery of the poison. Poisoning takes place by ingesting the animal material, particularly the tissue containing the poison. In poisonous animals, the poison may play only a small role in the animal's offensive or defensive activities. The toxin may be a by-product or a product of metabolism or a chemical that is passed along the food chain. Examples of the latter include barracuda, snapper, and other grouper fish, which can be a threat to human health because they have fed on smaller toxic fish and marine organisms such as dinoflagellates. The big fish eat the little fish that have consumed the toxicant and those who eat the big fish become ill.

Many plants also produce metabolic products (waste chemicals) or secondary products that can result in adverse effects if consumed in sufficient quantities. Plants did not evolve to be food for humans. There are far fewer species of plants used for food than those that are not. Many more plants are poisonous and therefore not safe to eat. In his studies in Africa, Leakey speculated that humans were first meat eaters until they learned how to use fire for cooking plant material to remove or inactivate toxic compounds. Many plants used for food contain small amounts of toxic chemicals. For example, potato and tomato, which are from the nightshade family, contain potentially toxic chemicals (alkaloids). The compound solanine is found in the eyes and peel of potato and if sunburned (green under the skin) or blighted, solanine levels can increase sevenfold, sufficient to harm a small child. Cooked potatoes with high concentrations of solanine have a bitter taste and can cause a burning sensation in the throat. Solanine has been shown to exhibit teratogenic effects in animals. It is likely that solanine serves as a natural pesticide to the beetle and leaf hopper. Another noxious chemical, tomatine, also an alkaloid, is found in tomato and may also serve as a natural plant pesticide. Psoralen, found in parsnip, carrots, and celery, is a chemical produced by a plant under stress. Psoralen is a skin irritant, causing rash and skin problems.

Overall, healthy individuals can tolerate naturally occurring toxicants. However, there are several conditions under which natural toxicants can create problems. Inborn errors of metabolism or certain drug interactions can make individuals prone to problems caused by natural toxicants. Whereas nutrients can be beneficial to most, they can be deleterious to some, e.g., consumption of lactose by lactose-intolerant people. Other examples include individuals with celiac sprue, sucrase deficiency, fructose intolerance, galactosemia, and phenylketonuria. Individuals taking drugs that inhibit monoamine oxidase enzymes can be affected when eating cheeses or drinking wines, which are high in tyramine. Individuals with sensitivities due to allergies can be affected by foods. Hypersensitivity to a particular substance produces anaphylactic shock. Examples of foods that cause allergies include milk, wheat, nuts, citrus, strawberries, fish (shellfish), and egg. Some individuals have bizarre food habits or diets because of which they may eat certain foods in abnormal amounts. Eating large amounts of rhubarb can result in renal damage because of the excess oxalate in rhubarb. Consumption of uncrushed bay leaves can physically damage the intestinal mucosa. Some people are prone to problems caused by natural toxicants because of abnormal food habits. Eating honey produced by bees that collect nectar from plants containing poisonous alkaloids, or eating puffer fish, can also cause people harm.

MARINE ANIMALS

For animals, in general, seafood poisons should be distinguished from marine venoms. Many seafood poisons are not limited to any single species and are likely to be affected by the environment. Some fish poisons (ichthyotoxins) are specific to a single species or genus. As illustrated in Table 12.1, seafood poisons can be categorized according to the tissues in which the toxin is found in the animal. Toxins localized in muscles, skin, liver, or intestine are known as ichthyosarcotoxins. Ich-

TABLE 12.1
Categories of Seafood Poisons

Type of Seafood Toxin	Location of Toxin
Ichthyosarcotoxin	Muscles, skin, liver, or intestines
Ichthyotoxin	Reproductive tissues
Ichthyohemotoxin	Circulatory system
Ichthyohepatotoxin	Liver

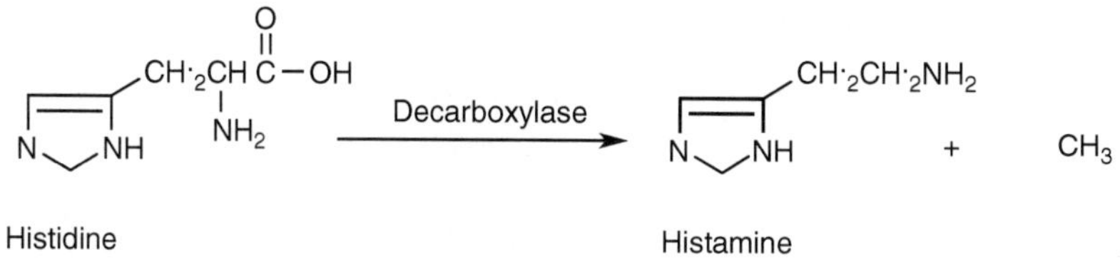

Animal Toxins and Plant Toxicants

$$\text{Histidine} \xrightarrow{\text{Decarboxylase}} \text{Histamine} + CH_3$$

FIGURE 12.1 Histamine formation in spoiled fish.

thyotoxins are toxic chemicals found in the testis or ovaries of animals. Toxins found in the circulatory system of animals are referred to as ichthyohemotoxins. Toxins localized in the hepatic system are known as ichthyohepatotoxins.

SCOMBROID POISONING

Scombroid poisoning occurs after the ingestion of tuna, skipjack, bonito, and mackerel-like fish. The clinical symptoms of this poisoning are different from those for poisoning by ciguatera toxins. If the scombroids are inadequately preserved, the toxic substance can continue to form in the musculature of the fish. Other products have also caused toxic effects, such as cheeses, the primary being Swiss cheese.

The toxin forms in a food when certain bacteria are present and time and temperature permit their growth. Distribution of the toxin within an individual fish fillet or between cans in a case lot can be uneven, with some sections of a product causing illnesses and others not. Cooking, canning, or freezing do not reduce the toxic effect. Common sensory examination by individuals cannot ensure the absence or presence of the toxin. The only reliable test for evaluating a product is a chemical test. Scombroid poisoning remains one of the most common forms of fish poisoning in the U.S. However, incidents of poisoning often go unreported because of the lack of required reporting, lack of information by some medical personnel, and confusion with symptoms of other illnesses. Hence there is underreporting of the actual number of cases, which is a worldwide problem.

Mode of Action

In part, the toxic symptoms are due to histamine formed by the action of enzymes and bacteria on the fish after death. The symptoms resemble allergic reactions due to histamine formation and are attributed to bacterial decarboxylation of histidine as the fish spoils. Figure 12.1 shows the reaction. Saurine, putrescine, and cadaverine are other noxious substances found in fish that may be involved in the toxic process. Keeping fish cold can slow down the spoilage; for example, at 32°F (0°C) fresh salmon remains unspoiled for 12 days, but at 60°F (15°C) it lasts only for a day. Any food that contains the appropriate amino acids and is subjected to certain bacterial contamination and growth may lead to scombroid poisoning when ingested.

Clinical Symptoms

People usually remember that the offending fish had a peppery taste. After ingestion or within 2 h, the patient shows several gastrointestinal effects, such as nausea,

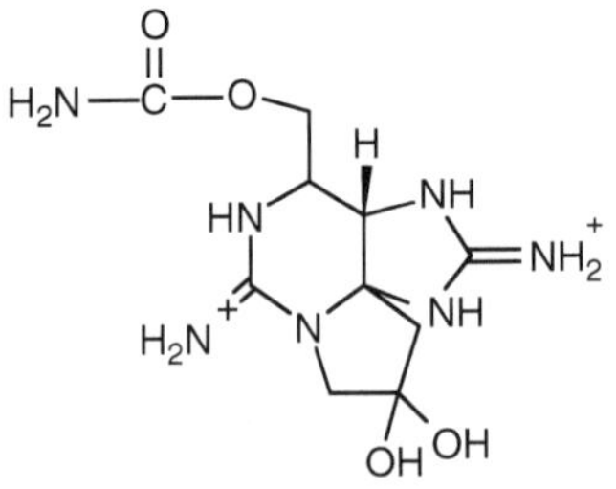

FIGURE 12.2 Saxitoxin.

vomiting, and diarrhea, as well as epigastric distress, headache, and burning sensation of the throat. This can be followed by neurological numbness, tingling, cutaneous flushing, and urticaria. Symptoms subside in ca. 16 h and generally there are no lasting ill effects. Diagnosis of the illness is usually based on the patient's symptoms, time of onset, and the effect of treatment with antihistamine medication. The onset of intoxication symptoms is rapid, ranging from immediate to 30 min. The duration of the illness is usually 3 h, but may last several days. To confirm a diagnosis, the suspected food must be analyzed within a few hours for elevated levels of histamine.

SAXITOXIN

Species of dinoflagellates, particularly *Gonylaux* sp., produce a toxin that accumulates in clams, mussels, and other shellfish that fed on the algae. The phenomenon of red tides or blooms can occur, resulting in rapid growth of the dinoflagellates. The danger of red tides was well known by the North American West Coast Indians, who refrained from eating shellfish during the first signs of colored water. The toxin has no ill effects on the shellfish, but can be dangerous to humans. Eating such fish can be a serious threat to public health and has been known as paralytic shellfish poisoning (PSP). PSP occurs throughout the world, particular at regions 30° or higher in latitude. The toxin cannot be removed by washing or destroyed by heating. All shellfishes (filter-feeding molluscs) are potentially toxic. However, PSP is generally associated with mussels, clams, cockles, and scallops.

Mode of Action

The active toxin is known as saxitoxin and the LD_{50} of an injection (IP) of saxitoxin in mice is 10 μg/kg. Twenty toxin derivatives make up saxitoxin and are responsible for PSP. The toxin has a curarelike action that prevents the muscle from responding to acetylcholine. Saxitoxin, whose structure is shown in Figure 12.2, has a direct effect on the heart and blocks action potentials in nerves and muscles.

Clinical Symptoms

Symptoms of the disease develop fairly rapidly, 30 min to 2 h after ingesting the shellfish, depending on the amount of the toxin consumed. In severe cases, respiratory paralysis is common, and death may occur if respiratory support is not provided.

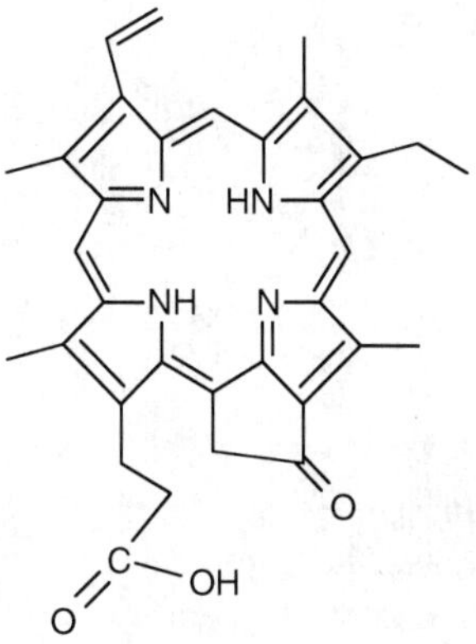

FIGURE 12.3 Pyropheophorbide-a.

When such support is applied within 12 h of exposure, recovery usually is complete, with no lasting side effects. In unusual cases, because of the weak hypotensive action of the toxin, death may occur from cardiovascular collapse despite respiratory support.

PYROPHEOPHORBIDE-A

Certain abalones (*Haliotis*) contain a toxin known as pyropheophorbide-a in the digestive gland or liver. This toxin is a derivative of chlorophyll, which can be ascertained by its blue-green pigment. It is thought that pyropheophorbide-a (Figure 12.3) is a toxin that is a metabolic product formed from chlorophyll in the seaweed on which the abalone feeds.

Mode of Action

The toxic reaction occurs when people eat the organs containing pyropheophorbide-a and are exposed to sunlight. Pyropheophorbide-a is photoactive, and this photosensitization in the body promotes the production of amine compounds from amino acids, histidine, tryptophan, and tryrosine. Such compounds produce inflammation and other toxic reactions. Two other compounds, murexine and enteramine (5-hydroxytryptamine), have been isolated and appear to have muscarinelike and nicotinelike activities.

Clinical Symptoms

Symptoms of photosensitized pyropheophorbide-a poisoning include appearance of facial and extremity redness and edema and dermatitis. The muscarinelike and nicotinelike activities cause cardiovascular changes with hypotension and increased respiration.

TETRODOTOXIN

There are about 90 species of puffer fish, which include blowfish, porcupine fish, toadfish, fugu (sold in Japanese restaurants), and molas. The California newt (*Taricha*

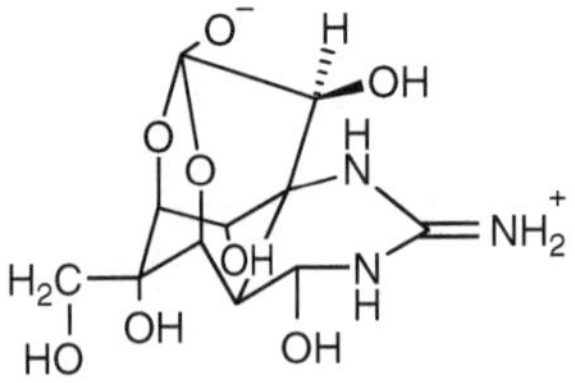

FIGURE 12.4 Tetrodotoxin.

torosa) and other amphibian species of the family Salamandridae also produce tetrodotoxin. Figure 12.4 shows the chemical structure of tetrodotoxin. In some cultures, the fish is considered a delicacy, and its consumption results in a tingling sensation. Specially trained individuals prepare the fish, but mistakes can happen. Poisoning may be caused by improper preparation or removal of ovaries, roe, liver, intestines, and skin, which contain the highest concentrations of tetrodotoxin. Actually, the toxin is found in nearly all tissues and is stable to boiling temperatures, unless made alkaline. The highest amounts are found during the spawning period of the fish.

Mode of Action

Tetrodotoxin, a neurotoxin, results in paralysis of the CNS and peripheral nerves by blocking the movement of all monovalent cations, increasing the early transient ionic permeability of the nerve. This causes the tingling sensation or prickly feeling of the fingers and toes. Tetrodotoxin, to a lesser extent, blocks the skeletal muscle membrane. It provokes hypotension and aversely affects respiration. The oral LD_{50} in mice is 322 µg/kg. It has been shown that certain bacteria can produce the toxin and may be the source of the poison. Two strains of bacteria belonging to genera *Alteromonas* and *Shewanella* have been isolated both from puffer fish and red algae.

Clinical Symptoms

The initial tingling sensations can be followed by malaise; dizziness; pallor; numbness of the extremities, lips, and tongue; and subsequent nausea, vomiting, ataxia, and diarrhea. Other symptoms include subcutaneous hemorrhage, desquamation, respiratory distress, muscular twitching, tremors, incoordination, muscle paralysis, cyanosis, and convulsions, and ca. 40 to 60% deaths can occur. Symptoms appear usually in 10 to 45 min; however, a lag time of 3 h or more has been observed.

CIGUATOXIN

Originally, ciguatera was applied to poisoning in the Caribbean resulting from the ingestion of the marine snail, *Livona pica* (cigua). Ciguatoxin, an ichthyosarcotoxin, is produced by more than 300 species of fish. Many fish caught for food have ciguatoxin because of their feeding habits. Fish ingest plant materials that contain the toxin. Photosynthetic benthic dinoflagellates are the likely organisms in ciguatera poisoning.

Mode of Action

Ciguatoxin inhibits cholinesterase, resulting in synaptic acetylcholine accumulation and disruption of nerve function. Death is usually attributed to respiratory paralysis. Ciguatoxin is a water-soluble and heat-stable hydroxylated lipid molecule whose structure is unknown. The toxin has been found to be antagonized by physostigmine.

Clinical Signs

Ciguatoxin poisoning begins with tingling of lips, tongue, and throat, and is rapidly followed by numbness in those areas. It may take up to 30 h following ingestion of the fish for symptoms to appear. Nausea, vomiting, abdominal pain with intestinal spasms, and diarrhea soon follow. Patients complain of headaches, which can be followed by muscle pain, visual disturbances, dermatitis, and even convulsions. Usually, poisoning is treated symptomatically. About 7% of the cases result in fatalities.

PLANTS

Approximately 700 species of some 30,000 species of North American plants are considered to be poisonous. Poisonous species are found throughout the plant kingdom, in algae, ferns, gymnosperms, and angiosperms. In some situations, groups of genera within a single family exhibit similar toxicity. On the other hand, some plants from the same genera differ vastly in toxicity. The nightshade, *Solanum nigrum,* is quite toxic, but *Solanum intrusum* is not known to be toxic. The latter is known as garden huckleberry or wonderberry, and recommended to home gardeners for its edible fruits. Poinsettia (*Euphorbia pulcherrima*) is another example. In the early 1900, poinsettia was responsible for a number of human mortalities in Hawaii. However, it appears that horticultural manipulation for longer-lasting and differently colored poinsettias may have resulted in a loss of toxicity, as determined by no toxic effects in rodents fed large quantities of the red bracts.

There is no easy way to classify toxic food components of plant origin. Some are low-molecular-weight endogenous toxins and others are products of secondary metabolism. Primary metabolism involves processes involved in energy metabolism, such as photosynthesis, growth, and reproduction. Macro- and micronutrients are the products of primary plant metabolism. Secondary metabolism is species specific and includes compounds such as plant pigments, flavors, or those that serve as protective compounds. Some of the secondary metabolic products are known as growth inhibitors, neurotoxins, mutagens, carcinogens, and teratogenes. Many are not tested because no government regulations require such testing and such testing would be extremely costly.

GOITROGENS

Human goiter, related to iodine deficiency, is an important health problem in certain parts of the world. In some areas, consumption of cruciferous plants can be a contributing factor to human endemic goiter. A goiter is produced when the seeds of various *Brassica* species are fed as part of the diet to animals. It is likely that

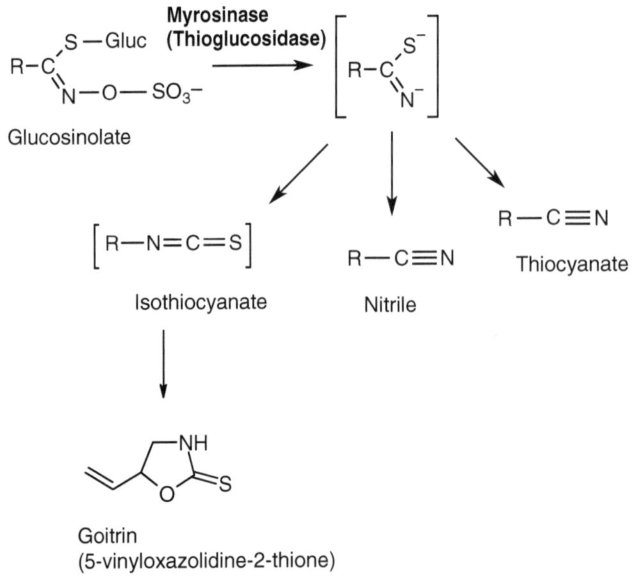

FIGURE 12.5 Goitrin formation.

consumption of unusually large amounts of *Brassica* species, such as cabbage, broccoli, turnip, rutabaga, and mustard greens, might cause thyroid enlargement, but not if consumption is as a normal part of an otherwise adequate diet.

Goitrin (Figure 12.5) is a goitrogenic substance formed from glucosinolate in Cruciferae. Glucosinolates are thioglucosides (sulfur-containing glucosides) and do not appear to be harmful until activated by myrosinase to isothiocynate, nitrile, and thiocyanate (Figure 12.5). Isothiocyanates are alkylating agents and thiocynates have antithyroid activity. Also, it is established that various nitriles are toxic to rats, and the product goitrin formed from isothicyanate is a thyroid-suppressing substance.

Cyanogenic Glycosides

These compounds are monosaccharide or disaccharide conjugates of cyanohydrins or precursors of hydrocyanic acid. Such compounds are natural herbicides. When the plant tissue is disrupted (macerated), hydrocyanic acid (HCN) is released. Amygdalin is a cyanogenic glycoside obtained from bitter almonds, kernels of cherries, apricots, and peach seeds. Amygdalin, also known as laetrile or vitamin B17 in the 1970s, was associated with the infamous treatment for cancer. Other cyanogenic glycosides include primasin, from bitter almonds and other fruit kernels; dhurrin, from sorghum and related grasses; and linamarin, from pulses, linseed, and cassava.

In populations where cassava is a staple crop, care is taken to soak, grate, and ferment the cassava, allowing the release of HCN before consumption. Lima beans can be a problem if cooked at low temperature, which is insufficient to destroy toxic glycosides. As few as 12 bitter almonds can potentially kill a small child. Table 12.2 lists the cyanide content that can be found in some common foods.

TABLE 12.2
Cyanide in Foods

Source	Cyanide (mg/100 g)
Sorghum (leaves, shoots)	60–240
Almond (kernel)	290
Apricot seed	60
Peach seed	160
Black beans	400
Pinto bean	17
Cassava	100

A lethal dose of cyanide is between 0.5 and 3.5 mg/kg body weight. Cyanide binds to ferric ions of mitochondrial cytochrome oxidase and halts cellular respiration. The symptoms of acute cyanide intoxication are mental confusion, muscular paralysis, and respiratory failure. As shown in Figure 12.6, the cyanide ion can be metabolically handled to produce thiocyanate, the reaction catalyzed by the enzyme rhodenase. Rhodenase is widely distributed in many tissues and it is unclear whether rhodanese's primary function is to detoxify cyanide. As Figure 12.6 illustrates,

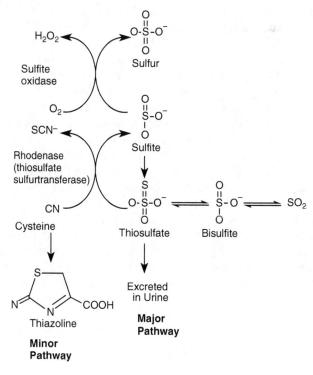

FIGURE 12.6 Cyanide metabolism.

TABLE 12.3
Phenolic Substances

Phenolic Substance	Subgroup
Flavonoids	Flavanone, flavone, anthocyanidin, isoflavanone, chalcone, aurone
Tannins	Hydrolyzable and condensed
Others	Coumarin, safrole, myristicin

thiosulfate plays a key role in detoxification of cyanide. Thiosulfate originates from sulfate metabolism.

Phenolic Substances

More than 800 phenolic substances are known in plants. Such compounds contribute to the bitter taste, flavor, and color of foods. Table 12.3 lists some classes of phenolic substances. Most of the phenolic substances are devoid of acute toxicity. Methods are available to detoxify them.

Tannins have evolved to be less desirable foods for herbivores, and they may protect the plant against microbial and fungal attack. There are two subgroups of tannins: the condensed and hydrolyzable compounds (Figure 12.7). Hydrolyzable tannins include gallic, digallic, and ellagic acid esters of glucose or quinic acid. Tannic acid is an example of a hydrolyzable tannin. Condensed tannins are flavonoids. They tend to polymerize at positions where carbon bonds link the monomers. Tannins such as gallic acid can tie up metals. Tannins are found in tropical fruits such as mangoes, dates, persimmons, and in tea, coffee, grapes, wine, and cocoa. Black tea contains oxidized tannins. Tannins have been reported to cause liver injury (necrosis and fatty liver). Tannins bind proteins or cause precipitation of proteins, inhibiting digestive enzymes. They also reduce the bioavailability of iron. In the Far East, betel nuts are often chewed after dinner, and because they contain 26% tannins, are believed to be responsible for high levels of cheek and esophageal cancers. In South Americans, the use of sorghum and heavy use of tannin-rich teas may be responsible for esophageal cancers.

Figure 12.8 shows the six subgroups of flavonoids. Most compounds within this group occur as β-glucosides. Flavones are abundant and many contribute to the yellow pigments in plants, such as in oil vesicles and the peel of citrus fruits. The well-known flavone quercetin, found in high amounts in onions, has been shown to be carcinogenic in mammals (two strains of rats) via oral routes. In contrast, flavonoids have been touted for their beneficial effects in preventing heart disease, particularly in populations with a high consumption of wine (French) and tea (Asians). One situation that has received some attention is referred to as the French Paradox. Despite having a diet rich in saturated fat and persistence for tobacco smoking, the French from Southern France, as a population, seem to have a lower mortality rate from cardiovascular disease. It has been suggested that this paradox

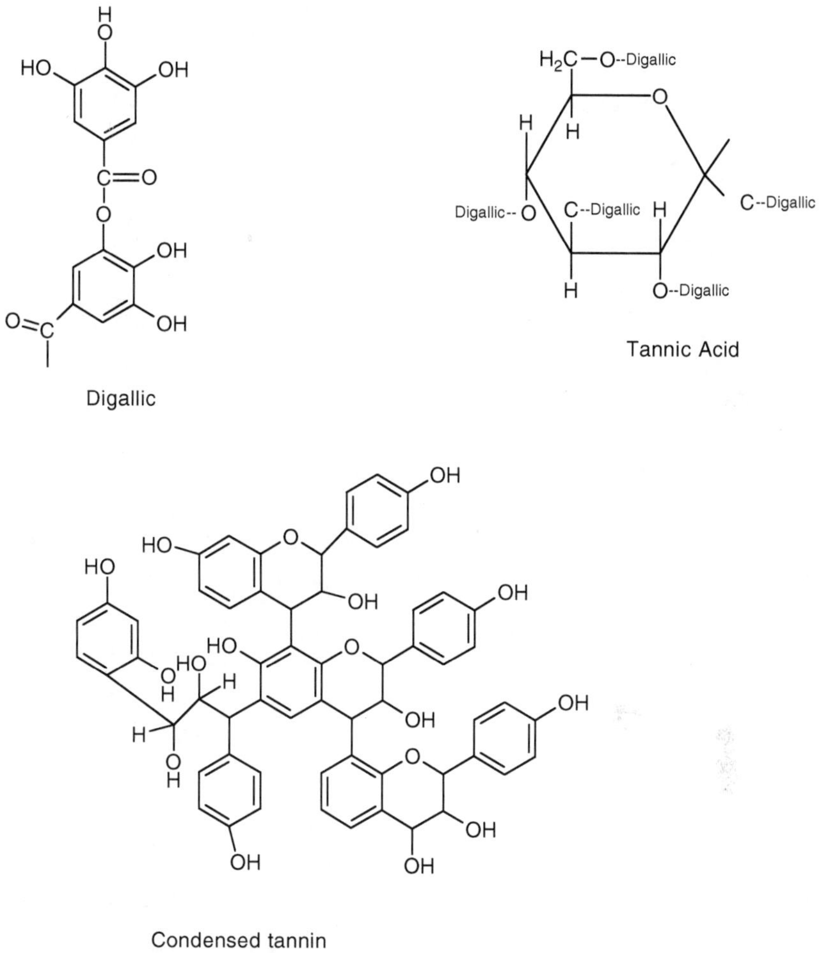

FIGURE 12.7 Condensed tannins.

might be explained by their consuming flavonoids in wine with their meals. A recent Danish study also reported that wine consumption was associated with a lower risk for heart disease compared to consumption of alcohol in other forms.

Tea consumption has also been reported to protect against cardiovascular diseases. Tea, particularly green tea, is rich in catechin, epicatechin, epicatechin gallate, gallocatechin, epigallocatechin, and epigallocatechin gallate. These flavanols may have health-promoting properties. Figure 12.9 shows the structures for two flavanols, epicatechin gallate and gallic acid.

Coumarin, safrole, and myristicin (Figure 12.10) are found as various flavor components. Coumarin occurs in citrus oils and impairs blood clotting and damages the liver. Safrole, a chemical found in oil of sassafras and in black pepper, causes liver tumors in rats. Safrole is a phenolic that makes up 80% of the essential oil extracted from the root and bark of the sassafras tree. It has been used in teas, tonics,

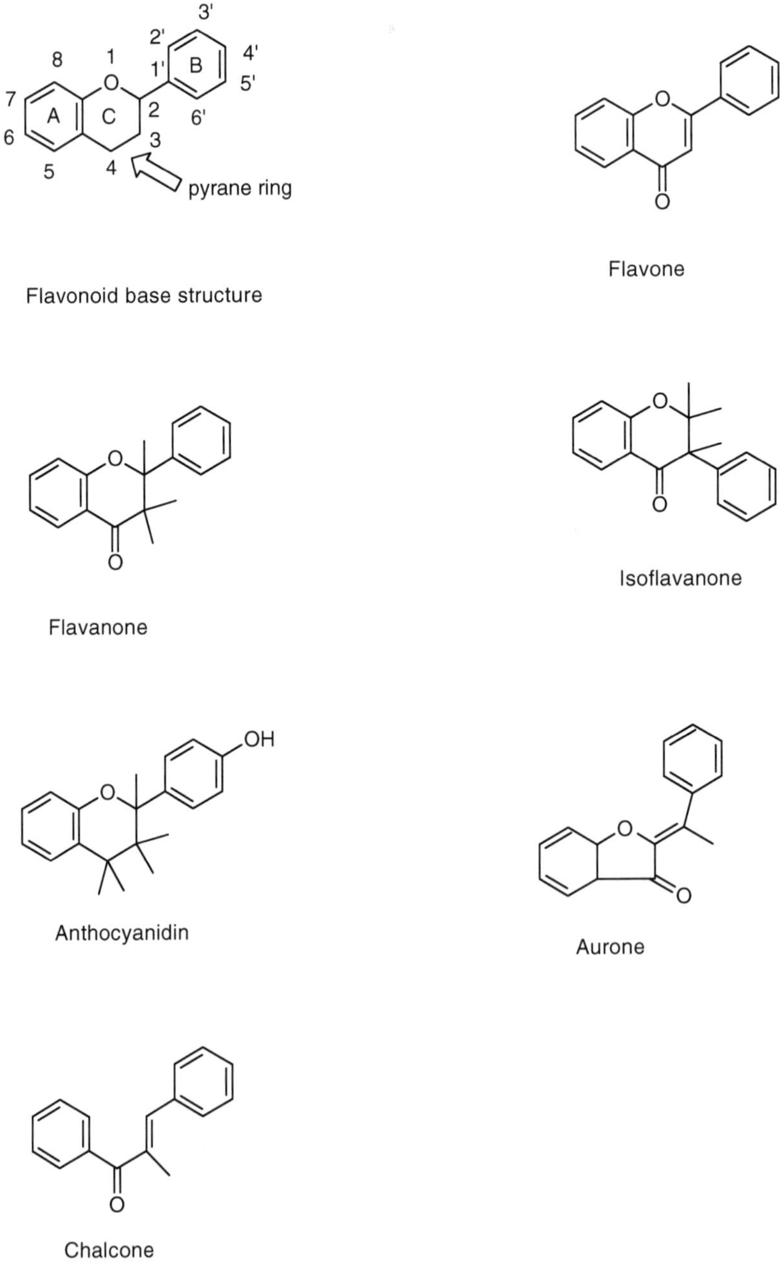

Flavonoid base structure

Flavone

Flavanone

Isoflavanone

Anthocyanidin

Aurone

Chalcone

FIGURE 12.8 Flavonoids.

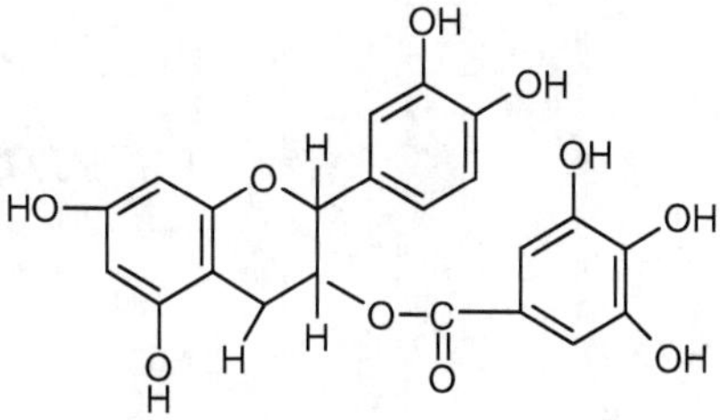

Epicatechin gallate

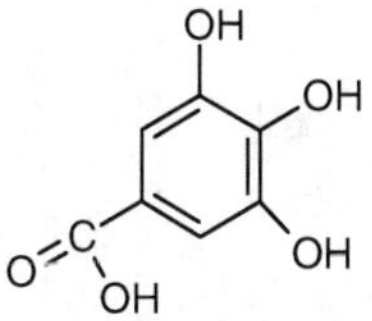

Gallic Acid

FIGURE 12.9 Flavanols, epicatechin gallate, and gallic acid.

and various cure-alls. It is a popular ingredient of New Orleans-style gumbo. Myristicin is found in spices and herbs such as black pepper, carrot, parsley, celery, and dill.

Gossypol is a toxic phenolic compound found in cottonseed. Cottonseed is a good source of protein, and through selective breeding, plants have been developed with less gossypol. However, the selective breeding has also resulted in plants more susceptible to mold growth and aflatoxin problems. Gossypol consumption results in loss of appetite, weight loss, diarrhea, anemia, diminished fertility, pulmonary

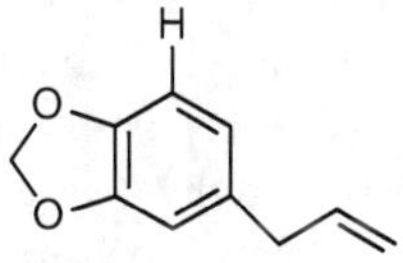

Safrole

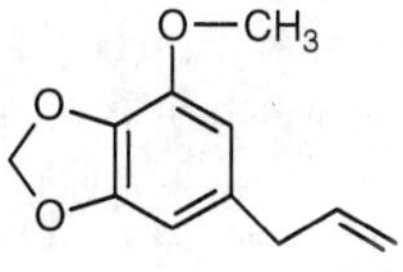

Myristicin

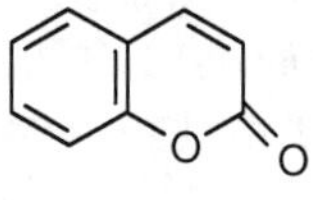

Coumarin

FIGURE 12.10 Coumarin, safrole, and myristicin.

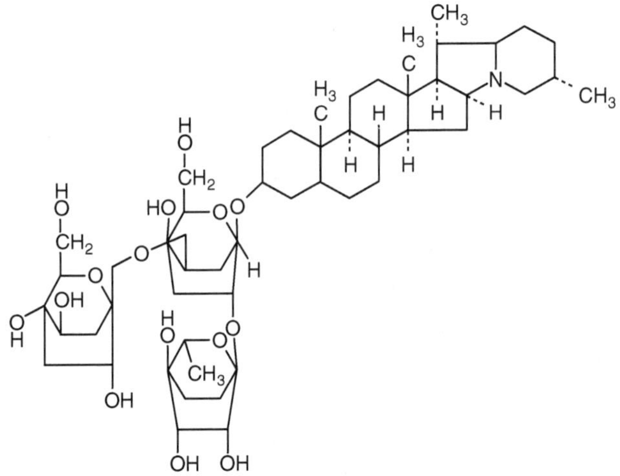

FIGURE 12.11 Solanine.

edema, circulatory failure, and hemorrhages of the GI tract. The phenolic compound inhibits the conversion of pepsinogen to pepsin and limits availability of iron.

CHOLINESTERASE INHIBITORS

The enzyme cholinesterase aids in the hydrolysis of acetylcholine, a substance released from vesicles at nerve synapses and responsible for transmission of nerve impulse across the synapse. After the nerve impulse is transmitted, the acetylcholine must be hydrolyzed so that the neuron can become ready for the next impulse. Physostigmine, which comes from the West African calibar bean, is a potent cholinesterase inhibitor. It was used as an ordeal poison in African witchcraft.

Solanine (Figure 12.11) is another anticholinesterase toxicant found in foods. Solanine and chaconine are glycoalkaloids or steroidal alkaloids that inhibit cholinesterase and irritate the intestinal mucosa. These compounds can be found in members of the genus *Solanum,* which includes potato, eggplant, and tomato. Large amounts of the toxicants can be found in potato, particularly if the potato has been exposed to light, fungal infection, or bruising. Solanine is heat stable and insoluble in water; therefore, cooking does not remove the toxicant. The commercial potato has about 2 mg of solanine/100 g, and greening increases the content to 50 to 100 mg/100 g. Greening is due to increased chlorophyll content, which in itself is not hazardous. Exposure to white fluorescent light can increase the total glycoalkaloid peel content of a Russet potato to 70 mg/100 g. One variety of potato, Lenape, specifically developed for potato chips, was discontinued because it had a total glycoalkaloid content of 30 mg/100 g fresh tuber. The FDA regulates the solanine content to be no more than 20 mg/100 g.

Clinical Symptoms

A few situations have resulted in illness or death due to solanine. Symptoms include increasing gastric pain followed by nausea and vomiting, respiratory difficulties, weakness, and prostration. In experiments using human volunteers, 0.3 mg/100 g of solanine caused drowsiness, itchiness and hyperesthesia, and labored breathing. Higher doses result in symptoms of organophosphate poisoning.

BIOGENIC AMINES

Many varieties of animal- or plant-based foods are sources of biogenic amines. Dopamine and tyramine are natural components of banana, cheese, and avocado, and bacterial action on the amino acids (see previously) found in meats and fish can produce putrescine and cadaverine. Also, histamine and b-phenylethylamine have been implicated as etiological agents in several outbreaks of food poisoning. These amines can affect the vascular system, resulting in vessel constriction and subsequently increased blood pressure (pressor amine effects). Norepinephrine and dopamine or catecholamines are pressor amines important as neutrotransmitters in adrenergic nerve cells. They cause diet-induced migraine headaches, and, in some cases, hypertensive crisis.

Usually, the added dietary load of bioactive amines is inconsequential, because such amines are carefully controlled by the action of the widely distributed enzyme monamine oxidase (MAO). Therefore, foods containing large amounts of biogenic amines are counterindicated in patients using MAO inhibitors, such as antidepressants (e.g., iproniazid).

Some specific examples include the fava bean, which contains dihydroxyphenylalanine (DOPA) that can be decarboxylated to dopamine. Tyramine content can be high in oriental preserved foods such as soy sauce, soybean paste, and various condiments. Swiss cheese has been implicated in outbreaks of histamine poisoning, attributed to *Lactoacillus buchneri*. Spanish wines have been shown to increase histamine and tyramine content within 5 d of manufacturing.

Clinical Symptoms

Marked pressor effects are seen when MAO is inhibited. Hypertension, palpitations, and severe headaches are common. In some cases, intracranial bleeding can occur, leading to death.

STUDY QUESTIONS AND EXERCISES

1. Give some examples of naturally occurring food toxicants that are deactivated, removed, or reduced by food processing.
2. Distinguish between primary and secondary metabolic products found in plants. What role do plant toxicants play in the physiology of plants?
3. Which subpopulations are most vulnerable to naturally occurring toxicants? What precautions should such populations take?
4. Fish is a very important source of protein and essential fatty acids; however, there are a number of potential hazards. Describe the hazards with respect to foodborne illnesses and the precautions individuals should observe.

RECOMMENDED READINGS

Committee on Food Protection, National Academy of Sciences, *Toxicants Occurring Naturally in Foods*, 2nd ed., National Academy of Sciences, Washington, D.C., 1973.

Dubick, M.A. and Omaye, S.T., Evidence for grape, wine and tea polyphenols as modulators of atherosclerosis and ischemic heart disease in humans, *J. Nutraceut. Func. Med. Foods,* 3, 67-93, 2001.

Leopold, A.C. and Ardrey, R., Toxic substances in plants and the food habits of early man, *Science*, 176, 512-513, 1972.

Liener, I.E., *Toxic Constituents of Plant Foodstuffs*, 2nd ed., Academic Press, New York, 1980.

Taylor, S.L. and Hefle, S.L. Naturally occurring toxicants in foods, in *Foodborne Diseases*, 2nd ed., Cliver, D.O. and Riemann, H.P., Eds., Academic Press, New York, pp. 193-210, 2002.

13 Fungal Mycotoxins

Molds and humans share a love–hate relationship. Certain molds have served humans by providing means to produce foods (ripening cheese) and medicines. Physical changes produced by mold growth have been recognized for many years. Molds are endowed with extracellular proteolytic and lipolytic enzymes, which catalyze reactions responsible for softening of foods. Mold growth gives flavor and odor to and changes the appearance of food.

Also molds, particularly filamentous fungi, produce metabolites (mycotoxins, *myo* meaning fungal) that can have adverse effects, such as estrogenic effects, carcinogenicity, mutagenicity, and teratogenicity, in humans and animals. Table 13.1 shows some health effects of mycotoxins. The genera *Aspergillus, Penicillium,* and *Fusarium* account for most of the hundreds of mycotoxins known to produce toxic syndromes (mycotoxicoses) in mammals. Many mycotoxins are unstable to cooking conditions or food-processing procedures. The ones of concern are chemically stable and resistant to cooking and can persist during food processing, despite the molds being killed. Absence of detectable presence of molds does not necessarily mean that there are no mycotoxins. Some foods with no visible evidence of molds may have mycotoxins. Dairy products can be contaminated if cattle are fed moldy feed. Any food on which molds have grown can potentially contain mycotoxins, which one cannot tell by appearance, taste, or smell. Mycotoxin production and contamination depend on environmental conditions (weather, moisture) and can occur in the field, during harvest or processing, and during storage and shipment. Although heat and high humidity sharply increase mold growth, many do well in limited amounts of moisture and require lower levels than those required to support the growth of bacteria. Molds can be found in the soil, and when the seed kernel is damaged, the fungus can invade and multiply. Drought situations or other forms of environmental stress to plants stimulate mold and insect damage. In the U.S. alone, $20 million are lost annually on one crop, peanuts, because of aflatoxin contamination.

Table 13.2 lists some means by which mycotoxins can be reduced in foods. Many mycotoxins are stable to heat and normal cooking. Moist heating, such as the roasting of peanuts, destroys 20 to 80% of some aflatoxins. In the U.S., refining practices are effective in removing aflatoxins; however, in the Orient, the flavor of crude peanut oil, which is because of the presence of significant mycotoxins, is preferred because of its taste. Force-air drying techniques help reduce moisture, preventing mold growth. During food production, prevention is the key in reducing the mycotoxin load of products. Some spices, such as peppers and mustard, inhibit mycotoxin production by molds.

TABLE 13.1
Adverse Effects of Mycotoxins

Mycotoxin	Health Effects
Ergot alkaloids	Ergotism
Aflatoxin	Acute toxicity, hepatic cancer, Reye's syndrome
Trichothecenes	Acute toxicity, cancer, alimentary toxic aleukia
Ocharatoxin	Cancer, kidney disorders, hepatic damage

TABLE 13.2
Processes for Reducing Mycotoxins

Refining of oils (peanut oil)
Milling of grains
Prevention of mold growth: sodium bisulfite, sorbate, propionate, nitrate
Ammonia and ozone treatment of grains

In addition, coping strategies against mold growth have been encouraged, such as taking care of crops in the field, during harvest, storage, and processing; having more inspections of crops after drought times, which may induce plant stress; and using dry heat to prevent moisture and reduce humidity. At home, individuals should discard moldy food and be aware that molds grow faster in baked goods not containing preservatives and that most toxins are heat stable.

ERGOT ALKALOIDS AND ERGOTISM

Mycotoxicoses have been known for a long time. Ergotism occurred in the Middle Ages, around the 14th century in Europe. Ergot is a fungus, *Claviceps purpurea*, that grows on rye, and the consumption leads to intoxications and episodes of hallucinations, delirium, and convulsion and causes arteriolar spasms and gangrene. The gangrenous effects are associated with alkaloids that are partial α-adrenergic agonists and promote vasoconstriction, and the hallucinogenic effects are because the ergot mold contains derivatives of the hallucinogen lysergic acid, with ergonovine (ergometrine) and ergotamine (Figure 13.1), being the most important. All are pharmacologically active compounds. Ergotamine causes constriction of vessels and has been used for migraines. Extensive use of ergotamine can result in gangrene. Ergonavine is a potent inducer of uterine constriction. In 1850, ergot alkaloids were associated with ergotism, then known as the holy fire or St. Anthony's fire. In 1951, an outbreak at Pont St. Esprit, France, affected a large part of the population after it ate bread made locally from ergot-contaminated flour.

Claviceps pupurea is a common preharvest grain mold and grows in the ears of grasses and cereals. Ergot formation is favored at 10 to 30°C and high relative humidity. During the hibernation stage, sclerotia are formed, which eventually end up in the cereal grain during harvest. As a modern-day problem, ergotism has almost

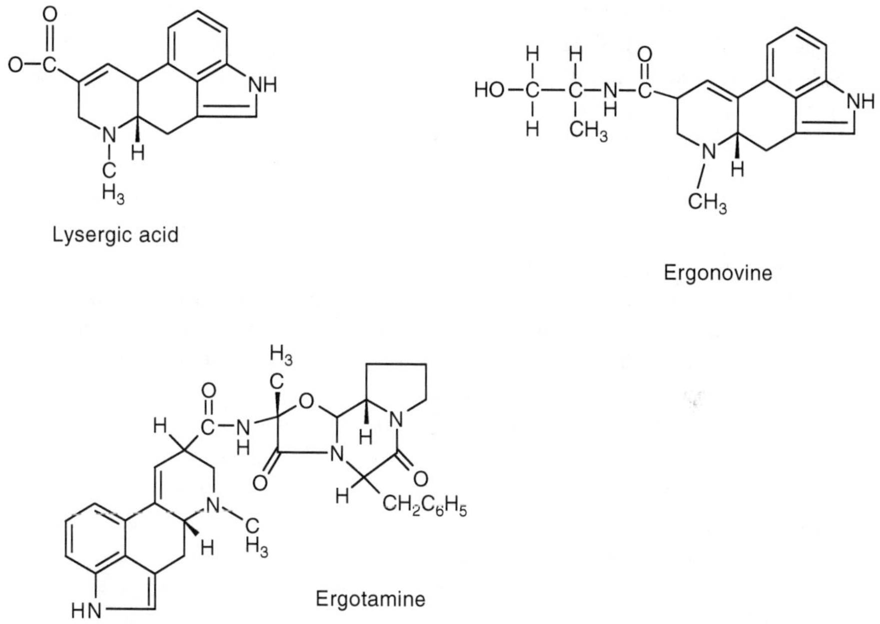

Fungal Mycotoxins

FIGURE 13.1 Lysergic acid, ergonovine, and ergotamine.

been eliminated, but in 1977 and 1978, several cases were reported in Ethiopia and the ergot alkaloid may still occur at low levels in rye. Current quality assurance systems prevent ergot from being a serious modern-day threat to humans and animals.

Mode of Action and Clinical Symptoms

Ergot alkaloids affect smooth muscles and result in peripheral artery constriction and neurological disorders. The early effects are characterized by intense tingling of the limbs followed by hot and cold sensations. Gangrenous effects of the extremities are due to long and intense peripheral vasoconstriction of the α-adrenergic ergot agonists. Central nervous system symptoms include itching, muscle cramps, psychological disorders, vomiting, headache, numbness, muscle spasm, and convulsion.

AFLATOXIN

Initially, the terms *mycotoxin* and *aflatoxin* were used interchangeably, because aflatoxin is probably the most important mycotoxin in food; however, mycotoxin has now become a generic term and is defined as any toxin of fungal origin. Aflatoxin refers to toxins produced by *Asperigillus flavus*. The mold is prevalent in nuts, cottonseeds, corn, and figs. Most animals, including humans, and poultry are particularly susceptible to aflatoxicosis. Interestingly, the mouse is totally resistant to aflatoxin's carcinogenic effects. In developing countries, there is a direct relationship between dietary aflatoxin and liver cancer, and human males are more susceptible. Incidences have been high in India and Africa, where populations have been forced to survive by eating moldy grains. Acute toxicity can occur within 3 weeks of ingestion. Epidemiological data indicate that exposure to aflatoxin B1 (AFB1) and hepatitis is required for populations to have a significant risk of cancer. In the U.S., liver cancer is low, as is hepatitis B.

Aflatoxins are highly substituted coumarins (Figure 13.2). The four major designated types of aflatoxins are B1, B2, G1, and G2, and their respective designations are based on blue or green fluorescence under ultraviolet light. The B-group contains a cyclopentanone ring and the G-group contains a lactone ring. AFB1 is the most potent carcinogen (LD_{50} = 0.3 to 9.0 mg/kg), followed, in order, by G1, B2, and G2. Some of the metabolites activated via cytochrome P450 to 2,3-epoxides of aflatoxin are the active carcinogens, and not the original parent compounds. These products are potent electrophiles that can covalently bind to proteins and DNA. The 4-hydroxyl derivative (aflatoxin M1) of AFB1 ingested by cows in their feed can be found in milk and may be a potential health hazard. The carcinogenic potency of AFM1 is about half that of AFB1.

Aflatoxins are heat stable and easily transformed to toxic products. Treatment with ammonia reduces and inactivates aflatoxins. Lactic fermentation at pH < 4.0 results in the conversion of AFB1 to AFB2a, which is less toxic. Other environmental conditions, such as the presence of organic acid, also irreversibly convert AFB1 to aflatoxicol B, which is 18 times less toxic than AFB1. Detoxification results in the opening of the lactone ring (see Figure 13.2) and can be monitored by reduced fluorescence.

The two concerns about aflatoxins are their acute toxicity and ability to produce cancer. The LD_{50} of aflatoxin is 0.5 mg/kg of the body weight, and death occurs within 72 h. Death is due to liver damage and hemorrhaging in the intestinal tract and peritoneal cavity. As animals mature, they become more resistant. Compared with a substance such as lead whose toxicity is about 500 mg/kg of body weight, aflatoxin is extremely toxic. Consumption of aflatoxin at sublethal concentration for several days to several weeks results in moderate to severe liver damage. Several forms of hepatic damage include biliary hyperplasia or excessive growth of cells in the bile duct region of the liver. Also prevalent are accumulation of fat and changes in appearance of the liver from purple-red to yellow-red.

AFB1 is a potent carcinogen in several animal species. In humans, epidemiological studies have shown a direct relationship between aflatoxin levels in the diet and primary hepatocellular carcinoma incidence in several parts of the world. The prevalence of hepatitis B virus is also correlated with liver cancer in many of the same areas around the world; thus, aflatoxin contamination may be an important etiological factor resulting in synergistic effects with hepatitis B virus exposure.

TRICHOTHECENES

During 1913, Russians near Siberia experienced extreme food shortage and were forced to eat grains of wheat, millet, and barley that had been left outside during the winter. The melting snow increased the moisture content, which favored mold growth and resulted in a large outbreak of mycotoxicosis. The disease, referred to

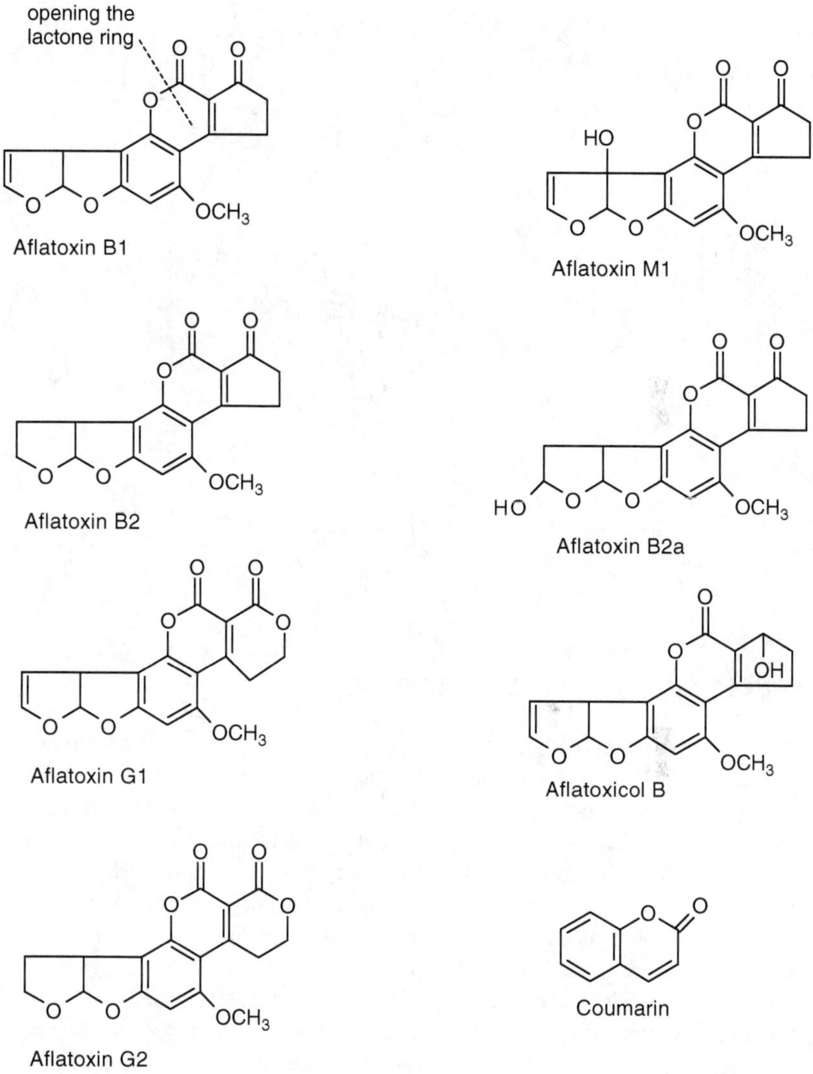

FIGURE 13.2 Aflatoxin

as alimentary toxic aleukia (ATA), reached epidemic proportions and was found to be related to the infection of grains by *Fusarium* species. ATA causes atrophy of the bone marrow, agranulocytosis, necrotic angina, sepsis, and death. The disease is manifested in three stages: (1) mouth and throat inflammation, gastroenteritis and vomiting; (2) an asymptomatic second stage when immunodepression sets in; (3) a fatal stage of pinpoint skin hemorrhages and necrotic ulcers over various parts of the body. The acute effects of toxicity are usually neurological, but the chronic effect of toxicity is characterized by massive necrosis of the GI tract, producing inflammation, hemorrhages, and leukopenia. Trichothecenes are the primary mycotoxins

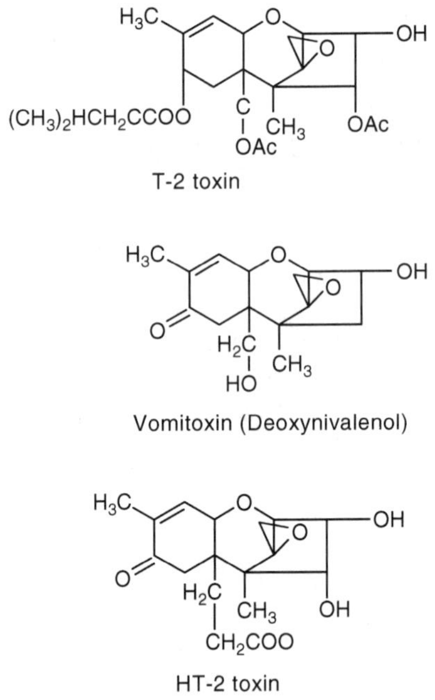

$$\text{(CH}_3\text{)}_2\text{HCHCH}_2\text{CCOO} \quad \begin{array}{c} \text{C} \\ | \\ \text{OAc} \end{array} \text{CH}_3 \quad \text{OAc}$$

T-2 toxin

Vomitoxin (Deoxynivalenol)

HT-2 toxin

FIGURE 13.3 T-2 toxin, vomitoxin, and HT-2 toxin.

produced by *Fusarium* and constitute a group of more than 80 sesquiterpenes, derivatives of 12,13-epoxytrichothecene. The main trichothecenes are T-2 toxin, vomitoxin (deoxynivalenol), HT-2 toxin, neosolaniol, and diacetoxyscirpenol (Figure 13.3). *In vivo*, these compounds can undergo hepatic and kidney deacetylation, hydroxylation, and glucuronidation, which may help reduce the risk of dietary trichothecenes. Acute toxicity (LD_{50}) is between 50 and 70 mg/kg. The toxicity is related to the epoxide ring found in their structure (see Figure 13.3). Toxic effects of trichothecenes are related to inhibition of protein synthesis, which can occur at the initiation, elongation, and termination phases of protein synthesis.

Vomitoxin levels of contamination can be generally high (>1 to 20 ppm) in barley, oats, sorghum, rye, and safflower seeds. Vomitoxin causes anorexia and emesis in animals and humans. Poisoning outbreaks in humans because of contamination of cereals with vomitoxin is a major concern for many countries. The lethal dose of vomitoxin is 50 to 70 mg/kg.

T-2 toxin produces neurobehavioral effects; is cytotoxic; and causes hemorrhage, edema, and necrosis of the skin. Neurological dysfunctions include refusal of feed, anorexia, and depression. The major devastating effect is on the hematopoietic system, with 10 to 75% rapid decreases in circulating white blood cells, platelets, and extensive cellular damage in the bone marrow, spleen, and lymph nodes. T-2 toxin is a potent immunosuppressant, causing lesions of lymph nodes, spleen, thymus, and the bursa of Fabricius. T-2 toxin is found naturally in barley, corn, oats, and wheat, but less frequently than vomitoxin. However, T-2 toxin is more toxic (LD_{50} = 2 to 4 mg/kg for mice).

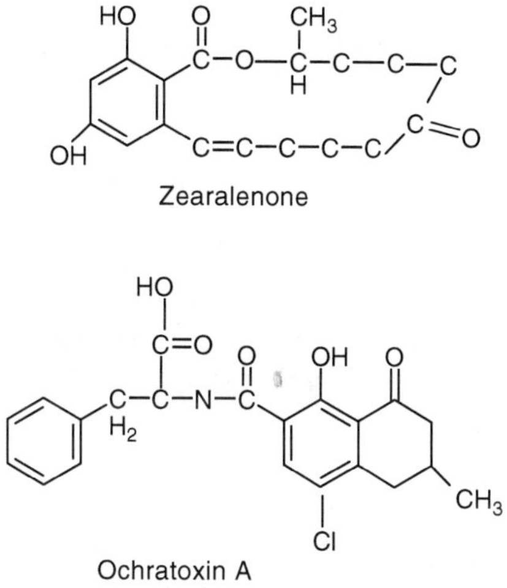

Fungal Mycotoxins

FIGURE 13.4 Zearalenone and ochratoxin A.

Nontrichothecenes mycotoxins produced by *Fusarium* include fumonisins, fusarochromanones, zearalenone, fusarins, moniliformin, and wortmannin. Fumonisins are associated with several animal and human diseases, e.g., animal toxicoses, including equine leukoencephalomalacia (ELEM) and swine pulmonary edema. Corn is the major staple associated with mycotoxin; in a 1990–1991 survey, 124 retail samples of corn-based human food from the U.S. and Africa contained significant amounts of fumonisin B1 and B2. High rates of human esophageal cancer have been associated with corn exposures, although the liver is the main site of toxicity, resulting in hepatocellular carcinoma and nephritis.

Zearalenone (Figure 13.4) can be found in moldy grains (maize, wheat) during times of high humidity and moderate temperatures. These mycotoxins exhibit estrogenic and anabolic properties, and pigs are very sensitive to the toxicity. *Fusarium* growth in feed grains can be a significant problem and feeding such grains to livestock can effect their health. *Fusarium* growth is favored by near-freezing conditions for an extended time. The estrogenic properties of the mycotoxins result in the uterus becoming enlarged and edematous and ovaries becoming shrunken. Pregnancy may be aborted in females and the males can acquire female characteristics.

PENICILLIA MYCOTOXINS

Penicillium notatum is the organism responsible for the highly used antibiotic penicillium, which effectively blocks the synthesis of bacterial cell walls.

RUBRATOXIN

About 40 years ago, a disease in swine and cattle was found to be due to consuming moldy corn. Swine died within a day after consuming about 0.5 lb of moldy corn (LD_{50} = 6.6 mg/kg of body weight, usually producing liver and kidney damage).

The mold responsible was *Pencillium rubrum*, producing a mycotoxin known as rubratoxin. The two forms of rubratoxin are designated as A and B.

PATULIN

Patulin is a mycotoxin produced by *Penicillum expansum*. The mold and mycotoxin are produced when the fruit deteriorates. Patulin is toxic to Gram-positive and Gram-negative bacteria and was once considered for use as an antibiotic. However, patulin was too toxic (LD_{50} of 15 to 35 mg/kg) and was shown to induce tumors. The mycotoxin is unstable in alkaline conditions but stable under acidic conditions, and adding ascorbic acid inactivates the mycotoxin.

YELLOW RICE TOXINS

Citrinin and citreoviridin are mycotoxins produced by penicillia that grow on rice, especially polished rice. The LD_{50} of citrinin is 50 mg/kg and the compound affects the kidneys and causes tubular damage. The LD_{50} of citreoviridin is 20 mg/kg and causes paralysis of hind limbs and respiratory disorders.

OTHER MYCOTOXINS

The formation of ochratoxin A by the microflora *Aspergillus ochraceus* is favored by humid conditions and moderate temperature and can be found in cereals. The mycotoxin has been associated with Balkan nephropathy in Bulgaria, Romania, and Yugoslavia, particularly in foods made from grains harvested after heavy rainfall. It can be found in grains, soybeans, peanuts, and cheese. Several years ago, the mycotoxin was found in pigs from Denmark, which carried over in tissues of bacon exported to various countries. The compound (LD_{50} of 20 to 50 mg/kg) exhibits nephrotoxicity in birds, fish, and mammals and is teratogenic in rats and chicken. Ochratoxin also targets the central nervous system. As noted in Figure 13.4, the structures of several ochratoxin A compounds involve a derivative of dihydroisocoumarin linked to phenylalanine by an amide bond, and in some situations include a chloride atom. Table 13.3 lists other mycotoxins.

TABLE 13.3
Other Mycotoxins

Mycotoxin	Source
Cyclopiazonic acid	Cheese, grains, peanuts
Kojic acid	Grains
3-Nitropropionic acid	Sugarcane
Citreoviridin	Rice
Cytochalasins	Corn, cereal grains
Sterigmatocystin	Corn
Penicillinic acid	Corn, dried beans, grains
Rubratoxins	Corn

STUDY QUESTIONS AND EXERCISES

1. Describe some measures that can be useful in reducing mycotoxins in the food supply.
2. Cite examples of mycotoxins that have been used in medicine. Describe the mechanism of action and counterindications for use of such compounds.
3. Explain how ruminants and mice as compared with humans can consume large amounts of aflatoxins with little or fewer adverse outcomes.

RECOMMENDED READINGS

Chu, F.S., Mycotoxins: food contamination, mechanism, carcinogenic potential and preventive measures, *Mutat Res.,* 259, 291-306, 1991.

Chu, F.S., Mycotoxins, in *Foodborne Disease*, 2nd ed., Cliver, D.O. and Riemann, H.P., Eds., Academic Press, New York, pp. 271-303, 2002.

Galvano, F., Piva, A., Ritienik, A., and Galvano, G., Dietary strategies to counteract the effects of mycotoxins: a review, *J. Food Prot.*, 64, 120-131, 2001.

Sinha, K.K. and Bhatnagar, D., *Mycotoxins in Agriculture and Food Safety*, Marcel Dekker, New York, 1998.

14 Toxicity of Nutrients

As noted before, many food chemicals are nutrients. Nutrients, as defined, are necessary for growth, maintenance, and reproduction of living organisms. In the overall scheme of nutrition, nutrients can be divided into macronutrients and micronutrients. Macronutrients include fats, carbohydrates, and proteins. Micronutrients can be divided into vitamins and minerals, the latter including trace elements. Several decades of nutritional research have been devoted to defining the intake levels of macro- and micronutrients necessary to meet the needs of people and levels safe for healthy individuals. Such information has been summarized in several publications emphasizing recommended dietary allowances (RDAs) and, recently, the dietary reference intake (DRI).

In addition to macronutrients, micronutrients, and nonnutrient substances, there is another group of substances found in food, known as antinutrients. Antinutrients are food substances that cause adverse effects without being active toxic agents themselves. However, the presence of such substances indirectly results in adverse effects, e.g., by causing a nutritional deficiency by interfering with the function or utilization of normal nutrients. Antinutrients may interfere with food components before intake, during digestion, and after absorption in the body. With regards to nutritional status and health, such substances can be a particular concern when they affect individuals with marginal nutritional status.

MACRONUTRIENTS

Carbohydrates, lipids, and proteins are related through their respective impacts as sources of energy. An increase in one constituent results in a decrease of one or both of the other constituents. Thus, a simplistic conclusion would be that the effects of macronutrient excesses are either toxicity magnifications or consequences of other macronutrient deficiencies or imbalances.

CARBOHYDRATES

This is a large and varied class of organic compounds. Carbohydrates consist of carbon, hydrogen, and oxygen in the ratio of 1:2:1. These compounds are usually discussed in terms of three classes: monosaccharides, disaccharides, and polysaccharides (Table 14.1). Carbohydrates are essential for providing glucose, and, if not provided for in sufficient amounts from food ingestion, the body must manufacture what it requires from other sources. However, essentiality is not without food safety concerns for carbohydrates — no food constituent is without such concerns.

TABLE 14.1
Classes of Carbohydrates

Classes	Examples
Monosaccharides	Simple sugars (galactose, fructose, glucose)
Disaccharides	Sucrose, lactose, maltose
Polysaccharides	Digestible starch, dextrins, indigestible starch

If healthy population groups around the world are studied, there are relatively few illustrations of toxic effects associated with carbohydrate intakes. If sufficient food is available, population groups whose diets consist mostly of carbohydrates do not suffer adverse effects. Some short-term effects such as intestinal problems and diarrhea can be attributed to marked changes in the amount or form of ingested carbohydrate, e.g., high-fiber foods.

On the other hand, there are subpopulations prone to significant adverse effects associated with carbohydrates, which include individuals with abnormal tolerances or intolerances (glucose, lactose). Milk sugar intolerance is prevalent in populations from the Far and Middle East and Africa. These individuals have difficulty digesting lactose, and, when they do ingest lactose, they experience gastric distress, cramping, and diarrhea. The intolerance is because such individuals lack the enzyme lactase to break down lactose to monosaccharides for absorption. Thus, the lactose remains in the GI tract, leading to osmotic catharsis and eventually fermentation to lactic acid in the colon, producing more diarrhea and gastric problems. Other forms of disaccharide intolerance as congenital defects, particularly in infants, exist in various subpopulations.

The popular notion is that dental caries is due to sucrose consumption. However, the etiology of dental caries is much more complex and multifactorial in nature, involving the susceptible teeth of the host, presence of viable microorganisms, lack of fluoride exposure, poor oral hygiene, and duration of time of exposure to media for the bacteria.

Natural foods with high carbohydrate levels can be carriers of naturally occurring toxicants. For example, honey can contain materials toxic to humans because of the varieties of plants the honey bees may visit. Honey producers take extreme care to see that their bees avoid potentially problematic plants and do not become contaminated with toxicants.

LIPIDS

These are organic compounds that usually contain a fatty acid or a fatty acid derivative. Lipids are a highly diverse and varied class of compounds soluble in organic solvents. Fat is obtained in the diet from either animal or vegetable sources as triglycerides. Triglycerides are composed of molecules of glycerol and three fatty acids. The fatty acids may be saturated, unsaturated, or contain multiple unsaturations (polyunsaturated fatty acids, PUFAs). In addition, lipids contain sterols, steroids, and fat-soluble vitamins. The steroid cholesterol is found in animal fats and plays an important role in health.

A number of plants used for natural foods may harbor lipids that can adversely affect consumers. Examples include erucic acid found in the oils obtained from a number of plants, such as rapeseed oil and mustard seed oil. Erucic acid has been shown to cause heart damage in experimental animals. Traditional rapeseed oil contains 20 to 55% erucic acid, whereas processed oil, i.e., canola, contains less than 2% of the fatty acid.

The primary toxicity issue for lipids is their role in chronic diseases such as heart disease and cancer. Heart disease is not only the dominant factor of death, but also a primary cause of permanent disability and reduced ability to be active. It leads to more days of hospitalization than does any other disorder. The relationship between fat and cholesterol and heart disease has led to many recommendations to make dietary changes.

PROTEIN

Protein, found in all living organisms, provides essential amino acids needed by the body for growth and tissue repair. Based on some 20 different amino acids, infinite combinations and arrangement possibilities explain the wide variety and characteristics of proteins in living organisms. Protein is a major constituent of enzymes, which in turn are required in a variety of metabolic reactions. Amino acids are essential because such compounds are not stored or made by humans. In a normal dietary intake of animal protein together with plant protein, individuals can easily obtain the required amounts of protein, as long as it is good-quality protein.

As in the case of other macronutrients, food safety problems are not generally associated with excessive intakes of natural sources of protein, the exceptions being those occurring because of allergic reactions or hypersensitivity. The wide availability of protein in the U.S. has led to higher consumption, well in excess of daily recommendations. Fad diets and misinformation about benefits of high-protein diets have further led to increased protein consumption. Regardless of the overt symptoms of protein toxicity, nutrition experts express caution. Animal studies have shown that excessive ingestion of protein can lead to liver and kidney hypertrophy. Studies on humans have shown that the ingestion of high-protein diets increases calcium excretion.

MICRONUTRIENTS

Vitamins and minerals make up the category of micronutrients. As such, they are essential and required to sustain life. The amount to satisfy requirements for micronutrients is much less than that described for macronutrients.

VITAMINS

Insufficient vitamin intakes can lead to the classical deficiency diseases, which if left unchecked can be fatal. The consumers' perception of the critical need of vitamins and current discussion about their role in health have led them to believe in high vitamin consumption, sometimes 100 times the recommended dietary levels. Fortunately, no substantial increase of toxicity effects is associated with excessive vitamin ingestion. But toxicity can readily be induced from large concentrations of vitamin supplements or by the misuse of specific foods.

To understand vitamin toxicity, it is important to differentiate between fat-soluble vitamins (A, D, E, and K) and water-soluble vitamins (B and C). Because fat-soluble vitamins have the ability to be stored in body fat depots, excessive intakes of such vitamins may result in their accumulation and accompanying toxic effects. More often, large or excessive consumption of water-soluble vitamins results in more body excretion of the compound, more in the urine and sweat. However, research over the past couple of decades has shown that serious side effects can be associated with excessive intakes of water-soluble vitamins.

Fat-Soluble Vitamins

Large intakes of vitamins A and D are known to cause the classical symptoms of toxicity. Excessive intakes of vitamin A compounds result in permanent liver damage and stunted growth. Usually, toxic symptoms are reversed when excessive intakes are ceased. Common foods do not present a problem; uncommon items such as polar bear liver, or shark, halibut, and cod liver oils, which may have up to 30,000 μg/g compared to the normal daily recommendation of 1000 μg/g, may cause problems. Acute toxicities in adult humans may not be easily achieved with common supplements; however, children can be at risk. Acute toxicity can appear in matter of hours. Symptoms include anorexia, bulging fontanelles, hyperirritability, vomiting, headaches, dizziness, drowsiness, and erythematous swelling. Chronic toxicity may take a few to several months to express clinical symptoms such as anorexia, headache, sore muscles, bleeding lips, hair loss, cracking and peeling skin, nose bleed, liver and spleen enlargement, and anemia.

Excessive vitamin D intakes have resulted in a variety of toxic effects, including death. Excessive ingestion of exogenous natural sources such as fish liver oils or supplements can lead to hypercalcemia, membrane damage, hypertension, cardiac insufficiency, renal failure, and hypochromic anemia. Often, withdrawing the vitamin can reverse the symptoms. Levels five times the recommended daily intake can be toxic, especially to children. Concentrations not more than 10 to 20 μg/d can be considered safe. Acute toxicity symptoms include anorexia, nausea, vomiting, diarrhea, headache, polyuria, and polydipsia, usually 2 to 8 d following ingestion. Chronic symptoms include weight loss, pallor, constipation, fever, hypercalcemia, and calcium deposition in soft tissues.

High intakes of vitamin E and vitamin K appear to be relatively nontoxic. Some studies show that intakes of vitamin E greater than ca. 500 mg/d (50 times the recommended daily intake) can impair functioning of white cells and the immune system. It also is known that excess amounts of vitamin E can antagonize vitamin K's role in the clotting mechanism. Although vitamin K is fat soluble, it is readily excreted from the body, making toxicity unlikely. However, one form of vitamin K known as menadione, which is water soluble, is extremely toxic at high concentrations, leading to jaundice and hemolytic anemia.

Water-Soluble Vitamins

As a group, these vitamins tend to have fewer toxic effects compared with fat-soluble vitamins, mainly because water-soluble vitamins are not retained in the body to the same extent as fat-soluble vitamins. When these vitamins reach urinary threshold levels, the excess is eliminated rapidly in the urine. Thus, discernible harm to the individual can be avoided because of these elimination factors preventing accidental or deliberate ingestion of water-soluble vitamins. Nevertheless, adverse effects associated with excessive intakes of some water-soluble vitamins are being reported with more frequency, which increases the need for more judicious use of supplements and for taking precautions to avoid adverse effects.

Niacin

Side effects are associated with large therapeutic doses of niacin. Nicotinic acid in large doses (100 to 300 mg oral or 20 mg intravenous) can result in vasodilative effects. Symptoms include flushing reaction, cramps, headache, and nausea. Therapeutic levels of niacin have been used successfully to reduce serum cholesterol, but with other reversible side effects such as pruritus, desquamation, and pigmented dermatosis. On the other hand, high doses of nicotinamide (used to therapeutically treat niacin deficiency) have no side effects. Nicotinamide does not lower serum cholesterol.

Folacin

The major concern with the use of high levels of folic acid is the masking pernicious anemia resulting from vitamin B12 deficiency. Prolonged masking can delay recognition of the neurological aspects of pernicious anemia arising from vitamin B12 deficiency, which if unnoticed can lead to severe neurological damage. High doses (>15 mg) of folic acid are associated with GI disturbance, irritability, malaise, hyperexcitability, disturbed sleep, and vivid dreams.

Vitamin B6 (Pyridoxine)

Pyridoxal hydrochloride demonstrates oral toxicity at ca. 2 g/kg body weight, or 20 times the therapeutic recommended dose, for peripheral neuritis. Such doses result in convulsive disorder and inhibition of prolactin secretion.

The remaining water-soluble B vitamins, pantothenic acid and thiamin, show few adverse effects, certainly none from dietary sources.

MINERALS AND TRACE ELEMENTS

As regards the toxic effects of minerals and trace elements, the absolute level of intake is not the only circumstance involved with either acute or chronic toxicity. Toxic intake levels can vary considerably with individual circumstances. An element that is easily stored may accumulate in tissues over time, and therefore ingestion of a lower concentration may produce a toxic effect that would not occur in an individual without any prior exposure. Other circumstances that may influence the toxicity of a mineral or trace element include absorption and excretion factors, immobilization or storage of the toxic element (bone storage), and detoxification mechanisms.

Magnesium

Excessive intake or administration of magnesium salts can result in hypermagnesemia. Such patients have concomitant renal failure. Neuromuscular symptoms are common. Nonspecific effects of magnesium intoxication include nausea, vomiting, and cutaneous flushing. Depressed respiration and apnea due to paralysis of the voluntary musculature and cardiac arrest may occur.

Iron

Iron overloads can be a serious problem for some individuals. The best-defined example of iron overload is hereditary hemochromatosis, an autosomally recessively inherited disease. In hemochromatosis, iron is absorbed in excess of what is needed, leading to accumulation of significant concentrations of nonprotein-bound iron and saturation of transferrin. Subsequent parenchymal iron loading results in clinical complications of diabetes mellitus, endocrine abnormalities, cardiomyopathy, arthritis, liver cirrhosis, and hepatic cancer. It is likely that lipid peroxidation and fibrogenesis play important contributory roles in the mechanism of iron-caused organ damage. Prospective evaluation of atherosclerosis shows that iron status in combination with serum low-density lipoproteins (LDLs) may be a significant risk factor. The findings suggest a concern regarding the appearance of a progressive increase in iron nutritional status of the U.S. population, as determined by comparisons between National Health and Nutritional Examination Surveys (NHANES) II and NHANES III.

Zinc

Long-term intakes of 6 to 20 times the RDA can produce overt zinc toxicity. Symptoms of zinc toxicity include impaired immune response, reduction in highdensity lipoprotein (HDL) cholesterol levels and induced copper deficiency (anemia). Acute effects of high zinc intake are vomiting, epigastric pain, fatigue, and lethargy. Particular concerns have been expressed regarding the popularity of zinc gluconate lozenges for the common cold. A lozenge contains 13 mg of zinc, which if taken every 2 h can approach toxic doses.

Copper

Once the capacity of the liver to bind copper is exceeded, toxicity may occur. GI distress has been seen with copper intakes of 5 mg/d. Weakness, listlessness, and anorexia are early signs of copper toxicity, followed by hepatic necrosis, vascular collapse, coma, and death.

Manganese

Oral toxicity is rare; however, airborne manganese (industrial or automobile emissions) can be very toxic, resulting in pancreatitis and neurological disorders similar to schizophrenia and Parkinson's disease.

Selenium

The range between adequate selenium and toxicity is narrow: 0.1 mg and 2 mg/kg of diet, respectively. Long-term intakes of dietary selenium at 4 to 5 mg/kg of diet are sufficient to cause growth inhibition and result in tissue damage of the liver. Selenium toxicity in humans brings on symptoms of nausea, weakness, and diarrhea, and eventually hair loss, changes in nails, mottling of the teeth, and lesions of the skin and nervous system.

ANTINUTRIENTS

The three board classes of antinutrients are antiproteins, antiminerals, and antivitamins.

ANTIPROTEINS

They are substances that interfere with the digestion, absorption, or utilization of proteins. Antiproteins occur in many plants and some animals. Various protease inhibitors inhibit proteolytic enzymes of the gut, usually by binding to the enzyme's active site. Lectins are antiproteins that have binding sites for cell receptors similar to what antibodies have. Consequently, lectins, also called hemaggulutinins, can agglutinate red blood cells.

Ovomucoids and ovoinhibitors are found in eggs and inhibit proteolytic enzymes. Egg whites contain chymotrypsin inhibitors. Many are sensitive to heat treatment and are inactivated at boiling temperatures for 15 min. Trypsin and chymotrypsin inhibitors are found in legumes, vegetables, milk, wheat, and potatoes. The trypsin inhibitor found in milk is only destroyed after heating 85°C for at least 1 h. Soybean has pancreatic enzyme inhibitors that have been shown in rodents to reduce growth. Elastase inhibitors have been isolated from soybeans, beans, and potatoes.

Lectins have been isolated from the legumes soybean, peanut, lima beans, kidney beans, fava beans, lentils, and pea, and potatoes, banana, mango, and wheat germ. These compounds bind avidly to intestinal mucosal cells and interfere with amino acids, thyroxine, and fat absorption; therefore, such lectins are goitrogenic. Ricin is a toxic lectin isolated from castor bean, and is notorious for causing deaths of children who eat raw castor beans as well for being a substance of concern as an instrument of bioterrorism. Ricin's mode of action is through intestinal cell necrosis. Most lectins are inactivated by moist heat; hence, steaming is an effective processing technique used to inactivate ricin in castor oil. However, dry heat is largely ineffective to deactivate lectins.

Antiminerals

Antiminerals are substances that interfere with absorption or metabolic utilization of minerals. Some examples are phytic acid, oxalic acid, glucosinolates, dietary fiber, and gossypol.

Phytic acid's negative effect on iron absorption has been known for decades. Phytic acid is found in bran and germ of many plant seeds and in grains, legumes, nuts and species. In addition, phytic acid can compromise the absorption of magnesium, zinc, copper, and manganese, usually forming precipitates. Formation of soybean protein–phytate complexes during processing has been associated with a reduction in bioavailability of minerals such as Ca, Zn, Fe and Mg. On the other hand, fermentation and other processing techniques are useful in reducing phytate levels.

Oxalic acid, like phytic acid, reduces the availability of bivalent cations. Sources of oxalate include rhubarb, spinach, beets, potatoes, tea, coffee, and cocoa. Tea drinking was associated with concerns for Ca deficits via complexes, which apparently can be counterbalanced by using milk with tea drinking.

Glucosinolates are goitrogenic and inhibit iodine uptake into the thyroid. Rutabaga, turnips, cabbage, peaches and strawberries are good sources for glucosinolates. Decreases in plasma thyroxin for glucosinolate intakes are found at the 15% dietary level in rodent studies.

Dietary fiber, even without phytate, can affect calcium, magnesium, zinc and phosphorus absorption. Collectively, dietary fiber refers to food components in plants cell walls that are not digested. Dietary fiber can act like ion exchangers and bind minerals.

Gossypol is a phenolic compound isolated from the cotton plant and is capable of chelating iron and binding up amino acids. This major toxic compound makes up 1% of the seed's dry weight. In the 1930s and 40s, outbreaks of infertility in some areas of China were traced to gossypol in cottonseed oil used as a cooking oil. Various processing techniques to isolate the protein can remove 90% of the gossypol. Gossypol also exerts genotoxic effects in mammalian cell cultures, possibly through production of superoxide anions and singlet oxygen induced strand breakage in DNA. It is not known whether any of these adverse effects of gossypol are related to effects on iron metabolism.

Antivitamins

Antivitamins are substances that inactivate or destroy vitamins or inhibit the activity of a vitamin in a metabolic reaction and increase an individual's need for vitamins. Again, the collection of compounds involved as antinutrients is diverse and does not lend itself to simple characterization. For example, ascorbic acid oxidase, an enzyme found in fruits and vegetables, can oxidize ascorbic acid. Hence, in addition to aerobic conditions, fresh juices lose 50% of the vitamin in less than 1 h. Raw fish contains thiaminase, which has antivitamin properties and splits the thiamin at the methylene linkage into two rings. Also, it is known that tannins found in plants destroy thiamin. Mushrooms contain vitamin B6 antagonists, and linatine found in linseed oil is an antipyridoxine factor. Finally, avidin, a heat-sensitive compound found in egg white, forms a complex with biotin.

STUDY QUESTIONS AND EXERCISES

1. List the potential health problems that could be associated with the consumption of raw fish.
2. Discuss the suggestion that overconsumption of macronutrients may cause chronic diseases or explain the consequence of macronutrient toxicity.
3. Look up the DRI and UL values for fat-soluble vitamins and the levels found in over-the-counter supplements. Is there a potential for toxicity with the abuse of such supplements?
4. Evaluate the effects of high-protein diets in humans and discuss how this impacts on diets that promote weight loss by the consumption of high protein and fats.

RECOMMENDED READINGS

Dietary Reference Intakes, http://www.nal.usda.gov/fnic/etext/000105.html.

Food Research Institute, University of Wisconsin, Madison, *Food Safety*, Marcel Dekker, New York, 1993.

Janssen, M.M.T., Antinutritives, in *Food Safety and Toxicity*, DeVries, J., Ed., CRC Press, Boca Raton, FL, 1997, pp. 39-52.

Omaye, S.T., Safety of megavitamin therapy, in *Nutritional and Toxicological Aspects of Food Safety*, Friedman, M., Ed., Plenum Press, New York, 1984, pp. 169-203.

Reddy, N.R. and Pierson, M.D., Reduction in antinutritional and toxic components in plant foods by fermentation, *Food Res. Int.*, 27, 281-290, 1994.

Tannenbaum, S.R., *Nutritional and Safety Aspects of Food Processing*, Marcel Dekker, New York, 1979.

15 Parasites, Viruses, and Prions

In the broadest definition of parasites, every infectious agent discussed up to this point, such as bacteria, fungi and viruses, can be included. However, traditionally the term has been reserved for an animal that derives its livelihood entirely from a larger animal or host. Our discussion here is limited to protozoa and worms and excludes anthropoids, which, except a few (e.g., body lice), are not strictly parasites but more often vectors for diseases (e.g., ticks). All parasites are pathogenic and the terms used to describe the diseases they produce end in the suffix *-iasis* (giardiasis) or *-osis* (toxoplasmosis). Some parasites are shed in feces and produce infection in those who ingest them with food or water. Other parasites are present only during a portion of their life cycle in animals used for food and subsequently eaten by humans, whereupon they carry out sexual reproduction and produce eggs that get shed in feces. None of the parasites transmissible through the food or water is capable of multiplying outside the host.

PROTOZOA

Protozoa (protozoon, singular) are one-cell animals. With respect to food or water sources, three types are important: *Entamoeba histolytica*, an ameba; *Giardia lamblia*, a flagellate; and *Toxoplasma gondii*, a coccidian. Each has at least one active feeding form, usually termed as trophozoite, and can reproduce by simple division, and a quiescent form in which it retains infectivity during periods outside the host.

E. HISTOLYTICA

Transmission is by fecal to an oral route. The major source of infection is usually an individual who is asymptomatic but excretes the protozoa via feces. Flies or roaches can be vectors, and the organism can be transmitted during sexual practices. Infection is a worldwide problem, usually related to poor hygiene and sanitation. It is estimated that 480 million infections exist. In the U.S., prevalence is about 2 to 3%, with higher rates localized in Southeastern states in male gay couples. The habitat is the colon, but the protozoa may move to other organs. The trophozoite is an active feeding form and reproduces by binary fission. The trophozoite can penetrate the mucosa, enter the blood stream, and be transported to other organs. The protozoa secrete enzymes capable of cell membrane lysis. For *E. histolytica*, the human host is the most important; however, the protozoa are found in dogs, cats, and other mammals. The cyst of *E. histolytica* is the infectious stage, and the protective cyst wall is resistant to many environmental conditions and is eventually excreted in feces.

Clinical manifestations can be grouped into four categories: (1) Asymptomatic carriers, in which the cyst can be passed via stools, but the individual is free of symptoms. (2) Nondysenteric colitis, in which the individual has nonspecific symptoms such as intermittent diarrhea, constipation, and abdominal pain. Cysts can be found in stools and trophozoites can be seen during diarrhea. (3) Dysentery, with symptoms of bloody diarrhea, mucus, low-grade fever, and colonic perforation with peritonitis. (4) Amebic liver abscesses, in which there is fever, pain in the right upper quadrant of the abdomen or the right lower chest, and the liver is enlarged, tender, and jaundiced. Metronidazole and chloroquine are effective drug treatments for *E. histolytica*.

GIARDIA LAMBLIA

These protozoa may gain access to the host by either ingestion of the cysts from feces or through sexual practices. The trophozoites attach to the mucosal surface of the small intestine and are confined to the lumen. They reproduce by simple division, and because of their adherence to the mucosal surface can interfere with nutritive absorption of the host. Many animals have *Giardia* and can infect humans. Beavers are a host for this organism. *Giardia* is a worldwide problem, particularly in areas of poor sanitation. High rates are seen in day-care centers in the U.S. Persons affected can be asymptomatic or show clinical symptoms of severe diarrhea (acute or chronic). Patients with immunoglobulin deficiencies are especially susceptible. The cysts are relatively resistant to chlorination, but treatment with metronidazole is effective.

TOXOPLASMA GONDII

This organism is an intracellular parasite, which multiplies within the intestinal mucosal cells of its host, the cat. The organism can eventually invade other cells in other parts of the body of the cat it infects. Entrance to the host is by ingestion of oocysts from cat feces or by inadequately cooked meat, particularly pork, lamb, or beef. The prevalence of *T. gondii* in cats is dependent on eating raw meat. In the U.S., 1 to 6 women per 1000 acquire toxoplasmosis that is associated with congenital diseases. In addition, *T. gondii* can affect the brain, skeletal muscle, and retina. Common problems include ocular and neurological problems, jaundice, abortions or stillbirths, and malformation. Immunosuppressed individuals or patients with AIDS are particularly at risk from this organism. The usual treatment includes the use of pyrimethamine and sulfa drugs; however, pregnant women should avoid cats.

WORMS

ROUNDWORMS

The life cycle of nematodes may occur entirely within a single host or be more complex. Reproduction is sexual and the female may lay eggs or give birth internally.

Trichinella spiralis

The transmissible form of *T. spiralis* is a larval cyst that can occur in pork muscles. Pork should be cooked till no pink color is visible in the meat. Microwave ovens can be a problem, as they do not cook the meat evenly. Education programs and livestock methods have been successful in reducing the incidence of trichinosis in humans. Unusual situations occur when people are infected by eating game meat, such as Alaskan grizzly bear meat. Following ingestion, the adult worm burrows into the lining of the intestine. Cysts that are eaten with meat liberate larvae, which undergo sexual differentiation. Adults penetrate the mucosa of the intestine to copulate, and later the males reenter the lumen of the intestine and are carried out. The female burrows deep into the mucosa and produces approximately 1500 larvae, and the newborns are carried via the lymph and blood to striated muscles, where they grow and encyst. The larvae burrow into striated muscles, causing edema, muscle and joint aches, and fever. Eventually, the high concentration of cysts in the striated muscle results in loss of efficiency of muscle contraction. In people who have died of trichinosis, more than 1000 cysts/g of muscle have been found.

Ascaris lumbricoides

These are large parasites that can be transmitted in the form of eggs. The incidence of infections is high for North America, affecting approximately 3 million people. Worldwide, about 7000 million individuals might be affected. The eggs of these worms are found in sewage-fertilizer and in soils. The eggs may contaminate crops grown in soil or fertilized with sewage. Infected food handlers may contaminate a wide variety of foods. People who consume uncooked vegetables and fruits grown in or near soil fertilized with sewage are vulnerable. Eggs of *Ascaris* have been detected on fresh vegetables (cabbage) sampled by inspectors.

These infections are more common in North America, and relative infection rates on other continents are not known. Infections may self-cure after the larvae have matured into adults or may require anthelmintic treatment. In severe cases, surgical removal may be necessary. Allergic symptoms are common in long-lasting infections or reinfection.

The worm is pathogenic because the larvae leave the blood and move into the lungs, causing hemorrhages and pneumonia. The worms can also access the pancreas and bile ducts, producing obstruction.

Anisakids

The worm is often referred to as herringworm, sealworm, codworm, or whaleworm. It has invasive larvae and commonly infests populations consuming raw fish, such as in Japan and the Netherlands where raw herring is often consumed. The life cycle involves warm-blooded sea animals, and humans are the accidental hosts.

Anisakiasis is often diagnosed when the affected individual feels a tingling or tickling sensation in the throat and coughs up the worm. Acute abdominal pain, similar to acute appendicitis, is accompanied by a nauseous feeling. Symptoms appear 1 h to about 2 weeks after consumption of raw or undercooked seafood. With their anterior ends, these larval nematodes from fish or shellfish usually burrow into the wall of the digestive tract to the level of the muscularis mucosae. (Occasionally, they penetrate the intestinal wall completely and are found in the body cavity.) Anisakids usually do not reach full maturity in humans and are eliminated spontaneously from the digestive tract lumen within 3 weeks of infection.

TAPEWORMS

These worms have complex life cycles and are relatively high order of species specificity. The three common types are *Taenia saginata*, found in beef; *Taenia solium*, found in pork; and *Diphyllobothrium latum*, found in fish. Tapeworms have been known to reside for many years in the intestine and grow to very long lengths. Reproduction is ultimately sexual, but adults have both sex organs. The tapeworm inhabits the intestine of the host by fastening itself by the head to the lining of the host's intestine. Anatomically, the worm is composed of a head (scolex), a short neck, and a tapelike body (stobila). The stobila is made up of many segments (proglottids) linked together by muscles and nerves. Each proglottid absorbs nutrients from the contents of the host's intestine. Eggs are released into the lumen and shed. Some individuals have been known to harbor tapeworms for up to 30 years. Problems can occur if the worm obstructs the intestinal tract. Embarrassment and distress can occur when a section of the proglottid exits the intestine without the host's participation.

VIRUSES

Viruses can be considered as obligatory intracellular parasites and are conceptually genetic elements of either DNA or RNA (usually not both), sometimes containing lipids, packaged in protein coats. Most RNA and protein coats can be antigenic, against which the host can mount an immune response. Viruses have no metabolic apparatus because they utilize the energy-processing components of the host. Viruses replicate within susceptible cells, and during replication there is an intimate mingling of viral components with the protoplasm of the host cells. Therefore, the host cell is induced to synthesize virus components at the host's expense. Replication of viruses occurs in four stages (Figure 15.1). The first stage begins when an infectious particle attaches to the surface of the host cell (attachment). The susceptibility of a cell to virus attachment depends on the presence of receptors on the host cell's plasma membrane. Receptors are glycoproteins set in the membrane of the host cell. The attachment sites of the virus and the viral receptors of the host cell are complementary. The next stage is referred to as penetration and involves engulfing (pinocytosis) of the virus particle by the host cell or by fusion of the cell membrane with the viral envelope, whereupon the viral coat is lost and the nucleic acid is released into the host cell, the process being termed uncoating. At this point, the infecting particle can no longer be recovered or be located by electron microscopy. In the third stage (synthetic), the viral nucleic acid directs the host cell to synthesize components of the progeny virus. Proteins are synthesized by using the viral RNA as messenger. This is followed by the assembly stage, in which the components

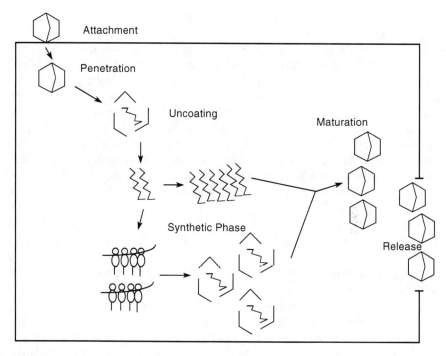

FIGURE 15.1 Replication of viruses.

synthesized are spontaneously assembled into progeny viral particles, also referred to as maturation. In the final release stage, bacterial viruses lyse the host cell and are released and animal viruses may stay within the host cell indefinitely.

Viruses can be pathogenic to cells because they kill cells, cause a loss of special function of cells, or proliferate in the cell. All the damages that viruses cause take place at the cell level. In cell lysis, cells may die or survive and even return to normal. During loss of special function, viral infection may induce the cells to relinquish their specialized functions. This can be a major problem if such cells have specialized activity and function in a vital organ. Proliferation at the expense of host cells can produce tumors or cancers in the host.

Another way of looking at the nature of virus infection on the host is to examine the impact on the organism. Tissue tropism (turning into) must be initiated, wherein because of receptors on the cell surface the virus can attach and begin to replicate, the process being called primary tropism. The progeny viruses are subsequently carried from the primary tropic site to other parts of the body, usually by the lymph and blood, resulting in the exposure of the virus to the host's defense mechanism. This results in secondary tropism, wherein other cells that have receptors for the virus interact with the virus. Secondary tropism is usually associated with symptoms of the disease, such as the spinal cord and meningitis or the liver and hepatitis. The host organism responds with both specific immunity and nonspecific immunity. The response of specific immunity is initially with IgM antibodies and for longer periods with IgG antibodies. Nonspecific immunity involves production of interferon, which is active against viruses in general. Nonspecific immunity mechanisms are likely to limit the duration of the infection.

For survival, the infecting virus must reach and infect another host immediately after its exit from the first host. The route of entrance of a virus to a new host and shedding from the current host are principally by mucous membranes. This is either through ingestion or inhalation, involving respiratory mucus and intestinal feces. Passage from host to host can be direct or indirect. Direct passage of enteric viruses can occur either through anal–oral contact or more commonly by way of soiled hands with feces residues. Respiratory sneezes aerosolize the viruses and expose new hosts. The indirect passage can be by vectors such as flies and mosquitoes. Also, foods may act as vehicles by which viruses are transmitted.

Viruses are transmitted as particles too small to be seen with conventional light microscopes and are a heterogeneous group of infectious agents that vary in diameter from 20 to 200 nm. The replication cycle of viruses takes place in a host cell and as the nuclear materials accumulate, the progeny eventually leaves that cell in blebs. Viruses exist either as inert or nebulous particles and are replicating intracellular parasites. Foodborne viruses can be transmitted through food and be infectious at the organism level. The particle is produced and occurs inside the host cell and is also the form in which the virus is transmitted from host to host.

All foodborne viruses contain RNA, usually single stranded and coated with structural protein. Foodborne viruses have no metabolism of their own, and therefore they cannot carry out any life process by themselves. They are transmitted enterically, shed with feces, and infect by being ingested. Viruses can enter the food supply in several ways, such as infected food handlers or contamination by sewage. More than 100 known enteric viruses are excreted and find their way to sewage. Table 15.1 lists the relatively few virus-induced foodborne diseases found in humans.

Preventive measures are the recommended means to avoid virus-induced foodborne diseases. The virus cannot grow in food, but appears to be more stable in food than water. For example, in water at neutral pH, viruses are destroyed by tempera-

TABLE 15.1
Foodborne Viruses and Human Diseases

Virus	Human Disease (Common Source)
Hepatitis A	Hepatitis A (shellfish, vegetables, milk)
Hepatitis E	Hepatitis E (clinically indistinguishable from hepatitis A disease, water-borne, person to person)
Norwalk-like	Gastroenteritis (salads, raw oysters, clams)
Rotavirus	Gastroenteritis (transmitted by the fecal–oral route, person-to-person spread through contaminated hands)
Caliciviruses	Acute nonbacterial infectious gastroenteritis and viral gastroenteritis (fecal–oral routes via person-to-person contact or ingestion of contaminated foods and water)
Astroviruses	Viral gastroenteritis is usually a mild illness characterized by nausea, vomiting, diarrhea, malaise, abdominal pain, headache, and fever (fecal–oral routes via person-to-person contact or ingestion of contaminated foods and water)

tures above 85°C but can survive pasteurization temperature in food. This is why shellfish that are steamed when open may be inadequately heated and unable to kill many viruses. A temperature of 85 to 90°C is required to adequately inactive viruses. In general, heat (30 min at 55°C) drying, freeze-drying, or irradiation inactivate some viruses. Chemical agents such as strong oxidizing agents, ozone, and chlorine, and acid conditions inactivate viruses. Before the advent of vaccines and pasteurization of milk, raw milk was a route of transmission for poliomyelitis.

Acute hepatitis is a common disease and is caused mostly by virus infections. At least five hepatitis viruses (A, B, C, D, and E) are pathogenic to humans. Hepatitis A is infectious hepatitis, transmitted via the anal–oral cycle. The incubation period is between 15 and 20 days. Hepatic infection produces a debilitating low-mortality disease. The liver becomes inflamed, enlarged, and tender, the symptoms usually subsiding after 2 to 4 weeks. Some outbreaks have been associated with food (including meat, poultry, and egg products) contaminated by infected food handlers. In the U.S., there has been an increased incidence related to contaminated shellfish consumption, particularly oysters and other molluscs. Another potential source is vegetables contaminated in the field via irrigation with water polluted with human excrements. Milk and other foods that require much handling are sources, and flies and cockroaches may also be vectors. The disease may be spread by persons with infection as early as 7 d before the onset of symptoms.

Hepatitis B induces hepatomas and can cause lifelong infection, cirrhosis (scarring) of the liver, liver cancer, liver failure, and death. About 30% of persons have no signs or symptoms. Signs and symptoms are less common in children than adults. Much less is known about hepatitis C, D, and E, except that they are similar to hepatitis B.

Hepatitis E disease is called hepatitis E or enterically transmitted non-A non-B hepatitis. Other names include fecal–oral non-A non-B hepatitis or A-like non-A non-B hepatitis. The disease is clinically indistinguishable from hepatitis A disease, with the following symptoms: malaise, anorexia, abdominal pain, arthralgia, and fever.

Hepatitis E is transmitted by the fecal–oral route. Waterborne and person-to-person spread has been documented and the potential exists for foodborne transmission. Hepatitis E occurs in both epidemic and sporadic-endemic forms, usually associated with contaminated drinking water. Major waterborne epidemics have occurred in Asia and North and East Africa.

The incubation period for hepatitis E varies from 2 to 9 weeks. The disease is usually mild and resolves in 2 weeks. Mortality is about 0.1 to 1%, but higher in pregnant women, who may have a fatality rate approaching 20%.

The Norwalk-like virus causes gastroenteritis with diarrhea and vomiting. Norwalk virus is a family of unclassified small, round-structured viruses that may be related to the caliciviruses. The family consists of several serologically distinct groups of viruses that have been named after the places where the outbreaks occurred. In the U.S., the Norwalk and Montgomery County agents are serologically related but distinct from the Hawaii and Snow Mountain agents. Common names of the illness caused by Norwalk and Norwalk-like viruses are viral gastroenteritis, acute nonbacterial gastroenteritis, food poisoning, and food infection.

The incubation period is 18 to 36 h, with the illness being mild and self-limiting. It is hard to establish a diagnosis because the virus only replicates in the host. The Norwalk-like virus appears to be responsible for several large outbreaks throughout the U.S., usually at large gatherings (banquets, picnics, etc.). The attack rate is high and those who consume the virus get sick. The disease is self-limiting, mild, and characterized by nausea, vomiting, diarrhea, and abdominal pain. Headache and low-grade fever may occur. The infectious dose is unknown but presumed to be low. The virus can be identified on early stool specimens by immune electron microscopy and various immunoassays. Norwalk gastroenteritis is transmitted by the fecal–oral route via contaminated water and foods. Secondary person-to-person transmission has been documented. Water is the most common source of outbreaks and may include water from municipal supplies, well, recreational lakes, swimming pools, and water stored aboard cruise ships. Shellfish and salad ingredients are the foods most often implicated in Norwalk outbreaks. Ingestion of raw or insufficiently steamed clams and oysters poses a high risk for infection with Norwalk virus. Foods other than shellfish are contaminated by ill food-handlers.

Rotavirus also is associated with gastroenteritis, particularly in infants and children under 5 years of age. The rotavirus is prevalent in developing countries. Rotavirus commonly causes seasonal diarrhea in infants and young children. In children aged 3 months to 2 years, rotavirus is one of the most common causes of gastroenteritis, and it often causes outbreaks of diarrhea in day-care centers and children's hospitals. Children with a rotavirus infection have fever, nausea, and vomiting, and often explosive, watery diarrhea. After 2 d, the fever and vomiting usually stop, but the diarrhea can continue for 5 to 7 d.

Other viruses have been implicated in foodborne outbreaks, including astroviruses and caliciviruses. Caliciviruses are classified in the family Caliciviridae. They contain a single strand of RNA surrounded by a protein capsid. Mature viruses have cup-shaped indentations, which give them a "Star of David" appearance in the electron microscope (EM). Astroviruses are unclassified viruses that contain a single positive strand of RNA of ca. 7.5 kb surrounded by a protein capsid of diameter 28 to 30 nm. A five- or six-pointed star shape can be observed on the particles under the EM.

The illnesses caused by these viruses are acute nonbacterial infectious gastroenteritis and viral gastroenteritis. Viral gastroenteritis is usually a mild illness characterized by nausea, vomiting, diarrhea, malaise, abdominal pain, headache, and fever. Viral gastroenteritis is transmitted by the fecal–oral route via person-to-person contact or by ingestion of contaminated foods and water. Astroviruses cause sporadic gastroenteritis in children under 4 years of age and account for ca. 4% of the cases hospitalized for diarrhea. Most U.S. children over 10 years of age have antibodies to the virus. Caliciviruses infect children between 6 and 24 months of age and account for about 3% of hospital admissions for diarrhea. By 6 years of age, more than 90% of all children develop immunity to the illness. The disease is mild, self-limiting, usually develops 10–70 h after contaminated food or water is consumed, and lasts for 2–9 days. The clinical features are milder but otherwise indistinguishable from rotavirus gastroenteritis.

Zoonoses are diseases transmitted from animal to other animals or to humans. Tick-borne encephalitis is an example of zoonoses. Virus is shed into the milk of goats and cattle that have been infected by tick bites. Ornithosis is a chlamydial (conjunctivitis) disease of poultry and is transmitted by the respiratory route of those who handle or kill infected birds. Q fever, a rickettsial disease of cattle and sheep, is transmitted to herdsmen and veterinarians by the respiratory route. More recently, prion-causing bovine spongiform encephalopathy (BSE, mad cow disease), responsible for the atypical Creutzfeldt–Jakob disease (CJD), can be categorized as zoonoses.

PRIONS (PROTEINACEOUS INFECTIOUS PARTICLES)

Early experiments demonstrated that an infectious agent was insensitive to treatments that inactivate DNA and RNA but whose infection was destroyed when subjected to protein denaturants. Stanley Prusiner, University of California, San Francisco, proposed that this unique infectious agent be called a prion (for proteinaceous infectious particle). Prions are found as a normal cellular form (PrP^C) and as an infectious form (PrP^{Sc}). PrP^C is expressed in most, if not all, cells. Conversion of PrP^C to PrP^{Sc} during the infectious process changes the protein structure from predominantly α-helical to a β-sheet form. Differences between prion forms are due to protein tertiary and quaternary structures. Conversion of PrP^C to PrP^{Sc} produces aggregates, resulting in a protease-resistant prion isomer. PrP^{Sc} may propagate its own conversion by acting as a template (seed), which results in self-replication (more conversion of PrP^C to PrP^{Sc}).

PrP^C isoform is a 33- to 35-kDa sialoglycoprotein with 208 to 220 amino acids, is expressed predominantly in the central nervous system, and is attached to the surface of neurons and other cell types by a glycophosphatidyl inositol (GPI) anchor. Two thirds of the molecule at the carboxyl terminal end is a helix bundle structure and the remaining 80 to 100 amino acids at the amino-terminal end contain a copper ion-binding motif. The normal function of PrP^C may be to traffic copper ions. PrP^C possesses superoxide dismutase activity and may play a role in cellular resistance to oxidative stress. Thus, the conformational shift from the helical cellular PrP^C to a sheet-rich pathogenic isoform PrP^{Sc} can result in loss of Cu-mediated antioxidant function and in a microenvironment (perhaps producing a metal ion prooxidant situation) that is more conducive to oxidative stress, which can trigger a neurodegenerative cascade. Use of antioxidants in PrP-related diseases has been proposed in Alzheimer's disease and other neurodegenerative diseases, but requires more research. In knockout mice studies, PrP-deficient brain cells die more rapidly in culture than wild-type cells. Programmed cell death can be suppressed under serum-free conditions by transfection with PrP or bcl-2 gene. PrP may be a member of the Bcl-2 family of proteins that modulate one of the molecular cascades leading to apoptosis.

The prototype of all prion diseases is the scrapie. Human prion diseases are rare (1 to 2 per million). Transmissible spongiform encephalopathies (TSEs) are a family of human and animal diseases, uniformly fatal, causing irreversible brain injury. The common form of TSE in humans is the CJD, manifested by progressive brain damage in the elderly (memory loss, loss in ability to think, with eventual loss of sight and ability to speak or feed themselves, lasting ca. 5 to 6 months). Kuru, a TSE neurodegenerative disease once common to the aboriginal tribes in New Guinea, was found to be transmitted by ritual cannibalism. Variant CJD (vCJD) is the form of CJD that is associated with BSE and is probably caused by dietary exposure of affected people to contaminated beef products. The belief has been recently supported by experimental evidence that the causative agent of BSE is identical to that of vCJD. The disease strikes young people, takes about 2 years or longer to kill, and symptoms involve psychiatric features, e.g., hallucinations.

PrP^C is encoded by an endogenous gene on Chromosome 20, and cases are attributable to point mutations that occur in the C-terminal half or N-terminal half of the PrP molecule. PrP expression is likely a prerequisite for a cell to support conversion to the infectious form. Transgenic models that lack PrP expression are resistant to PrP^{Sc} infection, and animals with overexpressed PrP have a shorter incubation time for PrP^{Sc} infection. Polymorphisms encoding amino acids at positions 129 and perhaps 219 of the PrP gene may play an important role in susceptibility to infection. In cell cultures, synthetic peptides that mimic the sequence transcribed at Codon 129 have been found to inhibit PrP conversion. The encoding alternatives, Met and Val, are distributed in the general Caucasian population in the following proportions: 50% Met/Val, 40% Met/Met, and 10% Val/Val. All vCJD patients tested are homozygous for Met. Thus, the infectious form may occur by exposure to exogenous PrP^{Sc}. In inherited prion disease, a pathogenic mutation is presumed to favor spontaneous conversion of PrP^C to PrP^{Sc} state, without needing contact with an exogenous infectious agent. Sporadic forms may be the consequences of an unusual conversion of wild-type PrP or presence of somatic mutations in PrP.

Sequence compatibility between exogenous PrP^{Sc} and host PrP^C facilitates the disease process; however, incompatible PrP sequences also result in disease transmission. Also another molecule besides PrP may be involved in the conversion of PrP^C to PrP^{Sc}. A molecule has been hypothesized, called cellular protein X, which acts as a molecular chaperone, binding to the carboxyl terminus of PrP^C and facilitating its conversion to PrP^{Sc}. Protein X is likely to be species specific, and if substantiated will account for the inefficiency of transmission across species.

The vCJD outbreaks in the U.K., attributed to consumption of contaminated products associated with BSE cattle, have shown only a modest increase during the past several years. However, there is the lingering uncertainty about the extent of the vCJD outbreak, because the incubation period of vCJD is largely unknown. Because of the measures to eliminate both animal and human exposure to BSE from 1987 to 1997, outbreaks of vCJD should remain low. Mathematical models predict that the total extent of the outbreak could range from a hundred to hundreds of thousands of cases. Human-to-human iatrogenic spread of vCJD may be very likely, i.e., via blood products, organ transplants, or contamination from surgical instruments (sterilization requires 1 N sodium hydroxide and autoclaving at 134°C). Thus, the U.S. and other countries have a blood donor policy that excludes donations from anyone who has lived in or visited the U.K. for a cumulative period of 6 months during 1980 to 1996. In 1996, with the report of 17 cases of atypical CJD, it was suspected that the patients obtained the infectious prion from eating contaminated beef. Since first recognized in 1985, mad cow disease has caused the destruction of over a million cows in the U.K. The cows were exposed to the infectious agent in their food, which had been contaminated with protein from sheep infected with scrapie (ovine spongiform encephalopathy). Twenty people in the U.K. and one person in France had the new CJD variant. Only one person survived. Currently, these diseases are seen in cattle, elk, mink, mule, deer, people, and sheep. In 1997, *The Lancet* reported on people in Kentucky with CJD associated with consuming squirrel brains. In rural Kentucky, people scramble squirrel brains with eggs or put them in stews. This observation requires confirmation by studies of larger populations and a search for a prion agent in the brains of squirrels.

With regard to the current food supply and world trade, BSE has not occurred in the U.S. or any other country that has historically imported few or no cattle or beef products from the U.K. However, there are concerns of whether the bovine-adapted scrapie agent has recrossed the species barrier to sheep, carrying its newly acquired ability to infect humans.

The emergence of BSE and vCJD has pointed at the magnitude of the problem and has propelled research in this area toward new frontiers. Yet, there is much more to do. Presently, determination is not possible of the actual number of people with vCJD in other countries where animals or animal products were exported before recognizing the threat of BSE to human health, e.g., in China, Eastern European countries, and the Mediterranean region. Better means are needed to detect infectious prions in human-derived medical products and perhaps in our food supply. The availability of sensitive and specific prion tests would enable a more effective worldwide surveillance program. To that end, WHO has coordinated a unified global surveillance. WHO also is developing partnerships with other organizations.

DIAGNOSING FOR BSE

BSE is one form of TSE, involving some rouge proteins, prions (PrP^{Sc}), that can replicate, resulting in various neurological disorders (mad cow disease, Kuru, CJD). There is a need to develop a sensitive and specific diagnostic test for the infectious PrP^{Sc}, apart from what is known as a normal prion (PrP^c). During the past few months, there has been a surge of research reports in this area, generating hope for more definitive tests in the near future.

Much has been said regarding the Europeans, and, more recently, both the Japanese and Chinese taking on enormous measures to initiate testing of cattle for BSE. Controversy has developed over the concern that the European Commission's (established by the European Union) reliance on BSE tests has not been properly validated. The tests authorized by the European Union use antibodies to detect the prions that aggregate in brains from necropsy cows. The oldest test is based on Western blots, whereas another uses immunocytochemical methods. Although some of the tests were subjected to validation studies by using them to identify cow brain tissues with or without BSE, no assessment was made of the tests' ability to detect infectious prions in cows incubating BSE. The current standard test for BSE is a bioassay in which samples taken from the brain tissue of the suspected cow are injected into the brains of mice. The mice are monitored for several months for development of the disease. One of the tests used in the study has shown more promise compared to the mouse bioassay in detecting the infectious protein diluted 1000-fold.

The goal for testing is to have a simple and rapid test on blood that could be used to test live animals or a test on other animal by-products used for food. Also, there is a growing clinical need regarding the concern about the infectious protein being transferred through blood donations and medical products derived from human tissues, iatrogenic CJD, or other TSEs. This may be difficult because there may not be enough prion protein in blood to be detected by conventional means. The feasibility of techniques for picking out the blood prions and then amplifying them to obvious detection levels must be considered. Approaches toward developing diagnostic prion tests include the use of prion binding to the blood protein plasminogen and the use of a competitive assay in which prion compete with fluorescently labeled synthesized PrP to bind antibodies.

Recent reports have been published alluding that new approaches may spin off diagnostic tests. One test may involve a genetic screen. A trait found in yeast that can spark the appearance of some known yeast prions may be capitalized for use in prion diagnosis. Another technique utilizes confocal, dual-color fluorescence cross-correlation spectroscopy and claims to have high specificity and sensitivity for prions in the cerebrospinal fluid. Another method based on modification of other tests exploits the combination of fluorescently labeled PrP and peptide antibodies and size-exclusion high performance liquid chromatography to separate free peptides from antibody-bound peptides (sensitive to detect 1 to 2 pg of PrP^{Sc}).

It is likely that advances in BSE diagnosis will assist in developing a better understanding about the biology and pathology of prions, which in turn can benefit human health with better ways to approach therapy and detect diseases. Also, the knowledge derived from BSE and TSE diagnostic research may help better understand other neurodegenerative diseases, e.g., Alzheimer's.

STUDY QUESTIONS AND EXERCISES

1. Describe the transmission clinical manifestations of toxoplasmosis. Why is it a foodborne illness problem? Which individuals are vulnerable?
2. Describe how viruses can produce foodborne illnesses and give some illustrative examples.
3. Describe the transmission of *E. histolytica*, *G. lamblia*, and *T. gondii*.
4. Do a literature search for Kuru, the TSE neurodegenerative disease once common to the aboriginal tribes in New Guinea and found to be transmitted by ritual cannibalism. Concentration on origin of the disease and how cultural practices contributed to the spread of the disease in New Guinea.
5. Document and discuss how diseases produced by prions may be examples of zoonoses.

RECOMMENDED READINGS

Baron, E.J., Chang, R.S., Howard, D.H., Miller, J.N., and Turner, J.A., *Medical Microbiology*, Wiley-Liss, New York, 1993.
Bieschke, J., Giese, A., Schulz-Schaeffer, W., Zerr, I., Poser, S., Eigen, M., and Kretzschmar, H., Ultrasensitive method for the diagnosis of prion diseases (Creutzfeldt-Jakob disease and BSE), *Proc. Natl. Acad. Sci.,* 97, 5468-5473, 2000.
Brown, P., Cervenakova, L., and Diringer, H., Blood infectivity and the prospects for a diagnostic screening test in Creutzfeldt-Jakob disease, *J. Lab. Clin. Med.,* 137, 5-13, 2001.
Bush, A.I., Metals and neuroscience. *Curr. Opin. Chem. Biol.,* 2, 184-191, 2000.
Campbell, W.C., *Trichinella and Trichinosis*, Plenum Press, New York, 1983.
Cliver, D.O. and Matsui, S.M., Viruses, in *Foodborne Diseases*, Cliver, D.O. and Riemann, H.P., Eds., Academic Press, New York, 2002, pp. 161-175.
Cohen, F. E., Prions, peptides and protein misfolding, *Mol. Med. Tod.,* 6, 292-293, 2000.
DeFrancesco, L., Quickening the diagnosis of mad cow disease, *The Scientist*, June 11, 2001, p. 22.
Doyle, M.P., Beuchat, L.R., and Montville, T.J., Eds., American Society for Microbiology Press, Washington, D.C., 2001, pp. 549-564.
Dubey, J. P., Murrell, K.D., and Cross, J.H., Parasites, in *Foodborne Diseases*, Cliver, D.O. and Riemann, H.P., Academic Press, New York, 2002, pp. 177-190.
Garcia, L.S. and Bruckner, D.A., *Diagnostic Medical Parasitology*, 3rd ed., American Society for Microbiology Press, Washington, D.C., 1997.
Giese, J., It's a mad, mad, mad, mad cow test, *Food Tech.,* 55, 60-61, 2001.
Glatzel, M. and Aguzzi, A., Peripheral pathogenesis of prion diseases, *Microb. Infect.,* 2, 613-619, 2000.
Harris, D.A., Prion diseases, *Nutrition,* 16, 554-556, 2000.
Omaye, S.T., Preventing BSE in the U.S., *Food Tech.,* 55, 26, 2001.
Ortega, Y.R., Protozoan parasites, in *Food Microbiology: Fundamentals and Frontiers*, 2nd ed., Doyle, M.P., Beuchat, L.R., and Monntville, J.J., Eds., American Society for Microbiology Press, Washington, D.C., 2001, pp. 515-531.
Wong, B.-S., Pan, T., Liu, T., Rullang, L., Petersen, R.B., Jones, I.M., Gambetti, P., Brown, D. R., and Sy, M.-S., Prion disease: a loss of antioxidant function? *Biochem. Biophys. Res. Commun.,* 275, 249-252, 2000.

Section III

Food Contamination and Safety

16 Residues in Foods

Through exposure from air, water, or land, a food supply may be contaminated with certain residues, which may eventually be consumed by humans. Some contaminations may be residues of compounds purposely used to protect crops from insects (insecticides) or destroy competing plants (herbicides). Other contaminations may be from industrial waste or pollution, by accident, ignorance, or recklessness. Some contaminations may be naturally found in the food supply, such as those derived from the soil as food plants are grown, e.g., some heavy metals. Residues or contaminants found in foods differ widely in chemical structure, but all possess toxic properties that may be a threat to human health. Some of these chemicals tend to accumulate in the food supply, being more toxic in higher-order mammals than in species of lower phylogenetic orders. For example, fish and crustaceans can tolerate much higher tissue levels of arsenic and mercury than can humans.

The objective of this chapter is to present how different residues affect our food supply and the potential health effects of such residues.

INSECTICIDES

Naturally occurring or synthetic pesticides are a diverse group of chemical agents used to control undesirable pests. The introduction of synthetic pesticides had an enormous impact on agriculture and human health. Dramatic increases in agricultural production, the so-called green revolution, in the U.S. in the past decades were achieved by the use of synthetic pesticides, herbicides, and fungicides. Insecticides and fungicides have been used and are being used to reduce postharvest losses of crops. Synthetic compounds that have been used for farming and food production have contributed to agriculture's success and affected our perception of the environment. For example, although current thinking has played down the usefulness of DDT (dichloro diphenyl trichloroethane), many lives were saved in Europe and Asia during and after World War II by controlling the mosquito vector of malaria transmission.

In the last few decades, attention has switched to the possible hazards to human health of pesticide residues in foods. Contamination of surface and groundwater by pesticides is recognized as a serious problem for agriculture. Most of the pesticides currently used degrade rapidly in the environment or are too insoluble to move through the environment. A few pesticides used in past years are persistent or mobile, or both.

DDT (1,1'-(2,2,2-Trichloroethylidene)bis(4-Chlorobenzene)

As a youngster growing up in Northern California in the 1960s, I have vivid memories of children running behind the DDT truck that sprayed the town streets to rid them of mosquitoes, which thrived because of the many adjacent rice fields near the town. DDT compounds were extensively used in the U.S. as pesticides before they were banned in 1973. In the 1960s, DDT production reached 170 million pounds (77 million kg), which were used in ca. 300 commodities. Subsequent to the ban, environmental exposure has declined substantially.

Dr. Paul Muller, a Swiss chemist, was awarded the Nobel Prize in Medicine in 1948 for his success in replacing a number of extremely dangerous chemicals then being used for pest control (arsenic, mercury, lead) with DDT, which he patented as a contact insecticide in 1939. Before the 1940s, because more than two thirds of the world's population lived in malaria-ridden areas, more than 200 million people worldwide were stricken yearly with malaria and 2 million malaria-related deaths occurred each year. DDT was heralded as one of the most important disease-preventing agents known to humans, highly lethal to insects and protecting field crops but remarkably harmless to human beings. DDT was used to dust people to kill lice, for which it was very effective. Figure 16.1 graphically shows the dramatic effect of DDT on saving lives. Ceylon, now Sri Lanka, provides examples of the positive impact of DDT on human health. Before the use of DDT, nearly 3 million cases of malaria were reported yearly in Ceylon (Table 16.1).

DDT application had an enormous impact on improving health in Ceylon. However, in 1964, the use of DDT was discontinued in Ceylon, which coincided with the publication of Carson's *Silent Spring*. By 1969, epidemic conditions reappeared in Ceylon.

Biologists linked DDT's increasingly indiscriminate use to the disappearance of songbirds and raptors. By then, the chemical had permeated the bodies of fish, livestock, and house pets. Some health officials expressed concerns, sometimes suggesting that the pesticide may be responsible for causing cancers in people who had applied it recklessly. Because of the advances in analytical chemistry and improved methods for detecting even minuscule amounts, it has been found that at present the bodies of most people carry at least traces of the compound. Time will tell whether the DDT ban was truly justified, particularly in terms of human lives lost.

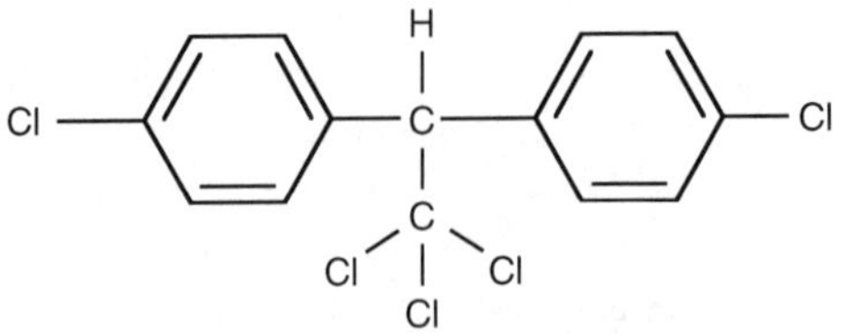

1,1'-(2,2,2-trichloroethylidene)bis(4-chlorobenzene) (DDT)

FIGURE 16.1 DDT (dichloro diphenyl trichloroethane).

TABLE 16.1
Malaria Cases in Ceylon between 1948 and 1969

Malaria Cases Reported	Year	Use of DDT
2,800,000	1948	No DDT
31	1962	Large-scale DDT usage
17	1963	Large-scale DDT usage
150	1964	Spraying discontinued
308	1965	
499	1966	
3466	1967	
16493	1968	
2,500,000	1969	

In retrospect, it is interesting to note that the attack on DDT and subsequent litigation has been based on three erroneous arguments. The first is that DDT was the cause of bird population diminution. Claims were made that DDT had caused the shells of bird eggs to become fragile, resulting in more breakage, contributing to the failure of birds to reproduce. Such claims were unfounded, and in one study DDT-laced worms fed to birds were unable to kill the birds or harm baby birds. Historical research has determined that bird eggshells have been becoming thinner long before DDT was used. The second argument was that DDT was so stable that it could never be eliminated from the environment. This argument was true and was the reason why DDT was so effective in the field. A single application could have long-lasting effects in preventing further insect infestation. The concern currently is whether the persistence of DDT in our bodies and the environment is a cause for alarm. Many studies have been done showing little in the way of adverse effects even with relatively high exposure levels to DDT. The third argument was that DDT might cause human diseases, including cancer. There is no evidence from human studies that DDT causes cancer. Individuals who have been occupationally exposed to high levels of DDT have been reported to only have transient effects such as tingling of the extremities. Some animal studies have reported the formation of hepatic tumors, but they appear to be artifactual.

Table 16.2 lists the LD_{50} of DDT for several animal species. Repeated administration of DDT to animals results in tremors, incoordination, muscular twitching, and weakness. It is likely that the effects are through repeated depolarization of the presynaptic nerve terminal. Repetitive discharge occurs in sensory, central, and motor neurons in DDT-poisoned insects. In dogs, rabbits, and monkeys, large doses of DDT produce convulsions, with changes confined mostly to the anterior horn cells. These effects have not been reported in humans.

In 1945, a scientist conducted a test on himself and inhaled 100 mg of pure DDT and drank water dusted at the rate of 3240 mg/m^2. He did not experience any ill effects. Oral doses of DDT to human volunteers were excreted as bis(p-chlorophenyl)acetic acid (DDA), which is promptly excreted in the urine.

TABLE 16.2
Acute Oral LD_{50} of DDT in Animals

Species	Oral LD_{50} (mg/kg)
Rat	500–2500
Mouse	300–1600
Guinea pig	250–560
Rabbit	300–1770
Dog	>300
Cat	100–410

With the current concern about other diseases that may be transmitted by mosquitoes and the lack of effective ways to eradicate these insects, one wonders whether DDT will be reevaluated for its potential rather than continue to be condemned. Although DDT can kill mosquitoes, a new study suggests that it primarily protects by repelling them. Thus, comparing DDT's killing action with that of other pesticides used for malaria control — the standard practice for 55 years — may be the wrong measure of its value.

ORGANOPHOSPHATES

Organophosphates (OPs) are the oldest of the synthetic pesticides. OPs have several commonly used names: organic phosphates, phosphorus insecticides, nerve gas relatives, phosphate, phosphate insecticides, and phosphorus esters or phosphoric acid esters. All compounds are derived from phosphoric acid, and, generally speaking, are the most toxic to vertebrate animals. Organophosphorus insecticides containing the P=S moiety owe their insecticidal activity and their mammalian toxicity to an oxidative reaction in which the P=S group is converted to P=O, thus changing from a compound relatively inactive to cholinesterases to one that is a potent cholinesterase inhibitor. Much of the research database came from Germany during World War II, because chemical structure and mode of action of OPs are similar to those of nerve gases. There are two distinct features of OPs. They are (1) more toxic to vertebrates than are the organochlorine insecticides, and (2) chemically unstable or nonpersistent. Thus, they have all the properties persistent organochlorines, particularly DDT, do not.

As noted, OPs exert their toxic action by inhibiting cholinesterases. Cholinesterases are responsible for removing acetylcholine in neurojunctions once electrical signals have been conducted across the gap by acetylcholine. Thus, OPs attach to cholinesterases in a way that prevents them from removing the acetylcholine, resulting in rapid twitching of voluntary muscles and eventually paralysis. Acetylcholine is the chemical transmitter of nerve impulses at the endings of postganglionic parasympathetic nerve fibers, somatic motor nerves to skeletal muscle, preganglionic fibers of both parasympathetic and sympathetic nerves, and certain synapses in the central nervous system. Signs and symptoms of organophosphorus insecticide poisoning that result from stimulation of these receptors include tightness in the chest and wheezing expiration due to bronchoconstriction and increased bronchial secre-

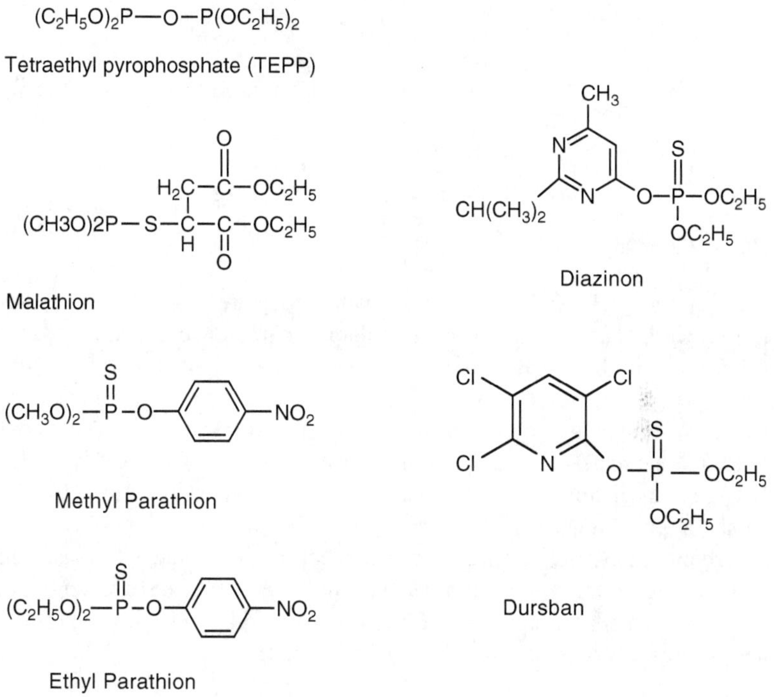

$(C_2H_5O)_2P-O-P(OC_2H_5)_2$

Tetraethyl pyrophosphate (TEPP)

Malathion: $(CH_3O)_2P-S-\underset{H}{\underset{|}{C}}-\underset{\parallel}{\underset{O}{C}}-OC_2H_5$ with $H_2C-\underset{\parallel}{\underset{O}{C}}-OC_2H_5$

Diazinon

Methyl Parathion: $(CH_3O)_2-\underset{\parallel}{\overset{S}{P}}-O-\text{C}_6\text{H}_4-NO_2$

Dursban

Ethyl Parathion: $(C_2H_5O)_2-\underset{\parallel}{\overset{S}{P}}-O-\text{C}_6\text{H}_4-NO_2$

FIGURE 16.2 TEPP, malathion, methyl parathion, ethyl parathion, diazinon, and dursban.

tions, and increased salivation and lacrimation. Sweating, increased gastrointestinal tone and peristalsis with nausea, vomiting, abdominal cramps, diarrhea, bardycardia, and contraction of smooth muscles of the bladder are other symptoms. The immediate cause of death in fatal organophosphate poisoning is asphyxia resulting from respiratory failure.

As a class of insecticides, OPs can be divided into three classes: aliphatic, phenyl, and heterocyclic derivatives (example illustrated in Figure 16.2). Aliphatic derivatives include tetraethyl pyrophosphate (TEPP), and malathion. Phenyl derivatives include parathion (methyl and ethyl) and heterocyclic derivatives include diazinon and dursban.

OPs are rapidly metabolized and excreted and do not accumulate in the body. Their structure accounts for their metabolism in insects and mammalian systems. The aromatic phosphate ester groups of parathion are resistant to enzymatic hydrolyses, but its metabolism in mammalian systems results in the activation to its toxic analog, paraoxon. On the other hand, malathion is easily metabolized by esterases and has low mammalian toxicity. The key to the usefulness of OPs is that residues on food products do not normally result in exposures sufficient to lead to health problems in humans.

CARBAMATES

These compounds are toxic alkaloids and analogs of physostigmine (Figure 16.3). The advantage of carbamate insecticides is that they target a narrower range of

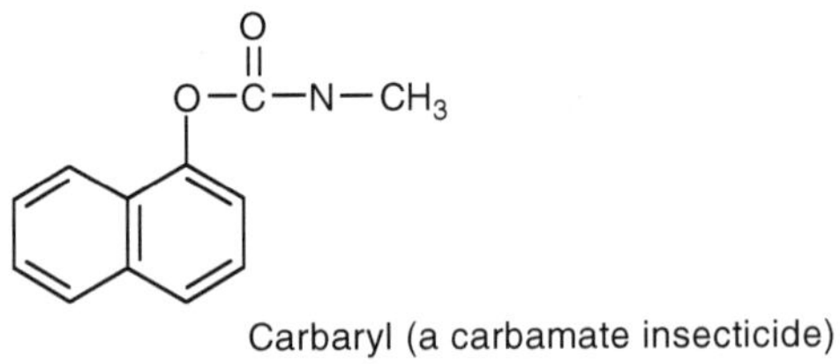

Carbaryl (a carbamate insecticide)

FIGURE 16.3 Carbaryl.

organisms than the OPs. The disadvantage is that they are highly toxic to beneficial insects too. Carbamates are quite water soluble and can accumulate to dangerous levels in foods with high water content. An example of such a problem occurred in California, where 250 individuals became ill as the result of contaminated watermelons. Thus, carbamates are not registered for use in food with high water contents, but their wide use makes contamination possible, as in the watermelon case.

Carbamate insecticides are cholinesterase inhibitors similar to OPs. Typical symptoms of poisoning include lacrimation, salivation, miosis, convulsion, and death. Carbamates are not considered broad-spectrum insecticides because some of the common household insects are relatively immune. Also, bees are very sensitive to these compounds. Carbamate insecticides are rapidly reversible inhibitors of cholinesterase with compounds such as atropine sulfate.

CYCLODIENE INSECTICIDES

This is an important group of chlorohydrocarbons, such as aldrin and dieldrin, the structures of which are shown in Figure 16.4. Cyclodienes are persistent insecticides and are stable in soil and relatively stable to the ultraviolet of sunlight. As a result, they are used as soil insecticides to control termites and soilborne insects whose larval stages feed on the roots of plants. The mode of action is neurotoxicity. Unlike DDT, cyclodienes have a positive temperature correlation, i.e., their toxicity increases with increase in the surrounding temperature. Cyclodienes act on the inhibitory mechanism mediated by the GABA (gamma-aminobutyric acid) receptor. This receptor operates by increasing chloride ion permeability of neurons. Cyclodienes appear to affect all animals in generally the same way, first with nervous

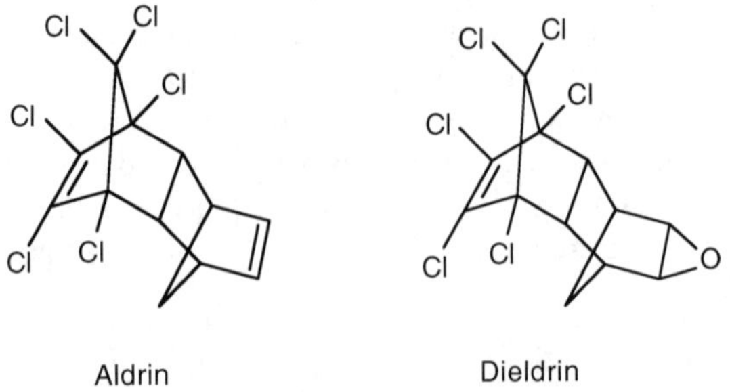

Aldrin   Dieldrin

FIGURE 16.4 Aldrin and dieldrin.

activity, followed by tremors, convulsions, and prostration. They, like DDT, are highly lipid soluble and quite stable and accumulate in animal tissues. Production and use of these compounds have been sharply curtailed.

HERBICIDES

Weeds and other nonfood plants can reduce yield by ca. 10%. Herbicides, or chemical weed killers, have largely replaced mechanical methods of weed control, especially where intensive and highly mechanized agriculture is practiced. The field hand with the hoe is gone because herbicides provide a more effective and economical means of weed control than cultivation, hoeing, or pulling weeds by hand. Many herbicides have been developed to control weed growth for not only crops but other areas too, such as industrial sites, roadsides, irrigation canals, fence lines, recreation areas, and golf fields. Many herbicides can be classified as selective, killing weeds without harming the crop, whereas others are nonselective, killing all vegetation. Other ways to classify herbicides include selectivity of herbicides, contact vs. translocation, timing, area covered, and chemical means.

Like insecticides, trace residues of herbicides can be found in final food products. However, the mere identification of a substance in food does not automatically imply that people are at risk. The list of herbicides is long, but this discussion limits the description to a few examples.

CHLOROPHENOXY ACID ESTERS (PHENOXYALIPATIC ACIDS)

Discovered in 1944, these compounds have the ability to mimic indole acetic acid, a plant hormone, which disrupts the growth of broadleaf weeds and woody plants. Figure 16.5 shows the structures of two typical chlorophenoxy herbicides, 2,4-D and 2,4,5-T. Chlorophenoxyl herbicides have complex mechanisms of action resembling those of plant growth hormones, or auxins. Their actions affect cellular division, modify nucleic acid metabolism, and activate phosphate metabolism. These compounds were the active ingredients in the defoliant Agent Orange used during the Vietnam War. Several reports note that 2,4-D and 2,4,5-T have been used for years on a large scale worldwide, with no apparent adverse effects on human or

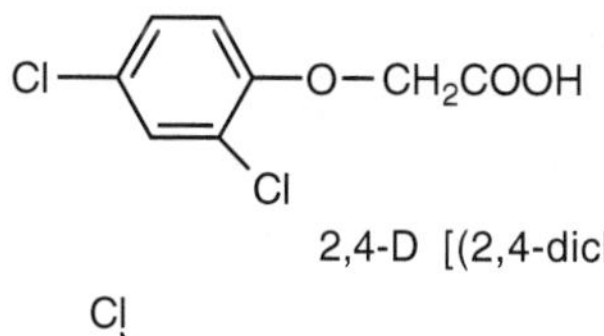

2,4-D [(2,4-dichlorophenoxy) acetic acid]

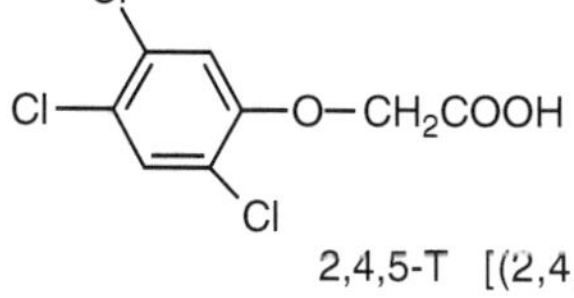

2,4,5-T [(2,4,5-trichlorophenoxy) acetic acid]

FIGURE 16.5 2,4-D and 2,4,5-T.

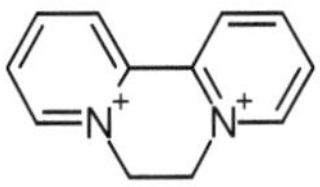

Diquat [6,7-dihydrodipyrido(1,2-alpha:2',1'-c)pyrazidinium]

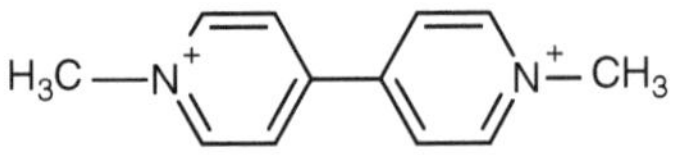

Paraquat [1,1'-dimethyl-4,4'-bipyridylium ion]

FIGURE 16.6 Diquat and paraquat.

animal health. It has been observed that 2,4,5-T used in Agent Orange contains excessive amounts of tetrachlorodioxin, a suspected toxic impurity.

The acute toxicities of chlorophenoxy acid esters are between 375 and 500 mg/kg, and they have relatively low toxicities in mammals. Some symptoms of toxicity include muscle weakness, ataxia, paralysis, and coma.

Bipyridyliums

This group of bipyridyl compounds fell from use because of its proven pulmonary toxicity. There are two important herbicides in this group: diquat and paraquat. On contact with the herbicides, plant tissues are quickly damaged, producing a frostbite appearance. The cell membrane is extensively damaged and photosynthesis is reduced. Both compounds (Figure 16.6) are not active in soils. The action on vegetation is spectacular and the application of the herbicide is available only to professional weed control specialists.

Cases of accidental or suicidal fatalities resulting from paraquat poisoning have been documented. Pathological changes observed are lung, liver, and kidney damage. The most striking change is a widespread cellular proliferation in the lungs. Ingestion of paraquat results in GI upset within a few hours of exposure, followed by the onset of respiratory symptoms and subsequently death by respiratory distress. The LD_{50} for paraquat in guinea pigs, cats, and cows is 30 to 50 mg/kg. Rats are more resistant, with an LD_{50} of 125 mg/kg. The LD_{50} for humans is estimated at about 40 mg/kg. Diquat produces acute and chronic effects that differ from those produced by paraquat in that the lung toxicity is not seen. Hyperexcitability leading to convulsions and distention of the GI tract and discoloration of intestinal fluids occur. Long-term ingestion of diquat at 0.05% causes cataracts. Studies have shown that the mechanism of action of dipyridyls is through free-radical–induced damage.

FUNGICIDES

Fungicides are chemicals used to kill or halt the development of fungi. There are hundreds of examples of plant diseases caused by fungi, such as storage rots, root rots, vascular wilts, leaf blights, rusts, smuts mildews, and seedling diseases. Early

$CH_3OCH_2CH_2HgCl$

Ceresan (2-methoxyethylmercuric chloride)

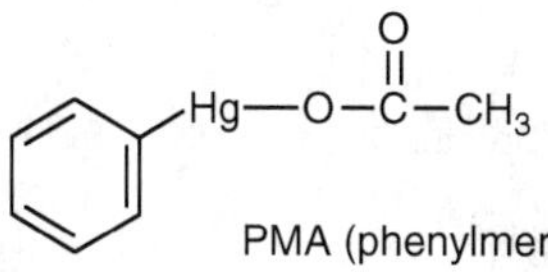

[Structure: phenyl–Hg–O–C(=O)–CH₃]

PMA (phenylmercury acetate)

FIGURE 16.7 Ceresan and PMA.

and sometimes continued application of selective fungicides can control fungi, but the problem with these diseases is that they occur either below ground and cannot be reached by fungicides or they may be systemic within the plant. Fungal diseases can be more difficult to control with chemicals than are insects. The major difficulty is to find a chemical that kills the fungus without harming the plant. It is also necessary that fungicides be applied to protect plants during stages when they are vulnerable to the pathogen, often before there is any evidence of disease, i.e., prophylactic application.

This class of pesticides is another heterogenous group of chemical compounds. Only a few fungicides have attracted some toxicological research. Although many of these compounds are used to control fungal diseases on plants or seeds of plants, they are rather nontoxic. The notable exception is mercury-containing fungicides. A host of organic mercury compounds that were developed several decades ago has been replaced by other organic fungicides. Ceresan and phenylmercury acetate (PMA) are typical examples. Ceresan was used for seed treatments, whereas PMA was useful for turf diseases (see Figure 16.7). The mode of action for the mercurials was the nonselective inhibition of enzymes, particularly those containing iron and sulfhydryl sites.

INDUSTRIAL AND ENVIRONMENTAL CONTAMINANTS

More than 40,000 chemical substances are logged by the Environmental Protection Agency (EPA) in its inventory of chemicals subject to the Toxic Substances Control Act. Most do not pose a threat to human health, but some certain incidents have indicated that they can be a potential hazard.

HALOGENATED HYDROCARBONS

Polychlorinated Biphenyls

PCBs (trade name Aroclor®) were first synthesized in 1881 and generically refer to several chlorinated isomers of biphenyl (two chemically bonded benzene rings and one or more chlorine atoms), shown in Figure 16.8. This family of ca. 200 chemical compounds exhibits physical characteristics ranging from light oily sub-

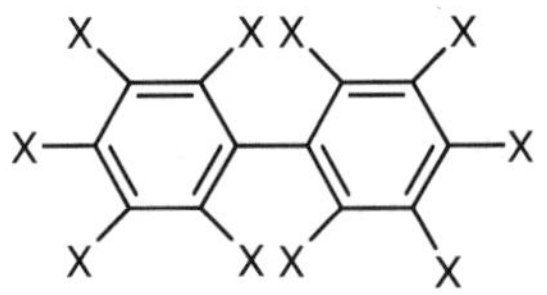

X = to H or Cl   Structure of polychlorinated biphenyls

FIGURE 16.8 Polychlorinated biphenyls.

stances to greasy and waxy substances. The molecular structure of PCBs has considerable resistance to acids, bases, high temperature, and electrical current, and is nonflammable. They were used as dielectrics (insulating fluids) in the electrical industry and in old transformers, capacitors, and hydraulic fluids. PCBs were used in food packaging material made from recycled paper. PCBs are also used in plasticizers, paints, lubricants, insulating tapes, fireproofing material, and inks. PCB production was discontinued in 1977; however, more than a billion pounds (0.5 billion kg) was produced in the U.S. It is estimated that about two-thirds was degraded or destroyed, but because of their high degree of stability, ca. 400 million pounds of discarded PCBs may be present in the environment.

Both acute and chronic effects of PCBs have been demonstrated in several animal species. Levels of 50 ppm in the diet of chicks result in depressed weight gain, edema, hyperparacardial fluid formation, internal hemorrhaging, increased liver size, and depression of secondary sexual characteristics. Levels as low as 2.5 to 5 ppm in the diet have been shown to produce severe acne-like skin eruptions (chloracne) and edema in female rhesus monkeys. In addition, the menstrual cycles are altered and pregnancies are problematic. The offspring delivered by the monkeys have lower birth weights and high contents of PCBs in their fatty tissues. Male monkeys exhibited no changes in reproductive function and only minor symptoms of toxicity. The symptoms exhibited by monkeys fed PCBs are similar to those documented in a case involving an industrial accident in Japan. In 1978, rice oil was contaminated with 3000 ppm of PCBs because of discharges from PCB heat-transfer agents into water used to irrigate rice fields. Over 1000 individuals had symptoms of chloracne, pigmentation of the skin and nails, edema, and weakness, and experienced vomiting, diarrhea, and weight loss (Yusho disease). Young children experienced growth retardation and 35.5% of the deaths in a 11-year period were traced to cancer. In the years after the poisoning episode in Japan, it has become less evident that PCBs were the cause of the health problems. Researchers claim that the original PCB fluid may have been converted to polychlorinated dibenzo-furans, which are far more toxic.

In rat studies, PCBs were shown to be involved in carcinogenesis. The liver is quite sensitive to the effects of PCBs, resulting in increased organ weight, hypertrophy, and proliferation of smooth endoplasmic reticulum. Also, microsomal cytochrome P450 increases markedly following exposure to PCBs, which may contribute to the metabolic activation of such compounds to active carcinogens. Long-term rat studies show that animals fed with PCBs at a level of 100 ppm developed hepatic preneoplastic lesions. However, a reevaluation of the rat studies found that the number of rats with benign or malignant liver tumors was less than that originally reported. Also, it was found that not all PCB mixtures are equal and that only PCBs with greater than 60% chlorination cause some cancer in rats.

Although PCB contamination in the environment in the U.S. is significant, liver cancer is relatively rare. Some of the highest levels of PCB contamination have been found in fish taken from the Great Lakes. Tissue levels range from 10 ppm to as high as 25 ppm, which has influenced local agencies to post warnings against consumption or tolerance levels of fish caught in their waters. Yet, an evaluation of health histories and current medical problems of those who ate the fish exposed to PCB did not reveal any significant differences. People who ate more fish had higher levels of PCB in the blood, but did not have any associated ill-health effects.

Extensive occupational studies of long-term exposure to PCBs in electrical-equipment workers showed no significant adverse health effect other than occasional skin irritations. Studies by both the National Institute for Occupational Safety and Health (NIOSH) and General Electric confirmed that even workers with PCB blood levels of up to 300 ppm, compared with levels of 10 to 20 ppb for nonworkers, did not exhibit any health effects, not even chloracne.

Although PCBs are persistent in the environment, no evidence exists that background levels or levels found among heavily exposed workers are a threat to health. It is preferable not to let PCBs or any other contaminant enter our bodies; however, the reaction to PCBs might have been overzealous. The EPA has reevaluated its position and has adopted a less stringent stance for cleanup. Unfortunately, other groups have been slow to grasp what science has found, thus costing taxpayers many millions of dollars for cleanups.

Dioxins

These are a large class of compounds that contain oxygen atoms held by ether linkages to carbon atoms, usually within a six-member ring. Trace amount of dioxins, such as chlorinated dibenzo-p-dioxins, occur in commercial chemical formulations, such as herbicides. Dioxins have been found in many reactions in which organic and chlorine-containing substances are burned together. Some of these compounds, such as tetrachlorodibenzo-p-dioxin (TCDD), are among the most potent toxicants known (Figure 16.9). TCDD is chemically very stable and binds strongly to solids or particulate matter in the soil, and is lipophilic but sparingly soluble in water or organic liquids.

The LD_{50} for TCDD in the guinea pig is under 1 mg/kg, although for the hamster it is more than 10 g/kg. Thus, the guinea pig is extremely sensitive to TCDD toxicity.

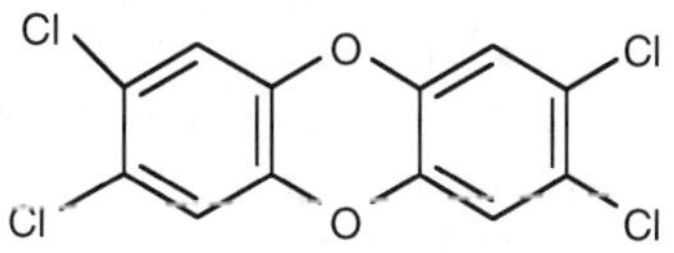

FIGURE 16.9 Tetrachlorodibenzo-p-dioxin (TCDD).

Liver lesions, adrenal atrophy, chloracne, and kidney abnormalities have been reported. Both skin and kidney effects appear in many species, which are likely targets for TCDD toxicity. In addition, TCDD is a promoter of carcinogenesis and is a carcinogen. Liver tumors and tumors of the mouth, nose, and lung have been found. TCDD may be three times more potent a carcinogen than is aflatoxin B_1. In addition, TCDD is a potent teratogen in mice and rabbits. Pregnancy ends in dose-dependent increased resorption and higher rates of postimplantation loss. TCDD is fetotoxic to the rhesus monkey, resulting in higher levels of abortion and death in pregnant females.

Based on the outcome of accidental TCDD exposures to humans, people seem to be less sensitive to the toxic effects of TCDD. Many hundreds of cases involving industrial accidents, and in one situation 37,000 residents of Seveso, Italy, had no fatalities. Documented toxic effects in humans include chloracne, fatigue, disturbances in the peripheral nervous system, and liver toxicity.

The most publicized health claim of neurological and particularly teratogenic effects made about TCDD was the exposure of Vietnam veterans to Agent Orange. Agent Orange was the military code name given to the fifty-fifty mixture of herbicides 2,4,5-T and 2,4-D. During the Vietnam War, Agent Orange was credited with saving many lives of the U.S. military by destroying enemy food crops. Dioxin was known to be a contaminant in 2,4,5-T, but dioxin has never been shown to be a human teratogen. In 1969, scientists reported a high rate of birth defects in laboratory animals exposed to 2,4,5-T and 2,4-D, which caused the suspension of the use of Agent Orange by the Department of Defense. In contrast to self-reported health problems by Vietnam veterans, studies by the National Cancer Institute and the American Cancer Society found no increased risk for most cancers and no links between birth defects and exposure to Agent Orange.

HEAVY METALS

Mercury

Mercury is a naturally occurring metal having several forms. Metallic mercury is a shiny, silver-white, odorless liquid. Mercury combines with other elements, such as chlorine, sulfur, or oxygen, to form inorganic mercury compounds or salts, which are usually white powders or crystals. Metallic mercury is used to produce chlorine gas and caustic soda, and is also used in thermometers, dental fillings, and batteries. Mercury also combines with carbon to make organic mercury compounds, such as methyl mercury, produced mainly by microscopic organisms in the water and soil. More mercury in the environment can increase the amounts of methyl mercury that the small organisms make.

The nervous system is very sensitive to all forms of mercury. Methyl mercury and metallic mercury vapors are more harmful than other forms, because more mercury in these forms reaches the brain. Exposure to high levels of metallic, inorganic, or organic mercury can permanently damage the brain, kidneys, and developing fetus. Effects on brain functioning may result in irritability, shyness, tremors, changes in vision or hearing, and memory problems. Short-term exposure to high levels of metallic mercury vapors may cause lung damage, nausea, vomiting, diarrhea, increases in blood pressure or heart rate, skin rashes, and eye irritation. There is inadequate human cancer data for all forms of mercury. Mercuric chloride has caused increases in several types of tumors in rats and mice, and methyl mercury has caused kidney tumors in male mice. Thus, the EPA has concluded that mercuric chloride and methyl mercury are possible human carcinogens.

Children are more sensitive to mercury than are adults, and mercury in the mother's body passes to the fetus. Mercury can also pass to a nursing infant through breast milk. However, most scientists agree that the benefits of breast-feeding may be greater than the possible adverse effects of mercury in breast milk. Children poisoned by mercury may develop problems in their nervous and digestive systems and suffer from kidney damage.

The EPA has set a limit of 2 parts of mercury per billion parts of drinking water (2 ppb). The Food and Drug Administration (FDA) has set a maximum permissible level of 1 part of methyl mercury in a million parts of seafood (1 ppm). Three major scientific arms (fishing industry, government agencies, and scientific bodies) may also be on a collision course. Fish are a good low-cost, low-fat source of nutrition, rich in healthy omega-3 fatty acids. However, there is strong indication that children *in utero* are more sensitive than adult humans. This stance is supported by two large controlled longitudinal studies of effects of prenatal mercury exposure from seafood consumption on child neurodevelopment (Seychelles Islands in the Indian Ocean and Faroe Islands near Scotland). Large, long-lived predatory ocean fishes, such as tuna, swordfish, king mackerel, and shark, bioaccumulate methyl mercury in the edible portions.

Some local and state agencies have had regulatory programs in effect for more than 20 years. In Wisconsin, women of childbearing years, nursing mothers, and children below 15 years have been warned only to eat one meal per week of bluegill, sunfish, crappie, yellow perch, or bullheads and only one meal per month of pike, catfish, sturgeon, carp, and bass.

It is well established that the organic forms, such as methyl mercury, are the more toxic mercury compounds. Their effects on the nervous system follow a sharp dose–response curve. The mechanisms of action involve the property of lipid solubility and the affinity of such compounds for protein sites rich in sulfhydryl groups. These same sites are frequently responsible for the functional properties of many proteins, such as enzymic activity and redox reactions. Methyl mercury is toxic to cerebral and cerebellar cortices, causing focal necrosis of neurons and destruction of glial cells. In addition, methyl mercury is a known teratogen.

The paradox becomes more complicated when one considers that several nutrients have a profound effect on mercury and methyl mercury toxicity (selenium, zinc, vitamins C and E). For more than 30 years, the protective effects of selenium against mercury have been known. Many marine organisms that have high tissue levels of mercury also have high tissue levels of selenium, or a mercury-to-selenium tissue ratio of 1:1 stoichiometrically. Thus, the apparent survival of certain species in the conditions of mercury intoxication may be related to a detoxification mechanism involving interactions between mercury and selenium. An interaction between the two elements may involve sequestering and neutralizing the toxic effects of either ionic mercury or organic mercury. Selenite (SeO_3) may act to both demethylate methyl mercury and form a molecular detoxification product of selenite and mercuric ion, which exhibits similarities to a synthetic Hg–Se–S species. Research in Europe has demonstrated the usefulness of a remediation process of adding selenium salts to mercury-contaminated lakes. The work has resulted in improving the ecology of such areas, including survival of endogenous aquatic organisms. However, U.S. agencies have not willingly grasped the concept of using a toxic element to remediate another toxic element.

Much more research is needed to develop a better understanding about the potential toxicant–dietary interactions and special susceptibilities. There are critical data gaps on exposure and neurological, immunological, and cardiovascular effects from toxicant–nutrient interactions. It is possible that such interactions result in overall better nutrition, health, and ecological stability.

Lead

Before the dangers of lead were established, this heavy metal was found in a variety of consumer products, e.g., lead solders, lead water pipes, lead-based paints, lead-glazed glasses, and automobile gasoline (antiknock gasoline additive tetraethyl lead). Thus, considerable concern has been expressed about contamination of food and water occurring over a long period of time. It is likely that the lead content of food has not increased because the soil retains lead effectively. Exposure of food to lead likely increases surface contamination of the food. However, lead-containing consumer products have made a major impact, particularly lead-based paints and gasoline, and children have been the most affected.

Weight reduction, anemia, renal function, and central and peripheral nervous system effects have been attributed to chronic ingestion of lead. Lead poisoning is usually due to occupational situations. Lead absorption in children is ca. 40% but in adults is only 10%. Distribution of lead is highest in the bone (95%), followed by soft tissues and blood. Anemia is a function of lead's inhibition of red blood cell heme synthesis. A sensitive indicator of hematological changes associated with lead intoxication is the enzyme δ-aminolevulinic acid (δ-ALA) dehydratase.

Neurological disorders may be related to low lead levels and may go unnoticed in the developing brains of children. Lead passes the placental and the blood–brain barrier of the fetus. Because children are highly vulnerable to the neurotoxic effects of lead, exposure has to be prevented, particularly by reducing intakes from dust and pica.

Federal and state regulatory standards and programs have helped minimize or eliminate the amount of lead in consumer products, occupational settings, and the environment; this decreased presence has contributed to remarkable reductions in lead poisoning in children in the U.S. Symptomatic childhood lead poisoning seen a decade ago in children with markedly elevated blood lead levels (>40 µg/dl) has almost disappeared as a clinical finding in the U.S., where the average blood lead level is currently 2.9 µg/dl.

The important concern currently is whether the continued focus on trace amounts of lead, such as in consumer products (e.g., cosmetics and dietary supplements), adequately takes into account the relative exposures these sources represent. It is likely that the lead in these products is not toxicologically significant and will not pose a health risk to humans. Claims of subtle neurobehavioral effects in children due to elevated blood lead levels are not based on firm evidence; many studies that attempt to link low-level lead exposure with learning disabilities, behavioral problems, attention deficit disorders, and lowered IQ are complicated by multiple confounding socioeconomic and familial factors. Unfortunately, there is a significant degree of public confusion regarding the Centers for Disease Control (CDC) action level of 10 µg/dl, which is the lowest level at which the CDC recommends initial action, limited to education and follow-up testing. Specific clinical intervention measures are not recommended until blood lead levels exceed 20 µg/dl.

Subsequently, targeted rather than universal screening for elevated lead levels is preferred in order to cost-efficiently identify children and other individuals with an increased risk of elevated blood lead levels. Lead abatement of homes should not be universally mandated, but be considered on a case-by-case basis; proper remediation techniques and attention to resident exposure during remediation are critical. Elimination or minimization of exposure to lead can be successfully achieved through alterations in personal habits, increased public education, and improvements in living conditions, particularly among population groups known to have higher likelihood of exposure.

Cadmium

Extensive industrial use has contributed to cadmium being widely distributed in the environment. Because organic cadmium compounds are unstable, most of the cadmium in foods is as inorganic cadmium salts. Cadmium may be electrolytically deposited as a coating on metals, chiefly iron or steel, on which it forms a chemically resistant coating. Alloys of cadmium with lead and zinc are used as a solder for iron. Cadmium salts are used in photography and to manufacture fireworks, rubber, fluorescent paints, glass, and porcelain. Cadmium sulfide is employed in a type of photovoltaic cell.

Cadmium is absorbed easily by and found in all parts of food plants. In animals and humans, cadmium can be found in the liver, kidney, and milk. Cadmium can be found in all foodstuffs, and particularly high amounts occur in organs of cattle, seafood, and some mushroom species. Although the absorption of cadmium is low in the GI tract, it has a long biological half-life because it accumulates in the body. In contrast, cadmium absorption by inhalation is four to five times more. Smokers can have an intake of 4 µg/d. Several factors impact on the amount of cadmium deposited in people. Absorption of cadmium from food varies and depends on age, nutritional status, and genetic factors. Adults accumulate less cadmium than do children. Cadmium absorption increases when the calcium or iron status is poor. Acute toxicity of cadmium affects the liver and the erythropoietic system. Chronic exposure of cadmium affects kidney and bones. High-fiber and low-fat diets interfere with the absorption of cadmium, and mineral levels of calcium, zinc, iron, and phosphorus lower the body retention of cadmium.

Accumulation of cadmium in the body of laboratory animals is associated with anemia, hypertension, and testicular damage. In Japan, chronic cadmium intoxication over a 12-year period has occurred in some populations that consumed rice contaminated with cadmium because of pollution. A painful disease (itai itai, meaning "ouch ouch," bone disease] developed, with symptoms of skeletal deformation and multiple fractures.

After absorption, cadmium binds to the protein metallothionein in cells of the intestinal tract wall and in the liver. Metallothionein is a key protein that contributes to the homeostasis of essential zinc and copper and in the detoxification of heavy metals. If people do not eat foods that contain enough iron or other nutrients, they are likely to take up more cadmium than the usual from their food. The general population and people living near hazardous waste sites may eat or drink cadmium in food, dust, or water.

Cadmium that enters the body stays in the liver and kidneys. Cadmium leaves the body slowly in urine and feces. The body keeps most cadmium in a form that is not harmful, but too much cadmium can overload the kidneys' storage system and damage health. Cadmium has no known good effects on health. However, one report suggests that rats have inhibited growth with very low intakes of the metal.

Breathing air with very high levels of cadmium severely damages the lungs and can cause death. Breathing lower levels for years leads to a build-up of cadmium in the kidneys, which can cause kidney disease. Long-term oral exposure to cadmium leads to nephrotoxicity. Renal effects always occur before or with other effects. Other effects that may occur after breathing cadmium for a long time are lung damage and fragile bones. Workers who inhale cadmium for a long time may have an increased chance of getting lung cancer. There is no proof about mice or hamsters getting lung cancer on breathing cadmium. However, some rats that breathe cadmium develop lung cancer. In humans, breathing cadmium can affect the ability to have children or can harm unborn babies. Female rats and mice that breathe high levels of cadmium have fewer litters and the pups may have more birth defects than usual. Breathing cadmium causes liver damage and changes in the immune systems of rats and mice. Eating food or drinking water with very high cadmium levels severely irritates the stomach, leading to vomiting and diarrhea. Eating lower levels of cadmium over a long period of time leads to a build-up of cadmium in the kidneys. This cadmium build-up causes kidney damage and also causes bones to become fragile and break easily. Animal studies have shown a relationship between cadmium in the drinking water and hypertension, iron-deficient blood, liver disease, and nerve or brain damage. Studies on humans and animals that had high intakes of cadmium did not show an increase in cancer. The International Agency for Research on Cancer has determined that cadmium is probably carcinogenic to humans. The EPA has determined that cadmium is a probable human carcinogen by inhalation. However, skin contact with cadmium is not known to cause health effects in humans or animals.

Arsenic

Populations have always been exposed to high arsenic levels in food, drinking water, wine, and other sources. Arsenic is found as inorganic and organic compounds. It is found naturally in rocks and soil worldwide, and industrial effluents contribute significant amounts. Arsenic is used in large quantities in the manufacture of glass to eliminate a green color caused by impurities of iron compounds. Arsenic is sometimes added to lead to harden it and is also used in the manufacture of such military poison gases as lewisite and adamsite. Until the introduction of penicillin, arsenic was of great importance in the treatment of syphilis. In other medicinal uses, it has been displaced by sulfa drugs or antibiotics. Lead arsenate, calcium arsenate, and Paris green are used extensively as insecticides. Arsenic is abundant in seafood, but in an organic form, arsenobetaine, that is not toxic and rapidly absorbed and excreted in the urine and bile.

Exposure to inorganic arsenic in drinking water is associated with health risks related to the duration and level of exposure, particularly above 300 ppb. Acute poisoning is associated with vomiting, bloody diarrhea, abnormal heart rhythm, esophageal and abdominal pain, and sometimes death because of cardiopulmonary collapse. Classical syndromes of chronic arsenic exposure include hyperkeratosis, corns, and warts on the feet (blackfoot) and hands. Studies from Taiwan and Japan strongly suggest that high arsenic intake is associated with cancers of the bladder, kidney, lung, and liver, which may be dose-related. Arsenic may be an indirect carcinogen.

In contrast to adverse effects of arsenic, small amounts of the metal may be essential to the body. Approximately 10 to 50 ppb might be necessary to maintain homeostasis of the body. In laboratory animals, low levels of arsenic fail to support normal weight gain and decrease the ability to become pregnant. Also, arsenic (arsenic trioxide) has been used successfully to treat patients with acute promyelocytic leukemia (APL).

The EPA recently reduced the standards for arsenic in drinking water from 50 ppb to 10 ppb. This will impact significantly on municipalities, which must deal with the regulation and reduce arsenic in their drinking water.

STUDY QUESTIONS AND EXERCISES

1. Speculate on the likelihood of a resurgence of DDT use in the U.S. as well as around the world.
2. Why are animals deficient in vitamin E or vitamin C more sensitive to paraquat poisoning?
3. Heavy metals interact extensively with sulfur amino acids, and dietary selenium has been known to follow the sulfur pathway. Suggest a mechanism of action for selenium's purported usefulness in protecting against heavy metal toxicity. Search the literature for reports on the interaction of selenium and heavy metals.
4. Heavy metal toxicity seems to be aggravated by reduced antioxidant status. What mechanism may be responsible for this aggravation?

RECOMMENDED READINGS

Dietz, R. et al., An assessment of selenium to mercury in Greenland marine animals, *Sci Tot. Environ.*, 245, 15-24, 2000.

Ecobichon, D.J., *Occupational Hazards of Pesticide Exposure: Sampling, Monitoring, Measuring*, Taylor & Francis, London, 1998.

Gailer, J. et al., Structural basis of the antagonism between inorganic mercury and selenium in mammals, *Chem. Res. Toxicol.,* 13, 1135-1142, 2000.

Goldman, L.R. and Shannon, M.W., Mercury in the environment: implication for pediatricians, *Pediatrics,* 108, 197-212, 2001.

O'Dell, B.L. and Sunde, R.A., *Handbook of Nutritional Essential Mineral Elements,* Marcel Dekker, New York, 1997.

Underwood, E.J., *Trace Elements in Human and Animal Nutrition,* 3rd ed., Academic Press, New York, 1971.

Trebacz, W. R. et al., Methylmercury and total mercury in tissues of arctic marine mammals. *Sci Tot. Environ.* 218, 19-31, 1998.

Waxman, M.F., *The Agrochemical and Pesticides Safety Handbook,* Lewis Publishers, Boca Raton, FL, 1998.

Whitford, F., *The Complete Book of Pesticide Management: Science, Regulation, Stewardship, and Communication,* John Wiley & Sons, New York, 2002.

17 Food Additives, Colors, and Flavors

For some consumers, processed food conjures up images of a food dead of nutrients and stripped of vitamins and fiber, and replaced with chemicals and worthless filler, or technology toying with nature in the name of profit.

From the beginning of time, humans have invented ways to preserve food after harvest and slaughter to make it last longer, be more palatable, and, in recent times, be more readily available for use. Fire and root cellars were among the first forms of food processing humans tried. Drying and fermentation are ancient practices of food processing. There is evidence from Egyptian tombs that food was cooked, salted, and dried. Both beer and wine, products of fermentation, were part of daily meals. The ancient Chinese were likely the first to go beyond the traditional preservation methods. They discovered that placing fruit near a burning kerosene lamp caused the fruit to ripen. This method was an early use of what was later attributed scientifically to the effects of ethylene, a fruit-ripening factor. Drying and salting techniques were widely used, and in some countries salt for flavor and preservation became so valued that it was used as a form of payment.

The modern era of food processing came during Napoleon's quest for power in 1810. Driven by concerns about feeding his army far from home, Napoleon offered a prize of 12,000 francs to anyone who could develop a stable ration. The French chef Nicholas Appert found that one could fill bottles with food and after the bottles were sealed with corks, they could be heated in boiling water, and this process made foods last for some time. Thus was invented the food process of canning or appertization.

The objectives for food processing are to make food look, taste, and smell as though it has not been preserved and to allow the food to be safely eaten at a later date. In recent times, the objectives have been modified to include the development of totally new food products that offer a higher level of convenience to the consumer. To accomplish these objectives, food science has found means to stop microbial growth and chemical reactions, however, not without some destruction of flavor, color, texture, and nutritive value.

The advantages of food processing are that these methods make foods safer (inhibit microbes), enhance nutrient value of food (e.g., adding iodine to salt or skimming of fat from milk and enrichment or fortification of foods), allow choice (regular and reduced fat, reduced cholesterol, fat-free), increase sensory properties of food (air in ice cream), provide convenience, and offer variety (unusual and ethnic foods).

There are some drawbacks of food processing. Food processing causes some nutrient loss compared with the raw material. Some food products seem to have little by way of nutrient benefit for the consumer, but may provide a degree of consumer satisfaction. One concern, which may be a sign of our modern society, is that total reliance on processed foods may result in the loss of skills for food preparation. Finally, packaging of processed foods has created environmental and energy concerns; for example, potato, the common staple, requires little energy for storage unless it is processed and frozen, as demanded by consumers.

The use of additives is an important part of food processing. A food additive is any substance not normally consumed as food but added to food either intentionally or by accident. Intentional additives are substances put into foods on purpose, whereas accidental (incidental) additives are substances that may get into the food by accident before or during food processing. Some intentional additives include nutrients, preservatives, colors, and antioxidants, and incidental additives include packaging material, metals, veterinary drugs, and pesticides.

The 1958 Food Additives Amendment to the Food, Drug, and Cosmetic Act requires that if food processors wish to add a substance to food, they must submit a petition to the Food and Drug Administration (FDA) with documentation on chemistry, use, function, and safety. On careful review that the substance is safe, the FDA will authorize it with specific conditions. When this amendment was passed, many substances were exempted from complying with the FDA procedure because there were no known hazards in their use at that time. The list of substances became known as the GRAS (generally recognized as safe) list. Since 1958, some substances on the GRAS list have been reviewed, and a few, such as cyclamate and red dye #3, were removed because new information linked them to health problems. However, many of the chemicals on the GRAS list have not been rigorously tested and it is likely they will not be tested because of their long-time histories of use without any proof of harm or because their chemical structures do not suggest they could cause harm. One of the standards an additive had to meet in order to be placed on the GRAS list was that it must not have been found to be a carcinogen in any test on animals or humans. This cause was intended to prohibit intentionally adding to foods a substance that was introduced after 1958 that causes cancer. Over the years, the Delaney Clause had come under fire for not allowing for the difference in effects on the body of varying dose levels. The value of animal cancer tests was questioned. For example, when the artificial sweetener cyclamate was banned in 1969, it was estimated that a human would have to daily drink at least 138 twelve-oz bottles of soft drinks containing cyclamate in order to mimic the dose given to rats in the test to cause the ban. Clearly, the dose makes the poison.

Another broad way to classify additives is based on whether the substance is synthetic or natural. Natural additives refer to the group of substances of plant, or, in some cases, animal origin. Synthetic food additives must be extensively evaluated for toxicity before being allowed for use in food.

PRESERVATIVES

This is a group of substances added to food to keep them edible for an extended period of time, usually by preventing the growth of bacteria and fungi. Overall, preservatives are harmless at the levels ingested and beneficial for their ability to reduce or prevent the risks due to microorganism contamination.

BENZOIC ACID AND SODIUM BENZOATE (FIGURE 17.1)

These compounds have long been used as antimicrobial agents. They are found at concentrations of 0.05 to 0.1% in beverages, fruit salads, jams and jellies, preserves, margarine, various relishes, pies, soy sauce, etc. The sodium form is preferred because it is more water soluble than the free acid. The LD_{50} in rodents is 2700 mg/kg. The symptoms of toxicity include weight loss, diarrhea, internal bleeding, enlargement of the liver and kidney, hypersensitivity, and paralysis followed by death. Benzoic acid can be conjugated with glycine and appear in the urine as hippuric acid.

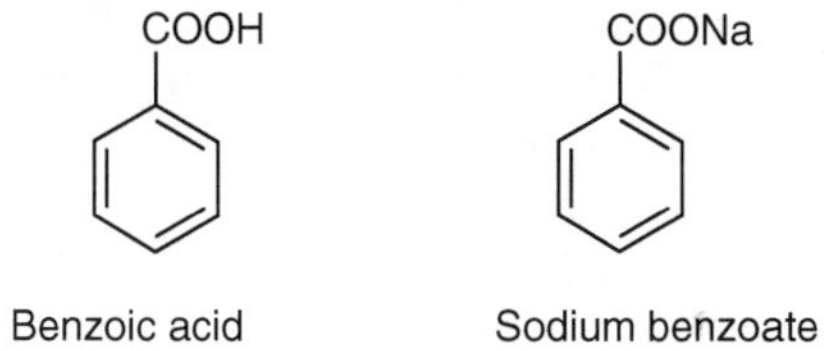

FIGURE 17.1 Benzoic acid and sodium benzoate.

SORBATE (FIGURE 17.2)

These compounds have broad-spectrum activities against yeast and molds. Sorbates have been used as preservatives in margarine, fish, cheese, bread, and cake. Sorbic acid is relatively nontoxic (LD_{50} = 10.5 g/kg). When dissolved in water, potassium sorbate ionizes to form sorbic acid, which is effective against yeasts, molds, and selective bacteria, and is widely used at 250 to 1000 ppm in cheeses, dips, yogurt, sour cream, bread, cakes, pies and fillings, baking mixes, dough, icing, fudges, toppings, beverages, margarine, salads, fermented and acidified vegetables, olives, fruit products, dressings, smoked and salted fish, confections, and mayonnaise.

In many food products, sorbate and benzoate are used together to provide greater protection against a wider variety of microorganisms (synergism). This is possible only if the pH of the product is below 4.5.

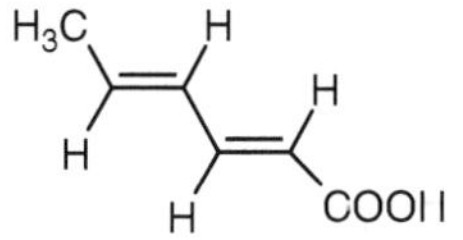

FIGURE 17.2 Sorbic acid.

$$H_2O_2$$

FIGURE 17.3 Hydrogen peroxide.

HYDROGEN PEROXIDE (FIGURE 17.3)

This compound has been used in the dairy industry as a substitute for heat pasteurization. It has also been used for its bleaching effect in cheese and fish-paste products. The LD_{50} in rats is 700 mg/kg.

NITRITE AND NITRATE

FDA food additive regulations for these compounds cover their uses in fish products and in preparations for curing of meats and meat products. These substances prevent growth of *C. botulinum*, the bacterium responsible for the highly potent botulinum toxin. However, a decrease in the incidence of botulism may be accompanied by increase in the formation of carcinogenic nitrosamines in meat products containing nitrite or nitrate. The acidic conditions in the stomach favor nitrosamine formation. Nitrosamines are known mutagens and carcinogens. They have been reported to induce a variety of cancers, such as those of the liver, respiratory tract, kidney, esophagus, stomach, and pancreas. Nitrosamine bioactivation is through cytochrome P450, involving oxidative N-dealkylation.

In addition to carcinogenic effects, nitrites and nitrates reduced by bacteria to nitrites can oxidize hemoglobin to methemoglobin. Methemoglobin poorly binds to oxygen and leads to a state of anoxia, which can be life threatening, particularly to children.

ANTIOXIDANTS

These substances are important because they are used to protect oils and fats against lipid peroxidation or oxidative rancidity. Foods rich in lipids and polyunsaturated fatty acids are extremely sensitive to oxidation, which results in changes of color, odor, taste, and nutritional value. Two types of antioxidants are recognized: (1) radical scavengers, which interfere with the propagation step, thereby terminating lipid peroxidation (e.g., BHT, vitamin E); and (2) synergists, which either regenerate the parent radical scavenging antioxidants from the radical formed in the interference with the propagation step, or act by chelating transition metals that are catalysts in the initiation and propagation steps of lipid peroxidation (e.g., vitamin C, ethylenediaminetetraacetic acid).

ASCORBIC ACID

Vitamin C (Figure 17.4) is not only a nutrient but also an important antioxidant in many foods. It is water soluble and can break down easily. Vitamin C is relatively nontoxic. Vitamin C may act as a radical scavenger or as a synergist. However, vitamin C in high levels and in the presence of metals such as iron and copper can cause oxidative damage.

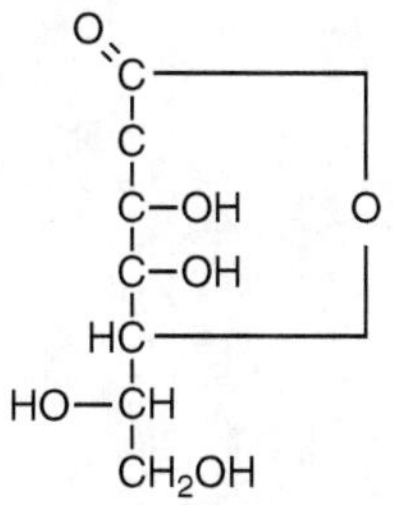

Food Additives, Colors, and Flavors

FIGURE 17.4 Ascorbic acid

TOCOPHEROL

Vitamin E (Figure 17.5) is an important lipid-soluble antioxidant. It is crucial in protecting unsaturated fatty acids from oxidative breakdown and preventing rancidity. The toxicity is low, but high concentrations (>2000 ppm) in oils promote prooxidant effects, particularly if metal ions are present.

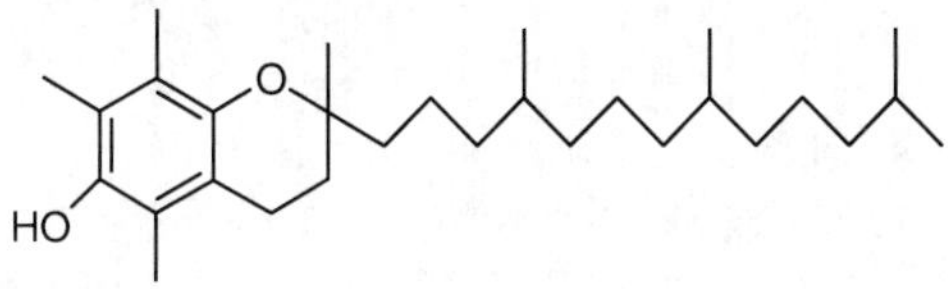

FIGURE 17.5 α-Tocopherol

PROPYL GALLATE

Propyl gallate, or *n*-propyl-3,4,5-trihydroxybenzoate, is used as an antioxidant in vegetable oils and butter. The bitter taste restricts its use in some foods. Figure 17.6 shows the structure of propyl gallate.

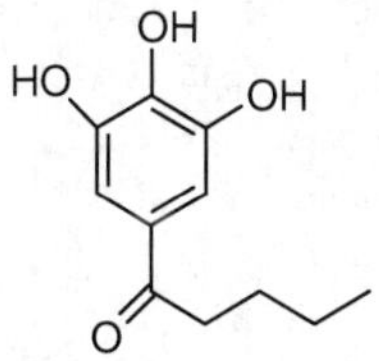

FIGURE 17.6 Propyl gallate.

BHT AND BHA

Butylated hydroxyanisole (BHA) and butylated hydroxytoluene (BHT; Figure 17.7) are very commonly used antioxidants in the food industry. Both are GRAS substances, limited by a total antioxidant content of not more than 0.02% of the oil or fat content of the food. They are also found as additives in dry cereals, shortenings, potato products, dessert mixes, and in beverages and desserts made from dry mixes.

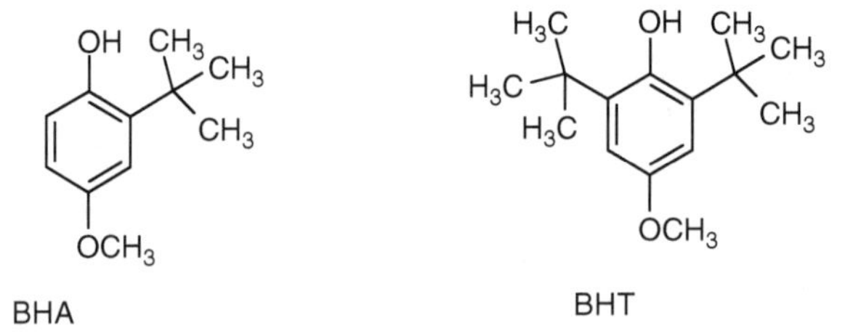

FIGURE 17.7 BHA and BHT.

BHT prevents degenerative oxidation of fats, which can lead to off-flavor and destruction of essential fatty acids and lipid-soluble vitamins. It also prevents the formation of toxic oxidation by-products. BHT was tested in the National Cancer Institute's Carcinogenesis Testing Program, which concluded that BHT was not carcinogenic for rats or mice.

SWEETENERS

SACCHARIN

It is not likely that saccharin (1,2-benzisothiazole-3(3H)-one 1,1-dioxide) would have been discovered today given the current emphasis on cleanliness and safety. The story goes that saccharin was discovered by a chemistry graduate student in 1879 at The Johns Hopkins University in Baltimore while working on the synthesis of a toluene derivative. Apparently, he was having lunch while working on the synthesis, and when he grasped his bread with unwashed hands, he discovered that it tasted very sweet. The sweet taste was found to be from one of the derivatives, saccharin. Saccharin (Figure 17.8) is ca. 500 times sweeter than sucrose.

This well-known nonnutritive artificial sweetener has very low toxicity. The saccharin molecule does not undergo metabolism, and several studies have shown that it is not genotoxic or carcinogenic. Very early studies using laboratory rats indicated that bladder tumors were produced in the offspring of dams fed 7.5% saccharin throughout pregnancy. The results were complicated by the presence of contaminants in the study saccharin.

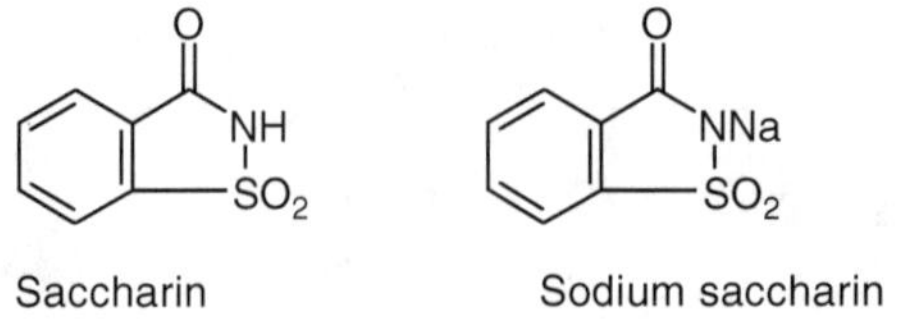

FIGURE 17.8 Saccharin and sodium saccharin.

SODIUM CYCLAMATE

This odorless, white crystalline powder is 30 times sweeter than sucrose. Two-year studies done in rats fed sodium cyclamate (Figure 17.9) resulted in bladder cancer.

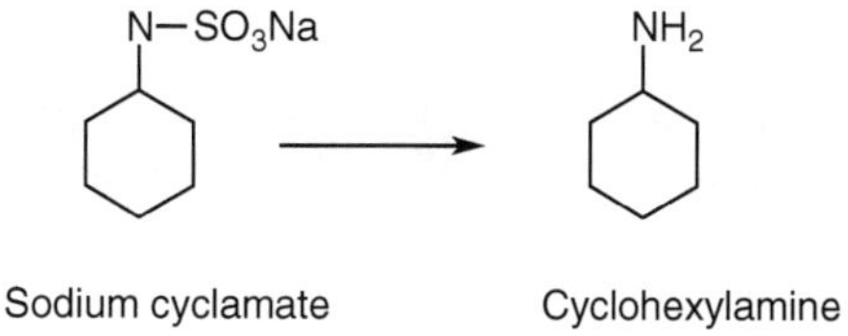

Food Additives, Colors, and Flavors

[Structures: Sodium cyclamate → Cyclohexylamine]

Sodium cyclamate   Cyclohexylamine

FIGURE 17.9 Sodium cyclamate.

Cyclamate can be converted to cyclohexylamine, which is extremely toxic. In 1968, studies completed by the FDA demonstrated that sodium cyclamate was a teratogen in rats and in 1969 the compound was banned.

ASPARTAME

This molecule is a dipeptide consisting of L-aspartic acid and the methyl ester of L-phenylalanine. Aspartame undergoes hydrolysis into three components, aspartic acid, phenylalanine, and methanol, in the gastrointestinal tract. Although shown to be safe, the released phenylalanine can lead to disturbances in individuals who are homozygous phenylketonuric. Such individuals lack the ability to hydroxylate phenylalanine. Figure 17.10 gives the structures of aspartame and metabolites of aspartame.

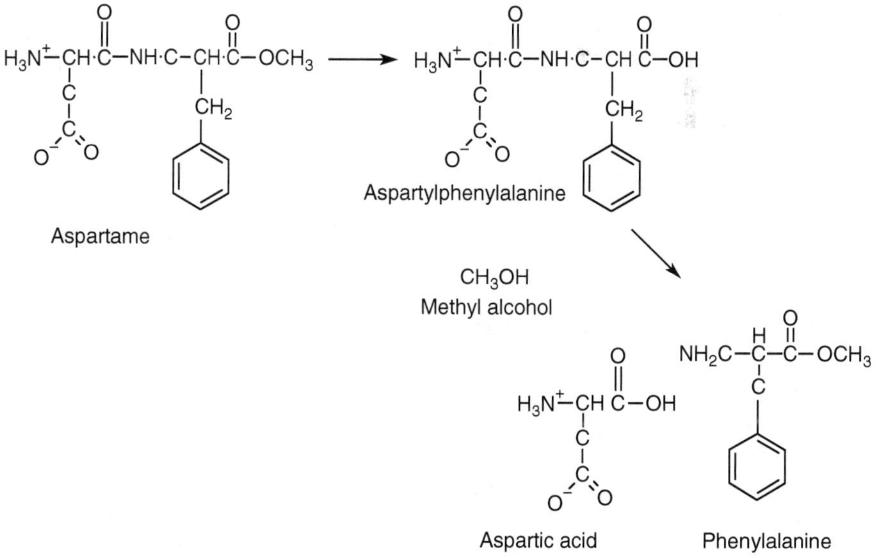

[Structures showing aspartame metabolism: Aspartame → Aspartylphenylalanine + CH₃OH (Methyl alcohol); Aspartylphenylalanine → Aspartic acid + Phenylalanine]

FIGURE 17.10 Aspartame metabolism.

ACESULFAME

Acesulfame was approved by the FDA in 1988 as an alternative sweetener. Acesulfame is 200 times sweeter than sucrose. It is not digested and contributes no energy to the diet.

Sugar Alcohols

The sugar alcohols sorbitol, mannitol, and xylitol are absorbed or metabolized to glucose more slowly than are simple sugars. They are often marketed to diabetic diets, but contribute to energy and affect blood glucose levels.

Alitame

Alitame, or Aclame™, is formed from two amino acids, L-aspartic acid and D-alanine, and is ca. 2000 times sweeter than sucrose.

D-Tagatose

D-Tagatose is a compound derived from lactose and is equal to sucrose in sweetness but with only half its energy value.

Sucralose

In sucralose, three of the hydroxyl groups of sucrose are substituted with chlorine atoms. Sucralose is 800 times sweeter than sucrose. Sucralose is a nonnutritive, high-intensity sweetener made from a process that begins with sucrose. It is a free-flowing, water-soluble white crystalline powder that, on average, is ca. 600 times sweeter than sugar.

Sucralose is being approved for use in baked goods, baking mixes, nonalcoholic beverages, chewing gum, coffee and tea products, confections and frostings, fats and oils, frozen dairy desserts and mixes, fruit and water ices, gelatins, puddings and fillings, jams and jellies, milk products, processed fruits and fruit juices, sugar substitutes, sweet sauces, and toppings and syrups. It can also be used as a tabletop sweetener, i.e., added directly to foods by consumers.

Sucralose is marketed under the brand name Splenda®. Preapproval research showed that sucralose caused shrunken thymus glands and enlarged liver and kidneys; however, the dose of sucralose in the experiments was high. The manufacturer claimed that sucralose was unpleasant for the rodents to eat in large doses. They said that starvation caused the shrunken thymus glands. Sucralose breaks down into small amounts of 1,6-dichlorofructose, a chemical that has not been adequately tested in humans.

In determining the safety of sucralose, FDA reviewed data from more than 110 studies in humans and animals. Many of the studies were designed to identify possible toxic effects, including carcinogenic, reproductive, and neurological effects. No such effects were found, and FDA's approval is based on its finding that sucralose is safe for human consumption.

COLORING AGENTS

Color additives have long been a part of human culture. Ancient Egyptian writings tell of drug colorants, and historians say food colors likely emerged around 1500 B.C. Through the years, color additives typically came from substances found in nature, e.g., turmeric, paprika, and saffron. But in the 20th century, new kinds of colors appeared that offered marketers wider coloring possibilities, many developed in the chemist's laboratory.

In the late 1800s, some manufacturers colored products with potentially poisonous mineral- and metal-based compounds. Toxic chemicals tinted certain candies and pickles, whereas other color additives contained arsenic or similar poisons. Thus, injuries, even deaths, resulted from tainted colorants. Food producers also deceived customers by employing color additives to mask poor product quality or spoiled stock. Color additives spread through the marketplace in all sorts of popular foods, including ketchup, mustard, jellies, and wine. Questions about safety were brought up, because many color additives had never been tested for toxicity or other adverse effects. In the 1900s, the bulk of chemically synthesized colors was derived from aniline, a petroleum product that in pure form is toxic. Originally, these were dubbed coal-tar colors, because the starting materials were obtained from bituminous coal. Manufacturers had strong economic incentives to use these products. Chemically synthesized colors were easier to produce, less expensive, and superior in coloring properties. Only tiny amounts were needed. They blended nicely and did not impart unwanted flavors to foods.

Although the 1938 law did much to bring color use under strict control, nagging questions lingered about tolerance levels for color additives. One incident in the 1950s, in which scores of children contracted diarrhea from Halloween candy and popcorn colored with large amounts of FD&C Orange No. 1, led FDA to retest food colors. As a result, in 1960, the 1938 law was amended to broaden FDA's scope and allow the agency to set limits on how much color could be safely added to products. FDA also instituted a premarketing approval process, which requires color producers to ensure before marketing that products are safe and properly labeled. Should safety questions arise later, colors can be reexamined. The 1960 measures put color additives already on the market into a provisional listing. This allowed continued use of the colors pending FDA's conclusions on safety.

The FDA certifies over 11.5 million pounds of color additives every year. Of all colors, straight dye FD&C Red No. 40 is by far the most popular. Manufacturers use this orange-red color in all sorts of gelatins, beverages, dairy products, and condiments. FDA certified more than 3 million pounds of the dye in fiscal year 1992, almost a million pounds more than the runner-up FD&C Yellow No. 5.

RED NO. 2 (AMARANTH)

In the early 1970s, data from Russian research raised concerns about the safety of Red No. 2. However, several subsequent studies showed no hazards, and FDA's own tests were inconclusive. The Toxicology Advisory Committee evaluated numerous reports and found that there was no evidence of a hazard. FDA scientists evaluated the biological data and concluded that at a high dosage Red No. 2 results in a statistically significant increase in malignant tumors in female rats. Although there was no positive proof of either potential danger or safety, the FDA ultimately decided to ban the color because it had not been shown to be safe. The agency based its decision in part on the presumption that the color might cause cancer. Although gone from U.S. shelves, products tinted with Red No. 2 can still be found in Canada and Europe. The industry can petition FDA to list Red No. 2 as a certifiable color if animal study data adequately show safety. Because of the cost, it is unlikely that industry will commission new animal studies to measure Red No. 2's safety.

Red No. 3

In 1990, FDA outlawed several uses of the strawberry-toned FD&C Red No. 3, invoking the Delaney Clause. The banned uses include cosmetics and externally applied drugs, as well as uses of the color's non-water-soluble form. FDA previously had allowed these provisional uses while studies were in progress to evaluate the color's safety. Research later showed large amounts of the color cause thyroid tumors in male rats. Though FDA viewed the cancer risk by Red No. 3 as low, ca. 1 in 100,000 over a 70-year lifetime, the agency banned provisional listings because of Delaney directives. At the same time, Red No. 3 has permanent listings for food and drug uses that are still allowed, although the agency has announced plans to propose revoking these uses as well. For now, Red No. 3 can be used in foods and oral medications. Products such as maraschino cherries, bubble gum, baked goods, and all sorts of snack foods and candy may contain Red No. 3.

According to the International Association of Color Manufacturers, Red No. 3 is widely used in the industry and hard to replace. It makes a very close match for primary red, which is important in creating color blends. It does not bleed, and therefore drug companies use it to color pills with discernible shades for identification.

Yellow No. 4 (Tartrazine)

Clinical symptoms of asthma, hyperactivity, and urticaria have been attributed to tartrazine. However, considerable controversy exists in the association between such symptoms and tartrazine.

Methyl Anthranilate

Methyl anthranilate is found in neroli oil and in citrus and other oils. It is prepared synthetically by esterification of anthranilic acid. It is a colorless to pale yellow liquid with a bluish fluorescence. It has a grape-like odor. The acute LD_{50} in rodents is 3000 to 4000 mg/kg. Also, methyl anthranilate, a biochemical pesticide, is exempt from the requirement of a tolerance when used in accordance with good agricultural practices on the following raw agricultural commodities: blueberry, cherry, corn, grape, and sunflower.

Safrole

Safrole (3,4-methylene-dioxyallylbenzene, $C_{10}H_{10}O_2$, mol. wt. 162.19) was once used as a flavoring ingredient in root beer; however, it was banned in the 1960s after reports that it was carcinogenic in rodent studies. Safrole is found in trace amounts in many species such as black pepper, cinnamon, and sweet basil. Safrole and related compounds are found in many edible plants, including sassafras. The FDA banned the sale of sassafras tea in 1976.

Monosodium Glutamate (MSG)

Monosodium glutamate (MSG) is the sodium salt of glutamic acid. It is derived from glutamate, an amino acid found in all protein-containing foods and one of the most abundant and important components of proteins. Glutamate occurs naturally in protein-containing foods such as cheese, milk, mushrooms, meat, fish, and many vegetables. Glutamate is also produced by the human body and is vital for growth, nerve metabolism, and brain function.

When MSG is added to foods, it provides a flavoring function similar to the glutamate that occurs naturally in food and has been used effectively to bring out meaty taste in foods. Many researchers also believe that MSG imparts a fifth taste, "umami," independent of the four basic tastes of sweet, sour, salty, and bitter. This taste in Japan is described as savory or meaty. It works well with a variety of foods such as meats, poultry, seafood, and many vegetables. It is used to enhance the flavor of some soups, stews, meat-based sauces, and snack foods.

The average adult consumes ca. 11 g of glutamate per day from natural protein sources and less than 1 g of glutamate per day from MSG. In contrast, the human body creates ca. 50 g of glutamate daily for use as a vital component of metabolism.

The U.S. FDA has found no evidence to suggest any long-term serious health consequences from consuming MSG. It is possible that some people might be sensitive to MSG, as they are to many other foods and food ingredients. There are some reports that mild, temporary reactions to MSG may occur in a small portion of the population, based on tests with a large dose of MSG in the absence of food.

STUDY QUESTIONS AND EXERCISES

1. Distinguish between intentional and incidental food additives. Provide a few examples of each and describe how incidental additives get into foods and why intentional additives (function of additives) are added to foods.
2. Discuss how the Delaney Clause has impacted on the use of food additives in foods and the implication this clause has on safety evaluation of additives. Put into perspective the benefits and risks of additives in foods.
3. List the common food-preservation techniques and provide examples of each.
4. The federal government reviews the safety of new food additives before they can be used in foods sold on the market. Describe the agencies involved and how laws in the U.S. assist promotion of food safety.

RECOMMENDED READINGS

Foulke, J.E., A fresh look at preservatives, *FDA Consum.*, 23-31, October 1993.
Hatchcock, J.N., and Rader, J., Food additives, contaminants and natural toxins, in *Modern Nutrition in Health and Disease*, Shils, M.E., Olson, J.A., and Shike, M., Eds., Lea & Febiger, Philadelphia, 1994.
Henkel, J., From shampoo to cereal — seeing to the safety of color additives, *FDA Consum.*, 14, December 1993.

Parke, D.V. and Lewis, D.F.V., Safety aspects of food preservatives, *Food Add. Contam.*, 9, 561-577, 1992.
Roberts, H.R., Food additives, in *Food Safety*, Roberts, H. R., Ed., John Wiley & Sons, New York, 1981, pp. 239-293.
Trebole, E., *Food Safety, Additives and Contaminants*, Nutrition Dimension, San Marcos, CA, 1991. Verhagen, H., Adverse effects of food additives, in *Food Safety and Toxicity*, DeVris, J., Ed., CRC Press, Boca Raton, FL, 1997, pp. 121-132.
Wuthrich, B., Adverse reactions to food additives, *Ann. Aller.,* 71, 379-392, 1993.

18 Food Irradiation

For many consumers, the phrase *food irradiation* conjures up images of devastation, debilitation, or concerns regarding danger to both life and the environment. Much of the unfounded fear is created by equating irradiation with its root word *radiation*. Food irradiation is a food preservation process or method that can protect food from microorganisms, insects, and other pests that can make our food supply unsafe or undesirable. Compared with other food preservation processes, food irradiation has many advantages, such as low energy consumption and low cost (even compared with conventional refrigeration and deep freezing). It is a cold process, which means that there are no changes in texture of the food, such as those that occur with canning or freezing. Food irradiation is an excellent alternative to chemical fumigants, such as the banned ethylene dibromide, and as a process is extremely effective to control many foodborne diseases, e.g., salmonellosis. Finally, as a process, food irradiation can reduce postharvest losses, which can be a vital tool in the war to eliminate world hunger. Currently, farmers lose as much as 30% of their harvest because of pests, and this loss can be reduced by food irradiation.

Irradiation is the process in which food is passed through a chamber, where it is exposed to gamma rays or x-rays. These high-energy rays are strong enough to break chemical bonds, destroy cell walls and cell membranes, and break down DNA. Thus, irradiation kills most bacteria, molds, and insects that may contaminate food. Irradiation also delays the ripening of fruits and sprouting of vegetables, permitting produce to be stored for longer periods of time. Because irradiation involves minimal heating, it has very little effect on the taste, texture, and nutritive value of food.

The Food and Drug Administration (FDA) first approved irradiation for use on wheat and wheat flour in 1963, and later approved its use on white potatoes, spices, pork, some fresh produce (onions, tomatoes, mushrooms, and strawberries), and poultry (Table 18.1). In 1997, in response to several foodborne illness outbreaks and increasing public concern over the safety of food supply, irradiation was approved for use on poultry products. In 1999 and 2000, irradiation was approved to curb pathogens in raw meats, including ground beef, steaks, and pork chops. Irradiation has also been used for more than 30 years to preserve some meals eaten by astronauts during long-term space missions. Some consumer groups have raised concerns that irradiation might cause the formation of toxic compounds in food. Because of these and other concerns, only a limited amount of irradiated food has been sold in the U.S. Irradiation gained notoriety in the winter of 2001, when the process was employed by the U.S. Postal Services to sterilize mail. After rejecting other methods, such as steam, heat, anthrax foam, and other toxic gases, the postal service was convinced that irradiation was the way to handle anthrax and other potential biot-

TABLE 18.1
Tracing the History of Food Irradiation

Year	Events
1905	First patents for the use of ionizing radiation targeting pests in foods
1920s	Irradiation used by French scientists to preserve foods
1921	U. S. patent to use x-ray irradiation to kill *Trichinella spiralis* in meat
1940	Testing to use irradiation of common foods by the U.S. Department of Army
1958	Amendment of the Food, Drug, and Cosmetic Act, defining source of irradiation for use in processing foods
1963	Irradiation approved for use to control insects in wheat
1964	Irradiation approved for use to extend shelf life of white potatoes
1966	U.S. Department of Army and U.S. Department of Agriculture petition FDA to approve irradiation of ham
1970s	Irradiation adopted by NASA to sterilize food for the space program
1980	U.S. Department of Army transfers food irradiation program to the U.S. Department of Agriculture
1983	Irradiation approved for use in spices and dry vegetables to kill insects and bacteria
1985	Low-dose irradiation approved to control *Trichinella* in pork
1986	Irradiation approved for use in fruits and vegetables to control insects and promote product maturation
1990, 1992	Irradiation approved for used in poultry to control *Salmonella* and other bacteria by FDA and USDA, respectively
1997	Irradiation approved for use in beef and other read meat
2000	Irradiation permitted for use in refrigerated and frozen uncooked meat and meat by-products and in fresh shell eggs to control *Salmonella*

errorism threats. The postal service handles more than 100 billion pieces of first-class mail every year, and the average mail carrier handles 2300 letters every day.

HISTORY OF FOOD IRRADIATION

As noted in Table 18.1, the benefits of ionizing radiation have been known since 1905. In addition to its potential to reduce the incidence of foodborne diseases, food irradiation can be used to eliminate pests such as the screw worm fly, which preys on cattle, the Mediterranean fruit fly, and the tsetse fly, by the release of sterile insects. Worries about nuclear weapons, combined with an antiprogress ideology, began to hinder food irradiation research after the war. Although there was at that time an adequate supply of gamma rays, the high-energy, short-wavelength rays given off by radionuclides, the antitechnology faction convinced the Congress to control the development of nuclear technology for treating foods.

In 1958, when the Food, Drug, and Cosmetic Act was passed by the U.S. Congress, there were many unanswered questions. Would irradiated food be made radioactive? What would be the effect of this additional radioactivity above that of the background on human health? Would irradiation of food produce new toxic products such as carcinogens? Would the process produce products with excessive loss of nutrients or changes in food taste, odor, color, or texture? In the killing of pathogens, would new microbiological problems evolve? Also, what would be the adverse effects, if any, on the environment should there be accidents? What sources of radiation (gamma) and what doses would be suitable for irradiation?

Successful lobbying by well-known public figures in the movie and entertainment circles convinced the Congress to keep food irradiation under tight control, i.e., treating ionizing radiation as a "food additive." This part of the 1958 law, known as the Delaney Clause, assured that no irradiated food could be approved for consumption without a lengthy drawn-out procedure, thereby singling out and stigmatizing foods so treated by requiring a long period for research and petition writing to the FDA and the U.S. Department of Agriculture (USDA) and then many months or years for evaluation.

After 1961–1962, the U. S. Department of Army's food radiation research and development program made it the top priority to try to sort out the diverse claims, either pro or con, about irradiated foods. The U.S. Army Medical Services completed studies for testing in rats, mice, and beagle dogs, using 21 foods representing all major food classes in the diets of U.S. people. In June 1965 in a hearing by the Joint Committee on Atomic Energy, the army surgeon general submitted a statement that all foods irradiated at sterilizing doses up to 5.6 Mrad (56 kGy) using cobalt-60, or electrons at energies below 10 MeV, were wholesome, i.e., safe to eat and nutritionally adequate.

Nutritional assessments showed that the irradiation process was no more destructive to nutrients than other processes then being used commercially. It was also demonstrated that there were no toxic products formed in quantities that would be hazardous to the health and well-being of consumers.

The microbiological standard for irradiation-sterilized foods was to use a radiation dose sufficient to reduce a theoretical population of spores of *Clostridium botulinum*. This standard, recommended by the National Academy of Sciences and the National Research Council Advisory Committee to the army's program on food irradiation, was adopted. In the ensuing years, there was no record of any problem with possible *C. botulinum* survivors, although this has continued to be one of the antinuclear arguments against food irradiation.

Thousands of irradiated components of meals have been served to volunteers. In every respect, the tested irradiated foods have passed with soaring results. Irradiated foods have been eaten by astronauts on the moon flights and on many other space missions, by immunocompromised patients, and by military personnel in several parts of the world.

Every conceivable possibility for harm has been carefully considered — none has been found. Nor have any chemicals formed that are unique to food irradiation. In the meantime, irradiated foods have been approved by the health authorities in 40 countries.

Between 1964 and 1997, the World Health Organization (WHO), in concert with the Food and Agricultural Organization (FAO) and the International Atomic Energy Agency (IAEA), held a series of meetings of experts from many countries to assess the quality and safety of foods. In a meeting in September 1997, they recommended the approval of irradiated foods without restrictions at all doses, up to the highest dose compatible with organoleptic properties. At each meeting, the internationally recognized health authorities have concluded that all irradiated foods are safe to eat without the need for further toxicological testing, at doses as high as those allowing an acceptable taste.

In view of the foregoing, food scientists believe that the FDA and the USDA should follow the WHO/FAO/IAEA recommendation that food irradiation is a process. Scientists have thought for three decades that the legal fiction designating ionizing radiation as a food additive, instead of a food process, unjustly penalized food irradiation and helped delay its implementation for more than 30 years. On the other hand, during these years, the additive designation has stimulated those working in the field to perform at the highest level of good science, thus convincing the scientific community worldwide that food irradiation has an important role to play in combating hunger and disease.

In totality, scientists have reached their objective in documenting that food irradiation is a safe and beneficial process. Now scientists need to educate government officials, as well as health workers, food processors, marketers, and the public, on the safety and advantages of food irradiation.

With approximately 9000 people dying annually from food poisoning in the U.S., and an estimated 30,000,000 cases of food infection each year, there is little doubt that the time has come to use food irradiation more widely for the benefit of human health. Ironically, in applying ionizing radiation to protect public health against foodborne pathogenic bacteria, public health officers currently face the same arguments that were voiced against pasteurization at the beginning of the century and later against canned and frozen foods. In the history of pasteurization, many voiced disbeliefs of pasteurization's benefits for sanitation, nutrition, physical and bacteriological quality, consumer health and safety, and economics. Loss of hair, skin tone, and general well-being, as well as potency, was also claimed. These mistaken beliefs are cited currently against the irradiation of food.

Food irradiation is now recognized as another method of preserving food and ensuring its wholesomeness by sterilization or cold pasteurization, and has wide application worldwide. If it had been in place in the U.S., recent foodborne disease outbreaks caused by *E. coli* O157:H7, which are found in food-producing animals, would not have occurred. There have been tens of thousands of *Salmonella, Campylobacter, Yersinia, Listeria,* and *Escherichia coli* foodborne disease outbreaks related to poultry and meat, the totals exceeding millions of human illnesses, over the last 40 years since the Delaney Clause established the travesty that gamma rays were a food additive.

We may never know how many thousands of deaths and illnesses could have been prevented if public health authorities had implemented food irradiation and educated the public about its benefits. The morbidity and medical expense of meat- and poultryborne diseases can be prevented, just as milkborne disease can be prevented by pasteurization. All the bacteria cited previously can be present in unpasteurized milk, even though the U.S. Public Health Service Grade A standards require that milk be free of disease-causing organisms. Imagine the public outcry if governments allowed the marketing of unpasteurized milk in which *Salmonella* or *E.*

coli virulent strains were found or soft cheese or Mexican-style cheese in which *Listeria* was found.

In 1984, Margaret Heckler, Secretary of Health, endorsed food irradiation, after lengthy studies had proven its safety. If public health officers had spoken out then for the irradiation of foods that are known to carry pathogenic bacteria, events such as the *E. coli* O157:H7 outbreaks from undercooked hamburger (3 deaths and more than 400 cases of illness) that occurred in the northwest U.S. in January 1993 could have been prevented. Even today, no national or state local health authority speaks in favor of requiring pasteurization by irradiation of hamburger meat patties, of which some tens of millions are consumed daily. The same attitude and apathy exist in Europe, where *Listeria*-contaminated pork meat and other food caused the death of 63 persons in France, as reported in 1993. Since then, *Listeria* has become a serious public health problem in the U.S.

TYPES OF IRRADIATION

What is irradiation? Irradiation is defined as exposure to radiation (rays). *Radius* is taken from Latin, meaning *ray*. The radiation used in the food irradiation process comes either from radioactive isotopes of cobalt or cesium or from devices that produce controlled amounts of x-rays, gamma rays, or high-energy electrons. The process exposes food to radiation but does not and cannot make the food radioactive. Gamma rays and x-rays emit waves of high frequencies and high energies. These waves produce enough energy to strip electrons from atoms, leaving ions (particles charged with electrical charge), or ionizing radiation. Ionizing radiation is the energy that exists in the form of waves and is defined by its wavelength. As the wavelength of energy gets shorter, the energy of the wave increases. The electromagnetic spectrum (Figure 18.1) identifies the kinds of energy that exist and how they are used. Visible light, radio and television waves, and microwaves are examples of nonionizing radiation. They cause molecules to move, but they cannot structurally change the atoms in the molecules. The energy is measured by frequency (Hz), which is the number of times per second that the wave completes its cycle in an electromagnetic field.

Simple cooking involves the absorption of infrared radiation or heat by the food. Early on, it was found that shortwave radiation could melt things such as a chocolate

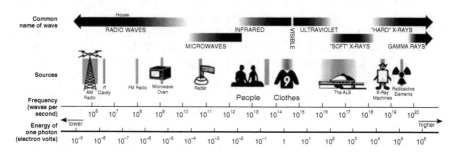

FIGURE 18.1 Electromagnetic spectrum.

bar. Shortwave radiation led to the invention of microwaves. In the microwave, radio waves, with shorter wavelengths and higher frequencies than those used for communication, cause water and other polar molecules within food to vibrate. Vibration can be up to 2.5 billion times/sec, which is enough vibration to cause heat by friction. Both cooking by heat and microwave are examples of the use of nonionizing radiation.

High frequencies constitute ionizing radiation. The radiation passes through the food without generating intense heat, disrupting cellular processes such as sprouting, ripening, or growth of microbes, parasites, and insects. Ionizing radiation has high energy — high enough to change atoms by knocking an electron from them to form an ion, but not high enough to split atoms and cause exposed objects to become radioactive. Therefore, the sources of radiation allowed for food processing (cobalt-60, cesium-137, accelerated electrons, and x-rays) cannot make food radioactive. Food irradiation makes use of high frequencies constituting ionizing radiation. In contrast, during a nuclear meltdown, incredibly high levels of ionizing radiation are emitted, because of which not only is the growth of microorganisms disrupted but the food itself can become radioactive. Thus, the difference is a matter of magnitude, owing to which people can enjoy the benefits of ionizing radiation with no worries about radioactive contamination.

Foods are processed in facilities designed for that purpose. Figure 18.2 shows the floor plan for a gamma irradiation facility. It consists of three areas. The outer area where food is received for processing and stored before and after processing is like any other food warehouse. If frozen or perishable foods are processed in the facility, it must have appropriate refrigeration facilities. No other requirements are unique to the area. The second area is the conveyor or other system used to transport the food to be processed. Food to be processed is loaded onto the conveyor and carried to the irradiation source, where it absorbs the energy needed to accomplish the desired effect. The third, the inner area, is the processing room. In this room, the source is stored until needed to process the food. In the case of gamma sources, a pool of water is used to store the source when it is not used to prevent radiation from escaping. When the source is raised into the room, concrete walls provide a shield to prevent the escape of radiation into the storage area. In the case of irradiation generated by a machine, the same shielding is used to prevent escape of radiation, but no other shielding is needed because no radiation is generated when the machine is turned off.

Processing facilities are safe for the employees who work there and for the surrounding environment. Facilities using gamma sources must be licensed by the U.S. Nuclear Regulatory Commission or an equivalent state agency to assure that they can be operated safely. All facilities must meet requirements of the Occupational Safety and Health Administration (OSHA) and the Environmental Protection Agency (EPA) to assure that workers and the environment will not be adversely affected in any way. In addition, when gamma sources are moved to or from the facilities, they are carried in special containers that have been proven safe for the purpose by the U.S. Department of Transportation. In more than four decades of transporting gamma sources in North America, there has never been an accident that has resulted in the escape of radioactive materials into the environment. Also, no radioactive waste is generated by irradiation; all spent sources are returned to the firm that supplied them for storage or further processing.

Food Irradiation

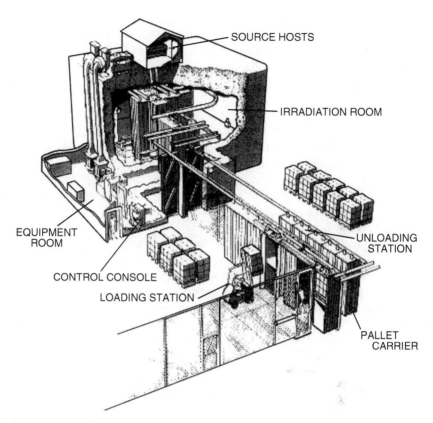

FIGURE 18.2 Facility used to irradiate foods.

During the process of food irradiation, ions are formed. The ions can cause chemical changes within the food, e.g., splitting of water molecules, which may recombine to form hydrogen peroxide. Such products may react with food to lower nutritional value or produce undesirable by-products. Food irradiation is a cold process, i.e., it achieves its effect with little rise in the temperature of the food. There is little, if any, change in the physical appearance of irradiated foods, because they do not undergo the changes in texture or color as do foods preserved by heat pasteurization, canning, or freezing. Food remains close to its original state. However, problems that have occurred include some off-flavors in meat and excess tissue-softening, which has been documented in fresh peaches and nectarines.

EFFECTIVENESS OF IRRADIATION

Currently, there are three dose levels of food irradiation, based on their applications. Low-dose applications, using less than 0.1 kGy, are effective against sprouting of infesting insects. Doses of 0.2 to 1 kGy kill infesting insects. Low-dose irradiation delays ripening and extends the shelf life of fruits, e.g., strawberries, bananas, mangoes, papayas, guavas, cherries, tomatoes, and avocados. Pasteurizing doses (radurized) of 1 to 3 kGy kill populations of microbes, and are effective against *Salmonella, Campylobacteria*, and parasitic liver flukes. Such doses destroy pathogenic microorganisms that might be present in milk and delay spoilage by significantly reducing the number of microbes responsible for spoilage. In Europe, irradiated milk has been used for years and is very popular because before opening it can be stored safely at room temperature. Sterilizing doses (reappertization) of 25 to 50 kGy decrease the number of nonsporing pathogenic organisms.

Early trails of irradiated foods resulted in undesirable changes both in taste and texture. Dairy products (cheeses) proved not to be good candidates for irradiation. There were also changes in aroma and texture of citrus crops.

Currently, the FAO and WHO allow only forms of ionizing energy for food irradiation that are unable to cause the food to become radioactive, i.e., x-rays and cobalt-60 or cesium-137 to produce gamma rays. Cobalt-60 and x-rays have been used many years in medical devices. Cesium-137 is a by-product of the nuclear industry and has become less popular. Each has its advantages and disadvantages. The 5-mEV x-ray machines offer the advantage of producing radiation only when desired. However, such machines are more complex technically and the electron beams are limited because they do not penetrate very far into the food. Cobalt-60 isotopes are problematic because they continuously emit radiation and cannot be turned off. The lives of the isotopes are limited and subject to regulatory controls. A typical facility using cobalt-60 has the isotopes doubly encapsulated in 18-in. stainless steel tubes. Food passes through the radiation on conveyor belts for exposure.

BY-PRODUCTS OF IRRADIATION

Previously, approximately 65 products were identified as unique compounds formed during food irradiation. Since then, all but six have been accounted for as naturally occurring or found in other food-processing situations. Free radical compounds are generated, but are not unique to food irradiation. One compound was traced to be a contaminant of a chemical used to sterilize the hooks from which carcasses were hung in slaughterhouses.

After several decades of research, including more than 1300 studies, no adverse effects have been found due to irradiation of foods. These include multigenerational feeding studies with rats, mice, dogs, and monkeys.

As with all preservation or cooking methods, some chemical changes occur in irradiated food. When high-energy particles strike matter, electrons are lost from atoms and ions are formed. Newly formed radiolytic products may then interact to create new compounds in the food that were not present before treatment, a few of which could produce off-flavors. In meat, this can be partly controlled by maintaining low product temperatures during the irradiation process. The most common chemical reaction during food irradiation is the conversion of water to hydrogen peroxide. Reactions such as these occur in all types of food preservation, and the few reactions unique to irradiation are not harmful.

The FDA concluded that "very few of these radiolytic products are unique to irradiated foods; approximately 90% of the radiolytic products...are known to be natural components of food." Some of these are fatty acids identical to those that result from the breakdown of triglycerides; amino acids that make up proteins; and compounds (hydrocarbons) commonly found in the waxy coverings of fruits such as apples, pears, and berries. Others are fatty compounds identical to those found from cooking meat by common methods such as grilling. The other 10% of radiolytic compounds are chemically very similar to natural components in food. The chemistry of irradiation is very predictable, and the products of an individual component such as proteins are not affected by the type of food or other food components present. Radiolytic products have been critically tested for toxicity and no evidence of hazards has been found.

Radiation does not impair the activity of certain nutrients, but overall nutrient retention in irradiated foods is similar to retention by other preservation methods. With regard to macronutrients, certain proteins are split or aggregated and the amino acid methionine is degraded. Also, double bonds of polyunsaturated fatty acids are broken down, producing off-flavors. Certain micronutrients are lost, such as vitamins C, E, K, B6, and riboflavin. Vitamin C (ascorbic acid) reduction has been reported, but it is attributed to a shift from ascorbic acid to dehydroascorbic acid, a change mostly insignificant from a nutritional standpoint. Tocopherol, which has vitamin E activity, appears to be very sensitive to irradiation in the presence of oxygen. Vitamin K seems relatively stable. These adverse effects of irradiation on vitamins can be reduced by excluding oxygen and light, keeping the food at a low temperature, and using the lowest dose needed to treat (process) food. However, improved processing techniques, such as excluding air from the radiation milieu or holding foods that can withstand freezing, have resulted in minimal losses and changes.

MISCONCEPTIONS

Consumer activist groups, such as the Health and Energy Institute and the National Coalition to Stop Food Irradiation, have made several unsubstantiated claims against food irradiation. They have claimed that there will be an increased risk of nuclear accidents. However, the half-life of cobalt-60 is such that there is no threat of meltdown because of the low energy. Activists are concerned about increased waste, but such sources to be used only constitute a minute portion of the 2.68 million ft^3. In addition, machine sources offer no waste. It is claimed that the food irradiation process is being pushed as a way to use radioactive waste from nuclear power and weapon production, but cobalt-60 is the isotope of choice created for use in medical centers. Concern has been expressed that irradiation will produce mutated microorganisms; however, it has been found that such organisms lack vigor and decrease in number because of competitive survivability. Finally, it has been expressed that more food irradiation will result in contaminated ground water; however, this is not likely because cobalt-60 is not water soluble.

REGULATIONS

Regardless of the fact that irradiation is a physical process and nothing is added to the food or leaves any residues, activists have lobbied for labeling of irradiated foods. This will be unusual, because typically labeling is not required for processed foods. For example, products such as frozen meals may be prepared from prepared tomato sauces before freezing, but such information is not required on the label. Many fruits and vegetables are treated with chemicals, such as ethylene oxide for ripening or isopropyl-n-chlorophenyl carbamate to prevent sprouting, and such chemicals do not appear on the label. On the other hand, certain soft cheeses are made with raw, unpasteurized milk, and labeling them may be useful for consumers so that they can choose whether to consume them. Labeling of irradiated food is not based on any of the traditional reasons for the need to label food, but rather on the need to ensure that the process, which has received so much controversial attention, is readily apparent to the public. It is hoped that eventually the consumer will view this label as a positive sign rather than a negative concern. Because irradiated foods can offer a greater degree of safety from foodborne disease, it is anticipated that the public will learn to seek out such products, similar to the Good Housekeeping Seal of Approval.

All irradiated foods sold at the retail level in the U.S. must be labeled with a radura, an international symbol for irradiation (Figure 18.3), and the words "Treated by Irradiation" or "Treated with Radiation." Products that contain irradiated ingredients, including spices, are not required to be labeled as such. The American Dietetic Association (ADA) supports the present labeling rules, including use of the radura and current wording on irradiated foods. Some professional agencies, such as the ADA, are concerned about statements that imply that irradiated food is free of pathogens, such as "Free of *Salmonella*," because food irradiation does not prevent recontamination of the irradiated food, which may occur following opening sealed containers of food previously treated by irradiation. Incentive labeling as specified by USDA regulations stipulates that elimination of a pathogen must be scientifically documented. There is continuing research to identify scientific detection methods to verify that unlabeled foods have not been irradiated and that foods have received the intended dose, apparently to detect fraud. An international general standard covering irradiated foods was adopted by the Codex Alimentarius Commission, a

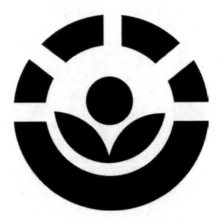

FIGURE 18.3 Radura, an international symbol for irradiation.

joint body of WHO and FAO. The standards are based on the findings of the Joint Expert Committee on Food Irradiation convened by FAO, WHO, and the IAEA.

Food irradiation has been identified as a safe technology to reduce the risk of foodborne illness as part of high-quality food production, processing, handling, and preparation. Food irradiation's history of scientific research, evaluation, and testing spans more than 50 years. The process has been approved by more than 40 countries worldwide and it has been endorsed or supported by numerous national and international food and health organizations and professional groups. Food irradiation (cold pasteurization) uses a source of ionizing energy that passes through food to destroy harmful bacteria and other organisms. Food irradiation offers negligible loss of nutrients or sensory qualities in food, because it does not substantially raise the temperature of the food during processing. In the U.S., manufacturers are required to identify irradiated food sold to consumers with an international symbol (radura) and terminology describing the process on product labels. When consumers are educated about food irradiation, many prefer irradiated products because of their increased safety.

STUDY QUESTIONS AND EXERCISES

1. What is irradiation and how does food irradiation work?
2. What kinds of foods are irradiated?
3. What are the benefits and problems of food irradiation?
4. What are the fallacies surrounding food irradiation?

RECOMMENDED READINGS

Animal and Plant Health Inspection Service (APHIS), Use of irradiation as a quarantine treatment for fresh fruits of papaya from Hawaii — final rule, *Federal Register*, 54, 387-393, January 1989.
American Dietetics Association, Food irradiation, *Jam. Diet. Assoc.*, 100, 246-253, 2000
Food Safety and Inspection Service (USDA), Pathogen reduction: hazard analysis and critical control point (HACCP) systems — final rule, *Federal Register*, 61, 38806, July 1996.
Josephson, E.S. and Dymsza, H.A., Food Irradiation, *Technology*, 6, 235-238, 1999.
Satin, M., *Food Irradiation: A Guidebook*, Technomic Press, Lancaster, PA, 1993.
World Health Organization, Safety and nutritional adequacy of irradiated food, WHO Report, Geneva, Switzerland, 1994.

19 Polycyclic Aromatic Hydrocarbons and Other Processing Products

Many cooking methods involve intense heat with limited availability of oxygen, both favorable conditions for mild browning or pyrolytic (300°C) decomposition of the food's fat and protein components. Pyrolytic decomposition is the breakdown of substances at high temperatures and in the absence of oxygen. Various browning products, polycyclic aromatic hydrocarbons (PAHs), and heterocyclic amines (HCAs) are the major decomposition products of such cooking. On the other hand, baking, using an oven, or deep fat frying (unless the oil is repeatedly used or extremely high temperatures are used) does not produce such decomposition. PAHs are produced during cooking, mainly by pyrolysis of fats, whereas HCAs are pyrolysis products of amino acids, especially tryptophan. Also, PAHs can be from environmental sources, such as those occurring in wood-burning stoves, diesel exhaust, and oil-burning heaters. PAHs are formed when fat from food drips into the hot coals and is incinerated. The resulting PAHs in smoke can subsequently adsorb to the cooking food. Table 19.1 lists some common PAHs found in the environment.

BENZO(α)PYRENE AND POLYCYCLIC AROMATIC HYDROCARBONS

A large number of PAHs have been identified as pyrolysis products of foods, and some examples are shown in Table 19.1. All three macronutrient categories have been implicated in the formation of PAHs, which proceeds largely by similar mechanisms in all three categories. PAHs most likely to pose human health problems are benzo(α)pyrene (3,4-benzpyrene, BP) and 7,12-dimethylbenzanthrene (DMBA), illustrated in Figure 19.1 with the base structure analog anthracene. Although most PAHs, particularly the low-molecular-weight compounds, are noncarcinogenic, both PAHs and many other similar compounds are potent carcinogens that are active after metabolic conversion to electrophilic epoxide derivatives. Benzo(α)pyrene has been identified in the charred crusts of biscuits and bread, broiled and barbecued meats (up to 200 ppb in charcoal-broiled meats), broiled fish, and roasted coffee. Broiled high-fat hamburger contains about 43 ppb of PAHs, whereas lean beef may have only 3 ppb of PAHs. Steaks cooked close to the charcoal to be well done can produce

**TABLE 19.1
Common PAHs Found in the Environment**

Acenaphthene dibenzo(a,h)anthracene
Anthracene fluoranthene
Benzo(α)anthracene fluorene
Benzo(α)pyrene indo(1,2,3-cd)pyrene
Benzo(β)fluoranthene naphthalene
Benzo(k)fluoranthene phenanthrene
Chrysene pyrene

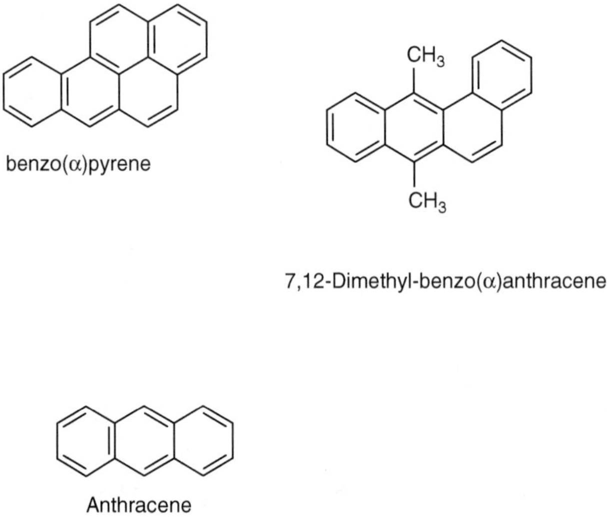

FIGURE 19.1 Benzo(α)pyrene; 7,12-dimethyl-benzo(α)anthracene; and anthracene.

up to 50 ppb of benzo(α)pyrene. The amount of contamination by PAHs falls off rapidly as the distance of the meat from the charcoal increases. On heating starch to temperatures promoting pyrolysis (390°C), detectable benzo(α)pyrene (<1 ppb) can be formed, usually at the surface, e.g., bread crust. Many foods have detectable levels, usually from environmental exposure via coal and petroleum products.

The major site for PAH-induced carcinogenesis is the skin. Tumors can be produced at other sites following ingestion, but the concentrations required are quite high. Synthetic DMBA is an exception, which serves as a model PAH and is a potent inducer of mammary tumors. Inhaled PAHs (tobacco smoke) have been implicated in cancer of the respiratory system, and the magnitude of this disease is likely to be more than that by the dietary route. PAHs can induce cytochrome P450, an enzyme responsible for their bioactivation. Thus, dietary exposure may substantially increase the sensitivity to subsequent PAH exposures.

The toxic effects of PAHs in tissues other than germ cells have been demonstrated to be due to its metabolite, an epoxide, which interacts with DNA, RNA, and other macromolecules. It has been suggested that a steady-state level of epoxides within the cells of a target organ is a function of the metabolites. Thus, the rates of epoxide-forming and -detoxifying enzyme activities in various tissues can be important determinants of tissue-specific toxicity.

Interactions of PAHs with DNA led to research on the interaction of carcinogens with DNA. Numerous carcinogens have since been found to bind to DNA. In PAHs such as benzo(α)pyrene, binding is by means of its activated form, the 7,8-dihydrodiol 9,10-epoxide, the reaction being through the 10-carbon of the benzo(α) metabolites to the 2-amino position in guanylic acid. Thus, considerable knowledge has accrued on the interaction with DNA of carcinogens collectively termed as genotoxic.

Long-term health effects of exposure to PAHs may include cataracts, kidney and liver damage, and jaundice. Repeated skin contact to the PAH naphthalene can result in redness and inflammation of the skin. Breathing or swallowing large amounts of naphthalene can cause the break down of red blood cells.

Long-term exposure to low levels of some PAHs has caused cancer in laboratory animals. Benzo(α)pyrene is the most common PAH to cause cancer in animals. Studies of workers exposed to mixtures of PAHs and other compounds have noted an increased risk of skin, lung, bladder, and gastrointestinal (GI) cancers. The information provided by these studies is limited, because the workers were exposed to other potential cancer-causing chemicals besides PAHs. Although animal studies have shown adverse reproductive and developmental effects from PAH exposure, these effects have generally not been seen in humans.

One of the greatest sources of exposure to PAHs is breathing these compounds in tobacco smoke. Smokers can lower their own exposure and the exposure of their families by stopping smoking. People can also reduce the use of wood-burning stoves and fireplaces. Additional steps to lower exposure to PAHs include decreasing consumption of smoked and char-broiled foods; decreasing the use of coal-tar-based cosmetics and shampoos; substituting cedar shavings or aromatic herbs for moth-balls, moth flakes, and deodorant cakes; avoiding skin contact by wearing protective clothing, such as long-sleeve shirts, long pants, and gloves, if handling creosote-treated wood products; and avoiding exposure to dust and fumes by wearing an appropriate respirator when working with products containing PAHs.

The U.S. Environmental Protection Agency (U.S. EPA) has established maximum contaminant levels (MCLs) for public water supplies to reduce the chances of adverse health effects from drinking contaminated water. MCLs are enforceable limits that public water supplies must meet. These standards are much lower than levels at which health effects have been observed. The U.S. EPA has not established MCLs for individual PAHs, but has set the MCL for total PAHs to 0.2 ppb. There are currently no standards for regulating levels of these chemicals in private wells. The U.S. EPA requires the reporting of any releases of PAHs exceeding 1 lb into the environment. There are no regulations for the PAH content of foods.

HETROCYCLIC AMINES

HCAs are produced by food pyrolysis products derived from tryptophan, glutamic acid, phenylalanine, and lysine. Also, pyrolysis products of carbolines, quinolines, and quinoxalines are implicated as important HCAs. In 1977, Japanese investigators found that extracts of charred surfaces of the meats and fish was quantitatively more mutagenic than could be accounted for by the presence of PAHs alone. These findings were confirmed and extended by others who showed similar mutagen contents produced under common household cooking conditions such as frying beef. We know that several of the major sources of cooked protein in the U.S. diet have significant mutagen content. Mutagenic activity has been found in cooked beef, pork, ham, bacon, lamb, chicken, fish, and eggs following broiling, frying, and barbecuing. Such substances are formed as a result of reactions involving proteins, amino acids, or other nitrogen-containing food constituents or proteinaceous foods. Very high temperatures of above 500°C are involved, resulting in incomplete combustion of the meat, especially the levels of creatine, or the cyclized form of creatinine, and carbohydrates. Creatine appears to be rate limiting with respect to mutagen formation. Tryptophan, a common amino acid, has been shown to be the precursor of such mutagens as 3-amino-1-methyl-5H-pyrido[4,3-b]indole (Figure 19.2). Protein-rich foods heated above 200°C produce heterocyclic mutagens such as quinolines and quinoxalines, also shown in Figure 19.2. Pan frying or broiling enhances formation of HCAs, compared with the much lower levels produced by deep frying or stewing. Cooking temperatures below 150°C (rare to medium rare) result in much lower amounts of amino acid pyrolysis. There is a positive correlation between the muscle level of creatine and production of mutagen. Roasting and pyrolysis of amino acids from fish (sardines) has been implicated in the high incidence of stomach cancer among the Japanese. Both carbolines and tryptophan pyrolysis products are more potent mutagens than BP and DMBA. All amino acid breakdown products can be detected in broiled beef, fish (in ppb), bread crust, toast, fried potatoes, and coffee. All the approximately 21 mutagenic compounds have been found to be carcinogens in laboratory animals, including monkeys.

All compounds are rapidly absorbed by the GI tract, distributed to all organs and tissues, and decline to undetectable levels within 72 h. The major target organs for HCAs are the liver, small and large intestine, oral cavity, lung, blood vessels, skin, and mammary glands. HCAs are activated through N-hydroxylation by cytochrome P450. The N-hydroxyl compound formed requires further activation by O-acetylation or O-sulfonation to react with DNA. DNA adducts can be formed with guanosine in various organs, including the liver, heart, kidney, colon, small intestine, fore stomach, pancreas, and lung. Unreacted substances are subject to phase II detoxification reactions and are excreted by the urine and feces. Rodents, monkeys, and humans have the capacity to activate HCAs. Studies using isolated hepatic microsomes showed that humans have a greater capacity to activate the majority of HCAs tested than do rodents of *Cynomolgus monkeys*.

Dietary fat appears to modulate the effects of HCA-induced mutagenic action. High-fat diets make rats more prone to activate HCA than do low-fat diets. Dietary fiber, particularly wheat bran, appears to absorb HCAs and make such compound less available for absorption.

Cooking processes can give rise to fumes containing air pollutants such as HCAs that are mutagenic and carcinogenic in animal tests. For example, the fumes generated by frying pork and beef have been found to be mutagenic. In contrast, no

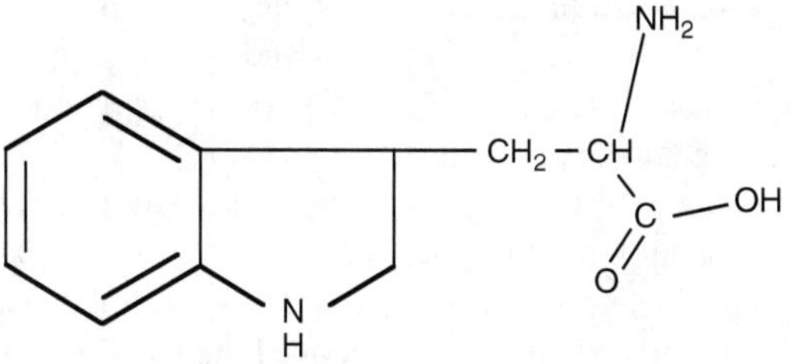

Tryptophan

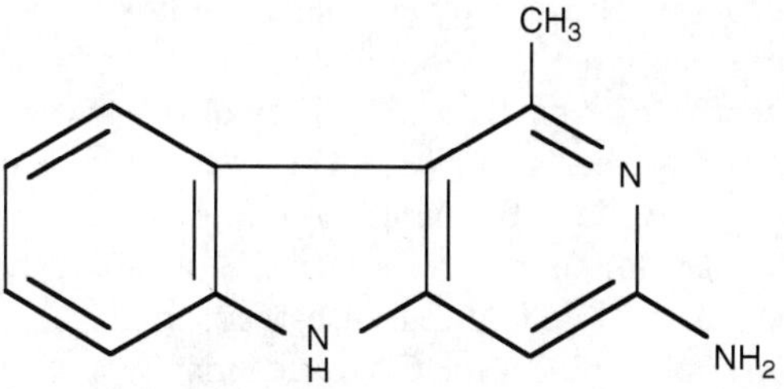

3-Amino-1-methyl-5H-pyrido (4,3-b) indole

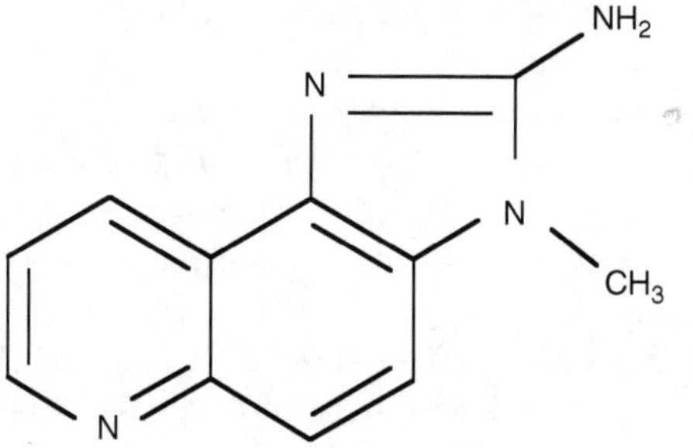

2-Amino-3-methylimidazo (4,5-f)quinoline

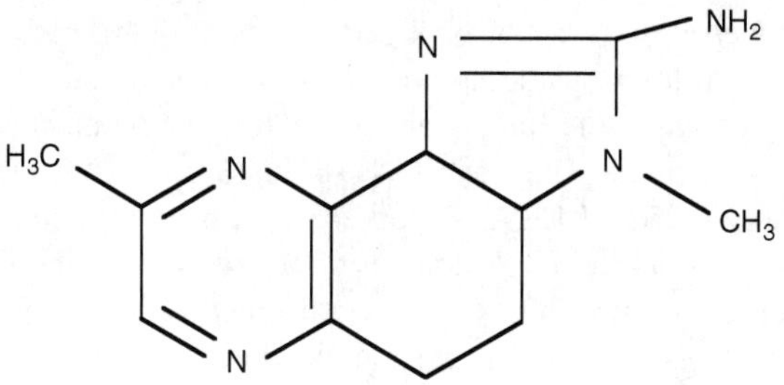

2-Amino-3,8-dimethylimidazole (4,5-f) quinoxaline

FIGURE 19.2 Tryptophan, 3-amino-1-methyl-5H-pyrido (4,3-b) indole; 2-amino-3-methylimidazo (4,5-f)quinoline; and 2-amino-3,8-dimethylimidazole (4,5-f) quinoxaline.

mutagenicity was detected in fumes from frying soybean-based food (tempeh burgers). Epidemiological studies on occupational exposed cooks and bakers, with respect to cancer, and case-control analysis also support the association between exposure to cooking fumes and cancers.

Recent studies have further evaluated the relationship between methods of cooking meat and the development of specific types of cancer. One study conducted by researchers from the National Cancer Institute found a link between individuals with stomach cancer and the consumption of cooked meats. The researchers assessed the diets and cooking habits of 176 people diagnosed with stomach cancer and 503 people without cancer. The researchers found that those who ate their beef medium-well or well done had more than three times the risk of stomach cancer than those who ate their beef rare or medium-rare. They also found that people who ate beef four or more times a week had more than twice the risk of stomach cancer than those consuming beef less frequently. Additional studies have shown that an increased risk of developing colorectal, pancreatic, and breast cancer is associated with high intakes of well-done, fried, or barbequed meats.

Thus, four factors influence HCA formation: type of food, cooking method, temperature, and time. HCAs are found in cooked muscle meats; other sources of protein (milk, eggs, tofu, and organ meats such as liver) have very little or no HCA content naturally or when cooked. Temperature is the most important factor in the formation of HCAs. Frying, broiling, and barbecuing produce the largest amounts of HCAs, because the meats are cooked at very high temperatures. One study conducted by researchers showed a threefold increase in the content of HCAs when the cooking temperature was increased from 200 to 250°C (392 to 482°F). Oven roasting and baking are done at lower temperatures, so lower levels of HCAs are likely to form; however, gravy made from meat drippings contains substantial amounts of HCAs. Stewing, boiling, or poaching is done at or below 100°C (212°F); cooking at this low temperature creates negligible amounts of the chemicals. Foods cooked for a long time (well done instead of medium) by other methods also form slightly more of the chemicals.

It is worthwhile noting that meats that are partially cooked in the microwave oven before cooking by other methods also have lower levels of HCAs. Studies have shown that microwaving meat before cooking helps decrease mutagens by removing the precursors. Meats that were microwaved for 2 min before cooking had a 90% decrease in HCA content. In addition, if the liquid that forms during microwaving is poured off before further cooking, the final quantity of HCAs is reduced.

Studies are needed to assess the amount of HCAs in the average U.S. diet, but at present the maximum daily intake of HCAs in food has not been established. At present, no federal agency monitors the HCA content of cooked meats, there is no good measure of how much HCAs would have to be consumed to increase cancer risk, and there are no guidelines concerning consumption of foods with HCAs. Further research is needed before such recommendations can be made.

People concerned can reduce their exposure to HCAs by varying the methods of cooking meats: microwaving meats more often, especially before frying, broiling, or barbecuing, and refraining from making gravy from meat drippings.

NITRATES, NITRITES, AND NITROSAMINES

Nitrates and nitrites in preserved meats (bacon, cold cuts) can prevent growth of *Clostridium botulinum*, the organism that can produce the potent botulinum toxin. However, nitrates and nitrites have been shown to have adverse effects, such as methemoglobinemia and carcinogenesis, the latter resulting from the formation of nitrosamines. Coincidentally, reduction of nitrate to nitrite is a common reaction for bacteria in the GI tract. Usually, the GI effect on nitrite is preceded by nitrate being reduced to nitrite by microflora of mouth saliva. The minimum nitrate intake for a person is estimated at 75 mg/d. The resulting nitrite can oxidize hemoglobin to methemoglobin, which results in the loss of oxygen-binding ability. Consequently, dietary or water sources of nitrate and nitrite can have life-threatening effects (methemoglobinemia), particularly in young children. NADH reductase is the major enzyme responsible for the reduction of methemoglobin. Because of a transient deficiency of NADH reductase, newborns are very sensitive to nitrate and nitrite toxicity.

The fatal dose of potassium nitrate for adult humans is 30 to 35 g consumed as a single dose; the fatal dose of sodium nitrite is 22 to 23 mg/kg body weight. There is no confirmable evidence in the literature on the carcinogenicity (cancer-causing capacity) of nitrate as such.

It is also notable that people normally consume more nitrates from their vegetable intake than from cured meat products. Spinach, beets, radishes, celery, and cabbages are among the vegetables that generally contain very high concentrations of nitrates. The nitrate content of vegetables is affected by maturity, soil conditions, fertilizer, variety, etc. It has been estimated that 10% of the human exposure to nitrite in the digestive tract comes from cured meats and 90% comes from vegetables and other sources. Nitrates can be reduced to nitrites by certain microorganisms present in foods and in the GI tract. This has resulted in nitrite toxicity in infants fed vegetables with a high nitrate level.

To obtain 22 mg of sodium nitrite/kg body weight (a lethal dose), a 154-lb adult will have to consume, in one intake, 18.57 lb of cured meat product containing 200 ppm sodium nitrite. (Because nitrite is rapidly converted to nitric oxide during the curing process, the 18.57-lb figure should be tripled at least.) Even if a person could eat that amount of cured meat, probably salt and not nitrite would be the toxic factor.

Nitrites react with secondary amines to form a variety of nitrosamines. Figure 19.3 shows the reactions for formation of some nitrosamines. Nitrosamine formation can occur under the acidic conditions of the GI tract. Also, the nitrosation reaction can occur during the frying of nitrite-cured bacon. The amines necessary for the nitrosation reaction occur widely in the human diet and many foods contain sufficient amounts of nitrosamines (see Table 19.2). Certain nitrosamines induce cancers in the liver, kidney, bladder, GI tract, pancreas, and respiratory tract. As shown in Figure 19.3, activation of nitrosamines is through cytochrome P450, involving oxidative N-dealkylation. The most common compound formed is diethylnitrosamine dimethylnitrosamine, a powerful carcinogen. Nitrosopyrrolidine is formed from the amino acid proline by nitrosation, followed by decarboxylation at elevated temperatures, such as in roasting or frying.

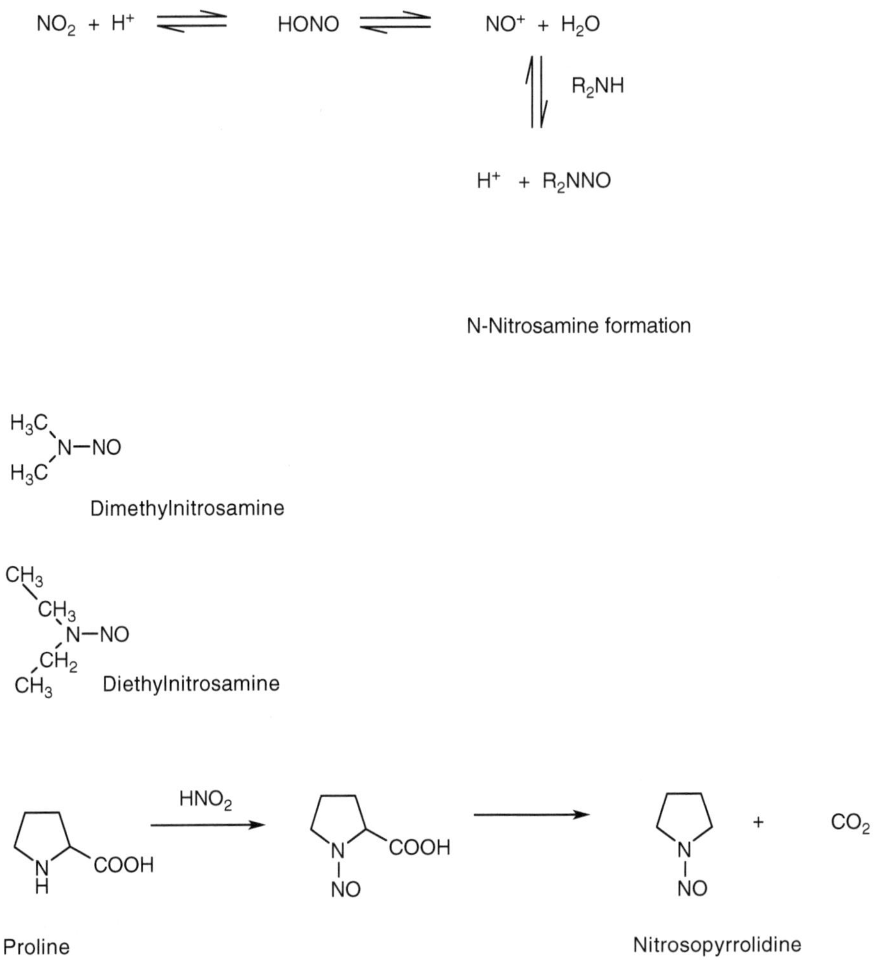

$$NO_2 + H^+ \rightleftharpoons HONO \rightleftharpoons NO^+ + H_2O$$

$$\updownarrow R_2NH$$

$$H^+ + R_2NNO$$

N-Nitrosamine formation

$$\begin{array}{c} H_3C \\ \diagdown \\ N-NO \\ \diagup \\ H_3C \end{array}$$

Dimethylnitrosamine

$$\begin{array}{c} CH_3 \\ \diagdown \\ CH_3 \\ \diagdown \\ N-NO \\ \diagup \\ CH_2 \\ \diagup \\ CH_3 \end{array}$$

Diethylnitrosamine

Proline → (HNO₂) → Nitrosopyrrolidine + CO₂

FIGURE 19.3 Formation of nitrosamines.

TABLE 19.2
Content of Nitrosamines in Food

Food	Content (μg/kg)
Hotdogs (frankfurter, franks)	0–84
Bacon and smoked meats	1–60
Ham (raw or roasted)	1–78
Salami	10–80
Fish (raw)	0–4
Fish (fried)	1–9
Fish (smoked, pickled)	4–26
Cheese (variety)	1–4

Not all cured meat products contain nitrosamines; when present, they usually are in very minute amounts. Many variables influence nitrosamine levels: amount of nitrite added during processing, concentrations of amines in meat, type and amounts of other ingredients used in processing, actual processing conditions, length of storage, storage temperatures, method of cooking, and degree of doneness. Inhibition of nitrosation reaction is possible. Nitrite is reduced to NO by the dehydro form of ascorbic acid. Likewise, tocopherols and other food antioxidants inhibit substitution reactions. Thus, the USDA now requires adding ascorbic acid (vitamin C) or erythorbic acid to bacon cure, a practice that greatly reduces the formation of nitrosamines.

The effects of heating meat products cured with nitrite have been investigated. When bacon was fried at 210°F for 10 min (raw), 210°F for 105 min (medium-well), 275°F for 10 min (very light), or 275°F for 30 min (medium-well), no conclusive evidence of nitrosopyrrolidine could be found. But when bacon was fried at 350°F for 6 min (medium-well), 400°F for 4 min (medium-well), or 400°F for 10 min (burned), nitrosopyrrolidine formation was conclusively found at 10, 17, and 19 ppb, respectively. Thus, well-done or burned bacon probably is potentially more hazardous than less-well-done bacon. Bacon cooked by microwave has less nitrosamine than fried bacon. The same study and others have shown that fat cookout or drippings usually contain more nitrosopyrrolidine than the bacon contains.

It is unknown at what levels, if any, nitrosamines are formed in humans after they eat cured meat products, or what constitutes a dangerous level in meat or in humans. Nitrosamines are found very infrequently in all cured products except overcooked bacon.

PRODUCTS OF THE MAILLARD REACTION

In the Maillard reaction, reducing sugars (pentoses > hexoses) condensate with amino acids, producing a mixture of insoluble dark-brown polymeric pigments, termed *melanoidins*. Aldoses and ketoses react with aliphatic primary and secondary amines of amino acids and proteins to form N-glycosides, which readily dehydrate to Schiff's base by the Maillard reaction (Figure 19.4). This is the basis for the well-known nonenzymatic browning reaction. In the early stages of the reaction, premelanoidins are formed, which are water-soluble mixtures of carbonyl and aromatic substances. The Maillard reaction of amino acids with sugars occurs during a variety of food processes, cooking, and in storage. Some products formed are volatile with strong odors. The development of Maillard reactions can result in the losses of essential amino acids (lysine and methionine) and undesired discoloration and off-flavor in food. Many Maillard reaction products, especially those with xylose or tryptophan in combination, strongly inhibit mutagenicity in model systems.

Premelanoidins have been shown to inhibit growth, cause liver damage, and interrupt reproduction in laboratory animals. Maillard products of fructose–glycine and fructose–arginine increase the mutagenicity of 3-amino-1,4-dimethyl 5H-pyridol-(4,3-b)indole. Antimutagenic effects seem to correlate well with antioxidant effects. However, mutagenicity of benzo(α)pyrene is moderately inhibited by such products. Some products of the Maillard reaction have been shown to induce allergic reactions.

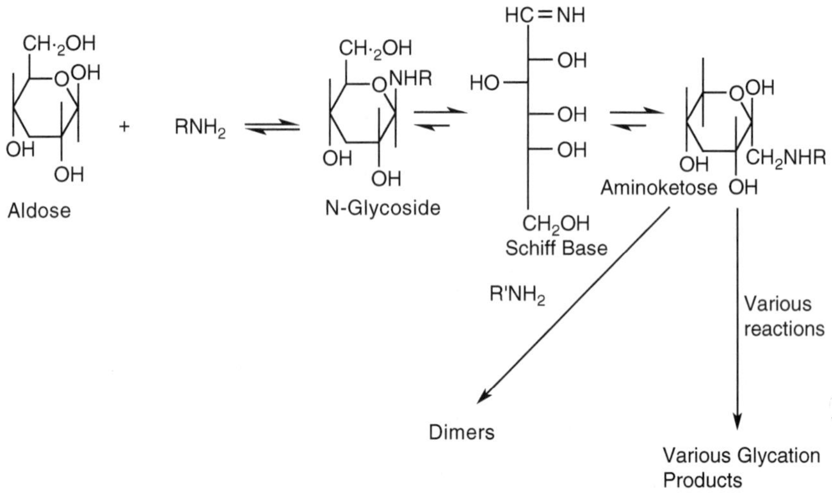

FIGURE 19.4 Maillard reaction of amines with aldoses.

Maillard reactions of sugars and amino acids and proteins lead to a cascade of reactions. The reaction end products have been observed in collagen-rich tissues *in vivo* and *in vitro*, and are associated with stiffening of artery walls and joints with aging. Plasma glucose reacts with hemoglobins via the Maillard reaction, which along with glycation of lens protein may contribute to complications of diabetes. The Maillard reaction can be prevented by adding carbonyl groups of reducing sugars and regulating the temperature, pH, and water content.

Amadori products result from early Maillard reactions. The products create brown pigments, giving the characteristic color of some cooked foods such as bread crust, as well as volatile compounds that give various odors such as roasting aromas. More than 2000 volatile compounds have been identified. The proportions and the amounts of different Maillard products depend on processing time, temperature, water activity, and pH, resulting in a variety of flavors and colors. Under- or overcooking can spoil the flavor of a meal, depending on the degree of Maillard products formed. Both stored and cooked foods contain Maillard products. The reaction can and does occur at room temperature, and many Maillard compounds are found in uncooked foods, though usually at lower concentrations than in cooked foods.

There has been a recent growing interest in studying the Maillard reaction *in vivo*, particularly in relation to diabetes and aging. It is thought that the cross-linking between long-lived proteins such as collagen and free sugars, especially fructose, which has a high cross-linking potential, produces glycation end products of Maillard reaction, which contribute to tissue degeneration. There is no reason to believe that Maillard reaction products consumed in food participate in any way in the body's own internal cross-linking reactions that contribute to aging, because the Maillard reaction products are produced as part of normal cellular metabolism and via a separate biochemical pathway.

Products from Maillard reactions have been found to possess antioxidant activity. Maillard reaction products are known to inhibit oxidative degradation of natural organic compounds. Not much is known about the structures of such Maillard reactions products or the mechanisms of their formation. They are found in most cooked foods and have a characteristic brown color. These antioxidant compounds have been found to be formed from histidine and glucose or arginine and xylose, with the amount produced depending on reaction time, initial pH, and molar ratio of reactants used.

STUDY QUESTIONS AND EXERCISES

1. Describe the conditions that promote the formation of PAHs and HCAs and their potential health consequences. What are the chemical characteristic structures of PAHs and HCAs?
2. How can the risk of exposure to PAHs and HCAs be avoided? What can be done to reduce the risk to exposure of HCA based on a physical characteristic of HCAs?
3. What is the relationship between consumption of nitrosamines and various antioxidants, such as vitamin C and vitamin E?
4. Describe the Maillard reaction. Describe the potential adverse effects and benefits that might be derived from ingesting such products.
5. What is the risk associated with nitrites and nitrates in drinking water or in food? Which populations are at risk of adverse effects associated with high intakes of nitrite and nitrate?

RECOMMENDED READINGS

Bjeldanes, L.F., Morris, M.M., and Felton, J.S., Mutagens from the cooking of food. 2. Survey by Ames salmonella-typhimurium test of mutagen formation in the major protein-rich foods of the American diet, *Food Chem. Toxicol.*, 20, 357-363, 1982.

Bjeldanes, L.F., Morris, M.M., and Timourian, H., Effects of meat composition and cooking conditions on mutagen formation in fried ground beef, *J. Agric. Food Chem.*, 31, 18-21, 1983.

Felton, J.S., Fultz, E., and Dolbeare, F.A., Effect of microwave pretreatment on heterocyclic aromatic amine mutagens/carcinogens in fried beef patties, *Food Chem. Toxicol*, 32, 897-903, 1994.

LaGoy, P.K. and Quirk, T.C., Establishing generic remediation goals for the polycyclic aromatic hydrocarbons: critical issues, *Environ. Hlth. Perspec.*, 102, 348-352, 1994.

Lee, K.-G. and Shibamoto, T., Toxicology and antioxidant activities of non-enzymatic browning reactions products: review, *Food Rev. Int.*, 18, 151-175, 2002.

Pariza, M.W., Ashoor, S.H., Chu, F.S. et al., Effects of temperature and time on mutagen formation in pan fried hamburger, *Canc. Lett.*, 7, 63–69, 1979.

National Academy of Sciences, *Polycyclic Aromatic Hydrocarbons Evaluation of Sources and Effects*, The National Academies Press, Washington, D.C., 1983.

Yang, W. and Omaye, S.T., Heterocyclic amines and Asian high temperature cooking: cancer and bacterial metagenicity, *Environ. Nutr. Interact.*, 1, 191-212, 1997.

20 Emerging Food Safety Issues in a Modern World

In addition to the concerns previously expressed about emerging foodborne pathogens, because of the ever-changing nature of the area, food safety is often faced with other new or reemerging issues. Science-based solutions should prevail for such issues; however, it is likely that the road to such solutions is long and tedious. The following discussion regarding issues of HACCP (Hazard Analysis of Critical Control Points), antibiotic resistance, and genetically modified organisms (GMOs) provides just a few examples of issues that have challenged, and continue to challenge, scientists in the field.

HACCP

HACCP was devised as a way to meet the nutritional needs of astronauts and ensure food safety. Since its early years, the National Aeronautics and Space Administration (NASA) has enforced a standard procedure for some canned foods, required for meat, poultry, and seafood, and is likely to become common for most of the food industry and programs with food service. The system is used to prevent, reduce, or minimize risks associated with foods by emphasizing on reducing or minimizing contamination. HACCP is a framework to produce food or food products safely and to prove that they were produced safely. Although there is no government mandate for HACCP, food industries are encouraged to voluntarily develop their own plans. HACCP is widely adapted by food service and industry in the U.S. and is gathering acceptance by many other nations.

HACCP was developed to alleviate the fear that an astronaut in space would contract a foodborne illness. The Pillsbury Company was chosen in 1959 to solve the problem and it determined that the standard quality assurance programs would not meet the more stringent requirements of NASA and began the search for new strategies. Pivotal to Pillsbury's plan was to develop a proactive system based on NASA record-keeping requirements and the U.S. Army's medical supply program, which encompassed two major factors: hazard analysis and establishment of critical control points. Hazard analysis is a systematic study of ingredients, food products, processing, handling, storage, packing, distribution, and consumer use for potential microbiological, chemical, or physical hazards. During hazard analysis, one explores

TABLE 20.1
The Seven Principles of HACCP

1. Conduct a hazard analysis. Prepare a list of steps in the process where significant hazards occur and describe the preventive measures.
2. Identify the critical control points in the process (risk assessment).
3. Establish critical limits for preventive measures associated with each identified CCP.
4. Establish CCP monitoring requirements. Establish procedures for using the results of monitoring to adjust the process and maintain control.
5. Establish the corrective action to be taken when monitoring indicates that there is a deviation from an established critical limit.
6. Establish effective record-keeping procedures that document the HACCP system.
7. Establish procedures for verifying that the HACCP system is working correctly.

how these problems could be prevented. Critical control points (CCP) are points anywhere in the process at which control can be applied and a food safety hazard can be prevented, eliminated, or reduced to acceptable levels.

HACCP principles were established for the NASA program and soon the concept spread to the industry. Some low-acid and acidified canned foods, particularly canned meats, have been made under HACCP procedures since the early 1970s, and the program has succeeded to such an extent that product recalls for canned products are rare.

During the mid-1980s, the National Academy of Sciences began to analyze how HACCP could be applied on a wider scale. The National Advisory Subcommittee on Microbiological Criteria for Food was designated to devise a plan, which subsequently became the seven major HACCP principles currently used and are listed in Table 20.1.

Establishment of good manufacturing practices (GMPs) underpins any HACCP program. Thus, as for the GMPs, establishment of sanitary standard operating procedures (SOPs) also helps provide a base to begin work. These practices control the environmental conditions to ensure safe food production and should be in place before implementing HACCP. The focus of HACCP is safety, and food quality is not an issue. The components of the food processing or service that affect safety are analyzed. Other necessary steps are a careful examination of the plant and equipment, written documentation of sampling and testing, and training of employees. Documentation is crucial to provide proof that the practices were indeed followed and as a defense against personal injury lawsuits by consumers.

It is relevant to note that in the application of HACCP, the use of microbiological testing is seldom an effective means of monitoring CCPs, because of the time required to obtain results. Waiting hours or days for test results is counterproductive. In most instances, monitoring of CCPs can be best accomplished by using physical and chemical tests and through visual observations. Microbiological criteria do, however, play a role in verifying that the overall HACCP system is working. Similar methods are employed for the assurance of food safety for chemical and physical hazards in addition to other biological hazards. For a successful HACCP program to be properly implemented, the management must be committed to an HACCP approach. A commitment by the management will indicate an awareness of the benefits and costs of HACCP and include education and training of employees. Benefits, in addition to enhanced assurance of food safety, are better use of resources and timely response to problems.

Developing an HACCP Plan

The format of HACCP plans varies. In many cases, the plans are product- and process-specific. However, some plans may use a unit operations approach. Generic HACCP plans can serve as useful guides to develop process and product HACCP plans; however, it is essential that the unique conditions within each facility be considered while developing all components of the HACCP plan.

In the development of an HACCP plan, the Food and Drug Administration (FDA) notes that it is important that five preliminary tasks be accomplished before applying the HACCP principles to a specific product and process.

Assemble the HACCP Team

An HACCP team should consist of individuals who have specific knowledge and expertise on the product and process. (The team should be multidisciplinary, with individuals from engineering, production, sanitation, quality assurance, and microbiology.) The team will develop the HACCP plan. An HACCP team may need assistance from outside experts who are knowledgeable in the potential biological, chemical, or physical hazards associated with the product and the process. It is recommended that experts who are knowledgeable in the food process either participate in or verify the completeness of the hazard analysis and the HACCP plan.

Describe the Food and Its Distribution

Describing the food consists of a general description of the food, ingredients, and processing methods. Description of the food distribution should include information on whether the food is to be distributed frozen, refrigerated, or at ambient temperature.

Describe the Intended Use and Consumers of the Food

The team is tasked with knowing for whom the food is intended. The intended consumers may be the general public or a subpopulation, such as the elderly, infants, or maybe immunocompromised individuals. Thus, it is important that the team consider any special needs of certain subpopulations for which the food may be intended.

Develop a Flow Diagram Describing the Process

The team is expected to develop a flow diagram that is a clear and simple outline of the steps involved in the process. It is crucial that the flow diagram covers all the steps in the process, which is directly under the control of the manufacturer's crew responsible for the process. Such a schematic outline of the facility is often useful to understand and evaluate product and processes flow.

Verify the Flow Diagram

An onsite review of the process operation to verify the accuracy and completeness of the flow diagram should be conducted. Modifications may be made to the flow diagram as necessary and documented.

After implementing the five preliminary tasks, the seven principles of HACCP are applied:

PRINCIPLE 1: HAZARD ANALYSIS

The hazard analysis process accomplishes three purposes: (1) identifies hazards of significance; (2) provides a risk basis for selecting likely hazards; (3) uses identified hazards to develop preventive measures for a process or product to ensure or improve food safety.

The first step is to identify hazards associated with the product. A hazard may be a biological, chemical, or a physical attribute that can cause a food to be unsafe. During analysis of hazards, two factors must be assessed with respect to any identified hazard: (1) the likelihood that the hazard will occur and (2) the severity if it does occur. Hazard analysis also involves establishment of preventive measures, elimination or reduction, for control. Numerous issues have to be considered, including factors beyond the immediate control of the food establishment. For example, how the food will be treated if taken by the consumer and how it will be consumed must be considered because these factors could influence how food should be prepared or processed in the establishment.

The flow diagram forms the foundation for applying the seven principles. The significant hazards associated with each step in the flow diagram should be listed along with preventive measures proposed to control the hazards. Such information should be used under Principle 2 to determine the CCPs. Each step in a process should be identified and observed to accurately construct the flow diagram. CCPs for biological, chemical, and physical hazards should be identified and preventive measures determined.

PRINCIPLE 2: DETERMINE CRITICAL CONTROL POINTS (CCPs)

A CCP is defined as a step at which control can be applied, and it is essential to prevent or eliminate a food safety hazard or reduce it to an acceptable level. The potential hazards that are reasonably likely to cause illness or injury in the absence of their control must be addressed in determining CCPs.

Complete and accurate identification of CCPs is crucial to control food safety hazards. The information developed during the hazard analysis is essential for the HACCP team in identifying which steps in the process are CCPs. A CCP decision tree can be useful in determining whether a particular step is a CCP for a previously identified hazard; however, it is merely a tool and not a mandatory element of

Emerging Food Safety Issues in a Modern World

HACCP. CCPs are located at any step where hazards can be prevented, eliminated, or reduced to acceptable levels. Also, CCPs must be carefully developed and documented. A specified heat process with a given time and temperature designed to destroy a specific microbiological pathogen is an example of a CCP. Other examples are refrigeration of a precooked food to prevent hazardous microorganisms from multiplying or the adjustment of a food to a pH necessary to prevent toxin formation.

PRINCIPLE 3: ESTABLISH CRITICAL LIMITS FOR PREVENTIVE MEASURES

This step involves establishing a criterion that must be met for each preventive measure associated with a CCP. Critical limits can be thought of as upper and lower limits of safety for each CCP and may be set for preventive measures such as temperature, time, physical dimensions, a_w, and pH. Critical limits may be taken from resources such as regulatory standards and guidelines, scientific literature, experimental studies, and consultation with experts.

An example is the cooking of beef patties. The process should be designed to eliminate the most heat-resistant pathogen that could be reasonably expected to be in the product. Criteria may be required for factors such as temperature, time, and meat patty thickness. The appropriate critical limits require accurate information on the probable maximum numbers of these microorganisms in the meat and their heat resistance.

PRINCIPLE 4: ESTABLISH PROCEDURES TO MONITOR CCPS

Monitoring is needed to assess whether a CCP is under control and to produce an accurate record for use in future verification procedures. Monitoring serves three main purposes. First, monitoring is essential to food safety management because it assists in tracking the operation. If monitoring indicates that there is a trend toward loss of control, then action can be taken to bring the process back into control before a deviation from a critical limit occurs. Second, monitoring is used to determine when there is loss of control and a deviation occurs at a CCP, i.e., exceeding or not meeting a critical limit. When a deviation occurs, an appropriate corrective action must be taken. Third, monitoring provides written documentation for use in verification.

Continuous monitoring is always preferred when feasible and continuous monitoring is possible with many types of physical and chemical methods. For example, the temperature and time for an institutional cook-chill operation can be recorded continuously on temperature-recording charts. If the temperature falls below the scheduled temperature or the time is insufficient, as recorded on the chart, the batch must be recorded as a process deviation and reprocessed or discarded.

When it is not possible to monitor a critical limit on a continuous basis, it is necessary to establish that the monitoring interval is reliable enough to indicate that the hazard is under control. Statistically designed data collection or sampling systems lend themselves to this purpose. When statistical process control is used, it is important to recognize that violations of critical limits must not occur. For example, when a temperature of 68°C (155°F) or higher is required for product safety, the minimum temperature of the product may be set at a target that is above this temperature to compensate for variation.

Most monitoring procedures for CCPs need to be done rapidly because the time frame between food preparation and consumption does not allow for lengthy analytical testing. Microbiological testing is seldom effective for monitoring CCPs because it is time consuming. Therefore, physical and chemical measurements are preferred, because they can be done rapidly and indicate whether microbiological control occurs.

Assigning responsibility for monitoring is an important consideration for each CCP within the operation. Specific assignments depend on the number of CCPs, preventive measures, and the complexity of monitoring. The most appropriate employees for such assignments are often directly associated with the operation, such as the person in charge of the food establishment, chefs, and departmental supervisors.

Individuals monitoring CCPs must be trained in the monitoring technique, completely understand the purpose and importance of monitoring, and be unbiased in monitoring and reporting so that monitoring is accurately recorded. The designated individuals must have ready access to the CCP being monitored and to the calibrated instrumentation designated in the HACCP plan.

The people responsible for monitoring must also record a food operation or product that does not meet critical limits and ensure that immediate corrective action is taken. All records and documents associated with CCP monitoring must be signed or initialed by the person doing the monitoring.

Random checks may be useful in supplementing the monitoring of certain CCPs. They may be used to check incoming ingredients, serve as a check for compliance when ingredients are recertified as meeting certain standards, and assess factors such as equipment. Random checks are also advisable for monitoring environmental factors, such as airborne contamination, and cleaning and sanitizing gloves.

With some foods containing microbiological sensitive ingredients, there may not be an alternative to microbiological testing. However, it is important to recognize that a sampling frequency adequate for reliable detection of low levels of pathogens is seldom possible because of the large number of samples needed. For this reason, microbiological testing has limitations in an HACCP system, but is valuable to establish and verify the effectiveness of control at CCPs (such as through challenge tests, random testing, or testing that focuses on isolating the source of a problem).

PRINCIPLE 5: CORRECTIVE ACTION WHEN A CRITICAL LIMIT IS EXCEEDED

Although the HACCP system is intended to prevent deviations from occurring, perfection is rarely, if ever, achievable. Thus, there must be a corrective action plan in place to (1) determine the disposition of any food that was produced when a deviation was occurring; (2) correct the cause of the deviation and ensure that the CCP is under control; and (3) maintain records of corrective actions.

The HACCP system for food safety management is designed to identify health hazards and to establish strategies to prevent, eliminate, or reduce their occurrence. However, ideal circumstances do not always prevail and deviations from established processes may occur. An important purpose of corrective actions is to prevent foods that may be hazardous from reaching consumers.

As a minimum, the HACCP plan should specify what is done when a deviation occurs, who is responsible for implementing the corrective actions, and ensure that a record is developed and maintained of the actions taken. Individuals who have a thorough understanding of the process, product, and HACCP plans should be assigned the responsibility of overseeing corrective actions. Experts may be consulted to review the information available and to assist in determining disposition of noncompliant products.

Principle 6: Effective Record-Keeping Systems

The principle requires the preparation and maintenance of a written HACCP plan by the food establishment. The plan must detail the hazards of each individual or a categorical product covered by the plan. It must clearly identify the CCPs and critical limits for each CCP. CCP monitoring and record-keeping procedures must be shown in the establishment's HACCP plan. The HACCP plan implementation strategy should be provided as a part of the food establishment's documentation.

The principle requires the maintenance of records generated during the operation of the plan. The record keeping associated with HACCP procedures ultimately makes the system work. One conclusion of a study of HACCP performed by the U.S. Department of Commerce is that correcting problems without record keeping almost guarantees that the problems will recur. The requirement to record events at CCPs on a regular basis ensures that preventive monitoring occurs in a systematic way. Unusual occurrences that are discovered as CCPs are monitored or that otherwise comes to light must be corrected and recorded immediately with a notation of the corrective action taken.

The level of sophistication of record keeping necessary for the food establishment depends on the complexity of the food preparation operation. A cook–chill operation for a large institution requires more record keeping than a limited-menu cook–serve operation. The simplest effective record-keeping system that lends itself well to integration within the existing operation is best.

Principle 7: Verify That the HAACP System Is Working

1. Verification procedures may include the following:
   - Establishment of appropriate verification inspection schedules.
   - Review of the HACCP plan.
   - Review of CCP records.
   - Review of deviations and their resolution, including the disposition of food.
   - Visual inspections of operations to observe whether CCPs are under control.
   - Random sample collection and analysis.
   - Review of critical limits to verify that they are adequate to control hazards.

- Review of written records of verification inspections that certify compliance with the HACCP plan or deviations from the plan and the corrective actions taken.
- Validation of HACCP plan, including onsite review and verification of flow diagrams and CCPs.
- Review of modifications of the HACCP plan.
2. Verification inspections should be conducted:
    - Routinely or on an unannounced basis, to ensure that selected CCPs are under control.
    - When it is determined that intensive coverage of a specific food is needed because of new information concerning food safety.
    - When foods prepared at the establishment have been implicated as vehicles of foodborne disease.
    - When requested on a consultative basis and resources allow accommodating the request.
    - When established criteria have not been met.
    - To verify that changes have been implemented correctly after an HACCP plan has been modified.
3. Verification reports should include information about:
    - Existence of an HACCP plan and the persons responsible for administering and updating the HACCP plan.
    - The status of records associated with CCP monitoring.
    - Direct monitoring data of the CCP while in operation and certification that monitoring equipment is properly calibrated and in working order.
    - Deviations and corrective actions.
    - Any samples analyzed to verify that CCPs are under control; analyses may involve physical, chemical, microbiological, or organoleptic methods.
    - Modifications to the HACCP plan.
    - Training and knowledge of individuals responsible for monitoring CCPs.

A periodic comprehensive verification of the HACCP system should be conducted by an unbiased, independent authority. Such authorities can be internal or external to the food operation. This should include a technical evaluation of the hazard analysis and each element of the HACCP plan as well as onsite review of all flow diagrams and appropriate records from operation of the plan. A comprehensive verification is independent of other verification procedures and must be performed to ensure that the HACCP plan results in the control of the hazards. If the results of the comprehensive verification identify deficiencies, the HACCP team should modify the HACCP plan as necessary.

Thus, HACCP is a systematic approach to food safety that will dramatically improve the level of food safety. The National Academy of Sciences has developed the seven HACCP principles discussed. The FDA recommends the implementation of an HACCP system throughout the food industry using these National Academy of Sciences recommendations.

An effective national food safety program from food production to consumer use is enhanced by the implementation of HACCP. The statistics from foodborne surveillance reveal that retail-level food establishments can significantly impact on the health of consumers.

Implementation of HACCP programs by the establishments will profoundly enhance their role in the protection of public health beyond the traditional emphasis on facility and equipment design and maintenance and adherence to the principles of sanitation, good manufacturing, and food preparation practices. Education and training of all personnel are critical to the success and effectiveness of any HACCP program. The *Food Code* stresses the application of HACCP principles and the knowledge and responsibilities of establishment management and employees. The *Food Code* is a reference document for regulatory agencies that oversee food safety in food service establishments, retail food stores, other food establishments at the retail level, and institutions such as nursing homes and childcare centers.

Specific HACCP plans for the products prepared and sold by retail food establishments should be developed and implemented for optimal food safety management. HACCP systems are recommended for use as a tool for regulatory inspections. The regulatory official should incorporate procedures in the inspection process that ensure record reviews and active monitoring.

Because the retail food establishment industry is composed of large, small, chain, and independent establishments, the level of food safety expertise varies widely and is not necessarily linked to size or affiliation. Regardless of the size and sophistication of the establishment, HACCP plans for safe food preparation and sales needs to be designed, implemented, and verified.

Studies have shown that a significant level of illness and mortality from foodborne disease in institutional feeding operations such as hospitals, nursing homes, and prisons is related to preventable causes. For populations that may be more vulnerable to foodborne disease, FDA and the National Advisory Committee on Microbiological Criteria of Foods (NACMCF) recommend that HACCP systems be immediately implemented by establishments and institutions preparing foods for these susceptible individuals.

Food-processing operations at retail food establishments such as reduced-oxygen packaging and curing and smoking under the *Food Code* are required to develop and implement an HACCP plan for that part of the operation. Food establishments have the primary responsibility for food safety. Development and implementation of HACCP programs are reliable and responsible steps to help ensure the safety of food offered for consumption.

ANTIBIOTIC RESISTANCE

Pathogenic bacteria that have become resistant to antibiotic therapy are an increasing public health problem. For example, tuberculosis, gonorrhea, malaria, and ear infections in children are just a few of the diseases that have become hard to treat with antibiotic drugs. Part of the problem is that microorganisms that cause infections are extremely hardy and can develop ways to endure drugs meant to kill or weaken them. This antibiotic resistance (antimicrobial resistance or drug resistance), is due largely to the increasing use of antibiotics. Ironically, antimicrobial resistance has been recognized since the introduction of penicillin nearly 50 years ago, when penicillin-resistant infections caused by *Staphylococcus aureus* rapidly appeared.

The 1990s has become known as the era of multidrug resistance. Bacteria causing several kinds of human infectious diseases have become resistant to multiple antibiotics and the different types continue to increase. Infections challenge and impede the treatment of some patients in hospitals and the community. In hospitals, organisms found include *Staphylococcus aureus, Escherichia coli, Pseudomonas,* and *Acinetobacter.* In the community, multidrug-resistant bacteria causing acquired infections include pneumococci, gonococci, streptococci, *E. coli,* and *Mycobacterium tuberculosis.* There is ample evidence that the antibiotic-resistance problem is global, confronting many communities worldwide. Also, it is known that resistant organisms are spreading from one country to another. Resistant organisms are making it difficult to treat sinusitis, urinary tract infections, pneumonia, septicemias, and meningitis. Two disease-causing organisms — enterococci in hospitals and *Mycobacterium tuberculosis* in the community and the hospital — have been linked to death because of their resistance to antibiotics.

The costs of antibiotic resistance continue to rise. Mortality and length of hospital stay are at least doubled for resistant strains of some organisms compared with susceptible ones. Treating resistant infections often requires the use of more expensive drugs or more drugs with significant side effects, resulting in longer hospital stays for infected patients. The Institute of Medicine, a part of the National Academy of Sciences, has estimated that the annual cost of treating antibiotic-resistant infections in the U.S. may be as high as $30 billion.

Besides the hospitalized and immunocompromised persons, children attending day-care centers and elderly patients in nursing homes are susceptible risk groups. To make the situation worse, about half of the pharmaceutical companies in the U.S. abandoned the once lucrative antimicrobial field in the mid-1980s. A key reason for the development of antimicrobial resistance is the ability of infectious organisms to adapt quickly to new environmental conditions. Microbes are, in essence, single-celled organisms that have a small number of genes. Subsequently, even a single arbitrary gene mutation can have a large impact on their disease-causing properties. Because of the high replication rates of microbes, mutations can evolve rapidly. Many mutations essentially help a microbe survive in the presence of an antibiotic drug, which could quickly predominate throughout the microbial population. Microbes commonly acquire genes, including those encoding for resistance, by direct transfer from organisms of their own species or from unrelated microorganisms. This inborn adaptability of microbes has been complicated by the widespread and inappropriate use of antimicrobials. Ideal conditions exist for the emergence of drug-resistant microbes when antibiotics are prescribed for the common cold and other conditions for which they are not required or when individuals do not complete or forget to take their prescribed treatment regimen. Hospitals can also provide a fertile environment for drug-resistant pathogens because of the close contact between sick patients and extensive use of antimicrobial force pathogens to develop resistance.

SCOPE OF THE PROBLEM

At present, hospital and nonhospital settings worldwide are facing unprecedented crises from the rapid emergence and distribution of microbes resistant to one or more antimicrobial agents. Strains of *Staphylococcus aureus* resistant to methicillin and other antibiotics are endemic in hospitals. Unfortunately, the number of useful drugs against these infections is limited. *S. aureus* strains with reduced susceptibility to vancomycin have emerged recently in Japan and the U.S., and this is a serious problem for patients and medical care workers. Currently, ca. 30% of *Streptococcus pneumoniae* isolates are resistant to penicillin, the primary drug used to treat this infection. Many penicillin-resistant strains are also resistant to other antimicrobial drugs. *S. pneumoniae* is responsible for thousands of cases of meningitis and pneumonia, and several million cases of ear infection in the U.S. every year. For sexually transmitted disease clinics that monitor outbreaks of drug-resistant infections, doctors have found that more than 30% of gonorrhea isolates are resistant to penicillin or tetracycline, or combinations of both.

About a half-billion people worldwide are infected with the parasites that cause malaria. Resistance to chloroquine, the drug of choice for preventing and treating malaria, has emerged worldwide. Also, resistance to other antimalarial drugs is widespread and growing.

Strains of multidrug-resistant tuberculosis have emerged over the last decade and pose a particular threat to vulnerable people, e.g., those infected with HIV. Drug-resistant strains are as contagious as drug-susceptible ones. Multidrug-resistant tuberculosis is more difficult and more expensive to treat, and patients may remain infectious longer because of inadequate treatment.

Foodborne diarrheal diseases cause almost 3 million deaths a year worldwide. Resistant strains of highly pathogenic bacteria such as *Shigella dysenteriae, Campylobacter, Vibrio cholerae, Escherichia coli,* and *Salmonella* are emerging. Recent outbreaks of *Salmonella* food poisoning have occurred in the U.S. A potentially dangerous strain, *Salmonella typhimurium*, resistant to ampicillin, sulfa, streptomycin, tetracycline and chloramphenicol, has caused illness in Europe, Canada, and the U.S.

New evidence that drugs used in poultry can cause antibiotic-resistant infections in consumers spurred the FDA's Center for Veterinary Medicine (CVM) to take action. CVM proposed to withdraw the approval of the antibacterial Baytril® (enrofloxacin) used to treat disease in chickens and turkeys. CVM had approved Baytril in 1996. Made by the Bayer Corporation, Baytril belongs to a class of antibacterials called fluoroquinolones, which have been used in humans since 1986. Poultry growers use fluoroquinolone drugs to keep chicken and turkeys from dying from *E. coli* infection, a disease endemic to turkeys. Because the size of flocks precludes testing and treating individual chicken, when a veterinarian diagnoses an infected bird, the farmers treat the whole flock via their drinking water. The drug may cure the *E. coli* infection in the poultry, but other kind of bacteria such as *Campylobacter*, may build up resistance to these drugs.

People who consume chicken or turkey contaminated with fluoroquinolone-resistant *Campylobacter* are therefore at risk of becoming infected with a bacterium that current drugs are ineffective against. *Campylobacter* is the most common bacterial cause of diarrheal illness in the U.S., according to the Centers for Disease Control and Prevention (CDC). It is estimated to affect more than 2 million people every year, or 1% of the population. *Campylobacter* does not make the birds sick, but humans who eat the bacteria-contaminated birds may become sick. *Campylobacter* can be life threatening in immunocompromised individuals. Undercooked chicken or turkey or other food that has been contaminated from contact with raw poultry is a frequent source of *Campylobacter* infection. People infected with *Campylobacter* may be prescribed a fluoroquinolone, but unfortunately the drug may or may not be effective.

Most researchers in the field of antibiotics agree that there is a need to develop molecular methods to detect resistance, and such research efforts need to be a priority. Also, surveillance systems need to be developed by using practitioners, hospital and private laboratories, and health maintenance organizations (HMOs) to detect new resistance mechanisms and to detect the development of resistance in normally susceptible organisms. This database will be useful to monitor trends in antibiotic resistance. Also, drugs and other means to deal with newly resistant organisms must be developed. Finally, it is crucial to enhance public awareness regarding the fact that the problem is real and that antimicrobial treatment is not always a good plan.

GMOs

It is estimated that about 40% of soybean and 30% of corn grown in the U.S. is genetically modified. For these crops, there are economic as well as environmental incentives to use the modified varieties. In addition to somewhat increased yields, lesser quantities of herbicides and pesticides are needed, which lowers production costs and decreases the addition of chemicals to the environment. It is estimated that the world's population will reach 9 billion within the next 50 years. Having enough food still remains a crucial issue worldwide. Advances in biotechnology provide the best hope of producing enough food to feed an ever-expanding population. If molecular biology is used with as much care as it has been till now, our food supply should remain abundant and safe long into the future.

Genetically modified (GM) foods have received a lot of bad publicity. There was a major issue of protesters, which has led to the ban of U.S. farm products by European markets. Critics have claimed that altered foods may be unsafe. Ironically, although many issues surround GM foods, safety and nutrition should not be among them. These foods are as safe and nutritious as their conventional counterparts. To the novice, manipulation of the genes of plants that are eaten may sound scary, but working with genes has not been all that mysterious because scientists unraveled their secrets years ago. Briefly, a gene, made of DNA, provides cells with instructions for making a specific protein. When DNA with a known structure is used by a cell to make a protein, the composition of the resulting protein is known with exact precision. Because of this precision, we were able to make a copy of DNA that served as the blueprint for human insulin. The copy was inserted into bacteria, which then produced human insulin. Such insulin has been used with absolute safety for years. This same precision is used to modify plant genes to produce proteins that the plant would not otherwise make. Because of such precision, one can make changes in the laboratory that might take decades to occur by the traditional breeding techniques.

In modern times, two modified crops have drawn the most fire from critics, probably because together they account for about 98% of GM crops grown worldwide: a soybean variety that is resistant to herbicides and a corn variety that has been altered to produce a protein that is toxic to the European corn borer. The soybean and corn varieties differ from their conventional parent in that each has an extra gene and each makes a protein that otherwise would not be made. Consuming the extra DNA will not produce adverse effects, because we consume DNA in our diet all the time. The protein made by the corn that is toxic to the European corn borer is not toxic to people. Like other proteins, the body will digest this protein too for its amino acid content. This will also be true for the extra protein made by the herbicide-resistant soybean.

Thus, modified soybean and corn are substantially equivalent to their conventional counterparts; that is, they are not different from the conventional product in terms of properties such as taste and nutritional quality or in use.

Critics of GM foods have expressed the concern that these types of hybrids could cause allergic reactions. However, more than 90% of food allergies are known to occur in response to specific proteins in eight foods: peanuts, tree nuts, milk, eggs, soybean, shellfish, fish, and wheat. The FDA is aware of the problem that can occur if allergenic proteins are transferred to other foods without consumer knowledge and has taken steps to prevent it.

Highly publicized controversial studies about the effects of GM corn pollen on monarch butterfly caterpillars have brought the issue of genetic engineering to the forefront of public consciousness in the U.S. In response to the public concern, the U.S. FDA held open meetings to solicit public opinions and begin the process of establishing a new regulatory procedure for government approval of GM foods.

The term *GM foods* or *GMOs* (genetically modified organisms) is most commonly used to refer to crop plants created for human or animal consumption by using the latest molecular biology techniques. These plants have been modified in the laboratory to enhance desired traits such as increased resistance to herbicides or improved nutritional content. The enhancement of desired traits has traditionally been undertaken through breeding, but conventional plant breeding methods can be very time consuming and are often not very accurate. Genetic engineering, on the other hand, can create plants with the exact desired trait very rapidly and with great accuracy. For example, plant geneticists can isolate the gene responsible for drought tolerance and insert the gene into a different plant, which will give the new GM plant drought tolerance as well. Not only can genes be transferred from one plant to another, but genes from nonplant organisms can also be used. The best-known example of this is the use of Bt, or *Bacillus thuringiensis*, genes in corn and other crops. Bt is a naturally occurring bacterium that produces crystal proteins lethal to insect larvae. Bt crystal protein genes have been transferred into corn, enabling the corn to produce its own pesticides against insects such as the European corn borer.

Ensuring an adequate food supply for the booming population is going to be a major challenge for the future. GM foods promise to meet this need in a number of ways.

Pest Resistance

Crop losses from insect pests can be staggering, resulting in devastating financial loss for farmers and starvation in developing countries. Farmers typically use many tons of chemical pesticides annually. Consumers do not want to eat food treated with pesticides because of potential health hazards, and run-off of agricultural wastes from excessive use of pesticides and fertilizers can poison the water supply and cause harm to the environment. The increasing number of GM foods such as Bt corn can help eliminate the application of chemical pesticides and reduce the cost of bringing a crop to market.

Herbicide Tolerance

For some crops, it is not cost effective to remove weeds by physical means such as tilling; therefore, farmers often spray large quantities of different herbicides (weed killers) to destroy weeds, which is a time-consuming and expensive process that requires care so that the herbicide does not harm the crop plant or the environment. Crop plants genetically engineered to be resistant to one very powerful herbicide could help prevent environmental damage by reducing the amount of herbicides needed. For example, a strain of soybean genetically modified to be not affected by herbicide product Roundup® has been developed. When grown, this soybean requires only a single application of a weed killer instead of multiple applications, reducing the production cost and limiting the dangers of agricultural waste run-off.

Disease Resistance

Many viruses, fungi, and bacteria cause plant diseases. Plant biologists are working to create plants with genetically engineered resistance to these diseases.

Cold Tolerance

Unexpected frost can destroy sensitive seedlings. An antifreeze gene from cold water fish has been introduced into plants such as tobacco and potato. With this antifreeze gene, these plants are able to tolerate cold temperatures that would normally kill unmodified seedlings.

Drought Tolerance and Salinity Tolerance

As the world population grows and more land is utilized for housing instead of food production, farmers will need to grow crops in locations previously unsuited for plant cultivation. Creating plants that can withstand long periods of drought or high salt content in soil and groundwater will help people grow crops in formerly inhospitable places.

Nutrition

Malnutrition is common in Third World countries, where impoverished people rely on a single crop such as rice for the main staple of their diet. However, rice does not contain adequate amounts of all necessary nutrients to prevent malnutrition. If rice can be genetically engineered to contain additional vitamins and minerals, nutrient deficiencies can be alleviated. For example, blindness due to vitamin A deficiency is a common problem in Third World countries. Researchers at the Institute for Plant Sciences, Swiss Federal Institute of Technology, have created a strain of golden rice containing an unusually high content of β-carotene (vitamin A). Plans are underway to develop a golden rice that also has increased iron content.

Pharmaceuticals

Medicines and vaccines are often costly to produce and sometimes require special storage conditions not readily available in Third World countries. Researchers are working to develop edible vaccines in tomatoes and potatoes. These vaccines will be much easier to ship, store, and administer than traditional injectable vaccines.

Phytoremediation

Not all GM plants are grown as crops. Soil and groundwater pollution continues to be a problem worldwide. Plants such as poplar trees have been genetically engineered to clean up heavy metal pollution from contaminated soil.

According to the FDA and the United States Department of Agriculture (USDA), more than 40 plant varieties have completed all the federal requirements for commercialization. Some examples of these plants are tomatoes and cantaloupes that have modified ripening characteristics, soybean and sugar beets that are resistant to herbicides, and corn and cotton plants with increased resistance to insect pests. Although there are very few GM whole fruits and vegetables available on produce stands, highly processed foods such as vegetable oils or breakfast cereals most likely contain a tiny percentage of GM ingredients because the raw ingredients have been pooled into one processing stream from many different sources. Also, the ubiquity of soybean derivatives as food additives in the modern U.S. diet virtually ensures that all U.S. consumers are exposed to GM food products.

Thirteen countries grew genetically engineered crops commercially in 2000, of which the U.S. produced the majority. In 2000, 68% of all GM crops were grown by U.S. farmers. In comparison, Argentina, Canada, and China produced only 23%, 7%, and 1%, respectively. Australia, Bulgaria, France, Germany, Mexico, Romania, South Africa, Spain, and Uruguay also grew commercial GM crops in 2000.

Soybean and corn are the two most widely grown GM crops (82%), with cotton, rapeseed (or canola), and potatoes trailing behind. Seventy-four percent of GM crops were modified for herbicide tolerance, 19% for insect pest resistance, and 7% for both herbicide tolerance and pest tolerance. Globally, acreage of GM crops has increased 25-fold in 5 years, from approximately 4.3 million acres in 1996 to 109 million acres in 2000 — almost twice the area of the U.K. Approximately 99 million acres were devoted to GM crops in the U.S. and Argentina alone.

In the U.S., approximately 54% of all soybean cultivated in 2000 was genetically modified, up from 42% in 1998 and only 7% in 1996. In 2000, GM cotton varieties accounted for 61% of the total cotton crop, up from 42% in 1998 and 15% in 1996. GM corn also experienced a similar but less dramatic increase. GM corn production increased to 25% of all corn grown in 2000, about the same as 1998 (26%), but up from 1.5% in 1996. As anticipated, pesticide and herbicide use on these GM varieties was slashed and, for the most part, yields were increased.

Environmental activists, religious organizations, public interest groups, professional associations, and other scientists and government officials have raised concerns about GM foods and criticized agribusiness for pursuing profit without concern for potential hazards and the government for failing to exercise adequate regulatory supervision. Most concerns about GM foods fall into three categories: environmental hazards, human health risks, and economic concerns.

ENVIRONMENTAL HAZARDS

Unintended Harm to Other Organisms

In 2002, a laboratory study was published in *Nature* showing that pollen from Bt corn caused high mortality rates in monarch butterfly caterpillars. Monarch caterpillars consume milkweed plants, not corn, but the fear is that if pollen from Bt corn is blown by the wind onto milkweed plants in neighboring fields, the caterpillars could eat the pollen and perish. Although the *Nature* study was not conducted under natural field conditions, the results seemed to support this viewpoint. Unfortunately, Bt toxins kill many species of insect larvae indiscriminately; it is not possible to design a Bt toxin that will only kill crop-damaging pests and remain harmless to all other insects. This study is being reexamined by the USDA, the U.S. EPA, and other nongovernment research groups, and preliminary data from new studies suggest that the original study may have been flawed. Currently, there is no agreement about the results of these studies, and the potential risk of harm to nontarget organisms will need to be evaluated further.

Reduced Effectiveness of Pesticides

Just as some populations of mosquitoes developed resistance to the now-banned pesticide DDT, many people are concerned that insects will become resistant to Bt or other crops that have been genetically modified to produce their own pesticides.

Gene Transfer to Nontarget Species

Another concern is that crop plants engineered for herbicide tolerance and weeds will crossbreed, resulting in the transfer of the herbicide-resistance genes from the crops into the weeds. These super weeds would then be herbicide tolerant as well. Other introduced genes may cross over into nonmodified crops planted next to GM crops. The possibility of interbreeding is shown by the defense of farmers against lawsuits filed by Monsanto. The company has filed patent infringement lawsuits against farmers who may have harvested GM crops. Monsanto claims that the farmers obtained Monsanto-licensed GM seeds from an unknown source and did not pay royalties to Monsanto. The farmers claim that their unmodified crops were cross-pollinated from someone else's GM crops planted a field or two away. Time and more investigation are needed to resolve this issue.

Human Health Risks

Allergenicity

Many children in the U.S. and Europe have developed life-threatening allergies to peanuts and other foods. There is a possibility that introducing a gene into a plant may create a new allergen or cause an allergic reaction in susceptible individuals. A proposal to incorporate a gene from Brazil nuts into soybeans was abandoned because of the fear of causing unexpected allergic reactions. Testing of GM foods may be required to avoid the possibility of harm to consumers with food allergies.

Unknown Effects on Human Health

There is a growing concern that introducing foreign genes into food plants may have an unexpected and negative impact on human health. A recent article published in *The Lancet* examined the effects of GM potatoes on the digestive tract in rats. This study claimed that there were appreciable differences in the intestines of rats fed GM potatoes and rats fed unmodified potatoes. Yet critics say that this paper, like the monarch butterfly data, is flawed and does not hold up to scientific scrutiny. Moreover, the gene introduced into the potatoes was a snowdrop flower lectin, a substance known to be toxic to mammals. The scientists who created this variety of potato chose to use the lectin gene simply to test the methodology, and these potatoes were never intended for human or animal consumption.

On the whole, with the exception of possible allergenicity, scientists believe that GM foods do not present a risk to human health.

Economic Concerns

Bringing a GM food to market is a lengthy and costly process, and agribiotech companies want to ensure a profitable return on their investment. Many new plant genetic engineering technologies and GM plants have been patented, and patent infringement is a big concern for agribusiness. Yet consumer advocates are worried that patenting these new plant varieties will raise the price of seeds to such an extent that small farmers and Third World countries will not be able to afford seeds for GM crops, thus widening the gap between the wealthy and the poor. Perhaps there needs to be a humanitarian gesture by more companies to offer their products at reduced cost to impoverished nations.

Governments worldwide are hard at work to establish a regulatory process to monitor the effects of and approve new varieties of GM plants. Yet depending on the political, social, and an economic climate within a region or country, different governments are responding in different ways.

In Japan, the Ministry of Health and Welfare has announced that health testing of GM foods will be mandatory. Currently, testing of GM foods is voluntary. Japanese supermarkets are offering both GM foods and unmodified foods, and customers are beginning to show a strong preference for unmodified fruits and vegetables.

India's government has not yet announced a policy on GM foods, because no GM crops are grown in India and no products are commercially available in supermarkets yet. India is, however, very supportive of transgenic plant research. It is highly likely that India will decide that the benefits of GM foods outweigh the risks, because Indian agriculture will need to adopt drastic new measures to counteract the country's endemic poverty and feed its exploding population.

Some states in Brazil have banned GM crops entirely, and the Brazilian Institute for the Defense of Consumers, in collaboration with Greenpeace, has filed a suit to prevent the importation of GM crops. Brazilian farmers, however, have resorted to smuggling GM soybean seeds into the country, because they fear economic harm if they are unable to compete in the global market with other grain-exporting countries.

In Europe, anti-GM food protestors have been especially active. In the last few years, Europe has experienced two major food scares: bovine spongiform encephalopathy (mad cow disease) in Great Britain and dioxin-tainted foods originating from Belgium. These food scares have undermined consumer confidence about the European food supply, and citizens are disinclined to trust government information about GM foods. In response to the public outcry, Europe now requires mandatory food labeling of GM foods in stores, and the European Commission (EC) has established a 1% threshold for contamination of unmodified foods with GM food products.

In the U.S., the regulatory process is confused because three different government agencies have jurisdiction over GM foods. To put it very simply, the EPA evaluates GM plants for environmental safety, the USDA evaluates whether the plant is safe to grow, and the FDA evaluates whether the plant is safe to eat. The EPA is responsible for regulating substances such as pesticides or toxins that may cause harm to the environment. GM crops such as Bt pesticide-laced corn or herbicide-tolerant crops but not foods modified for their nutritional value fall under the purview of the EPA. The USDA is responsible for GM crops that do not fall under the umbrella of the EPA, such as drought-tolerant or disease-tolerant crops; crops grown for animal feeds; or whole fruits, vegetables, and grains for human consumption. The FDA historically has been concerned with pharmaceuticals, cosmetics, and food products and additives, and not whole foods. Under current guidelines, a GM ear of corn sold at a produce stand is not regulated by the FDA because it is a whole food, but a box of cornflakes is regulated because it is a food product. The FDA's stance is that GM foods are substantially equivalent to unmodified, natural foods, and therefore not subject to FDA regulation.

The EPA conducts risk assessment studies on pesticides that could potentially cause harm to human health and the environment and establishes tolerance and residue levels for pesticides. There are strict limits on the amount of pesticides that may be applied to crops during growth and production, as well as the amount that remains in the food after processing. Growers using pesticides must have a license for each pesticide and must follow the directions on the label to accord with EPA's safety standards. Government inspectors may periodically visit farms and conduct investigations to ensure compliance. Violation of government regulations may result in steep fines, loss of license, and even jail sentences.

As an example of the EPA regulatory approach, consider Bt corn. The EPA has not established limits on residue levels in Bt corn because the Bt in the corn is not sprayed as a chemical pesticide but is a gene that is integrated into the genetic material of the corn itself. Growers must have a license from the EPA for Bt corn, and the EPA had issued a letter for the 2000 growing season requiring farmers to plant 20% unmodified corn and up to 50% unmodified corn in regions where cotton is also cultivated. This planting strategy may help prevent insects from developing resistance to the Bt pesticides as well as provide a refuge for nontarget insects such as monarch butterflies.

The USDA has many internal divisions that share responsibility for assessing GM foods. Among these divisions is the Animal Health and Plant Inspection Service (APHIS), which conducts field tests and issues permits to grow GM crops; the Agricultural Research Service, which performs in-house GM food research; and the Cooperative State Research, Education and Extension Service, which oversees the USDA risk assessment program. The USDA is concerned with potential hazards of the plant itself. Does it harbor insect pests? Is it a noxious weed? Will it cause harm to indigenous species if it escapes from farmers' fields? The USDA has the power to impose quarantines on problem regions to prevent movement of suspected plants, restrict import or export of suspected plants, and can even destroy plants cultivated in violation of USDA regulations. Many GM plants do not require USDA permits from APHIS. A GM plant does not require a permit if it meets the following six criteria: (1) the plant is not a noxious weed; (2) the genetic material introduced into the GM plant is subtly integrated into the plant's own genome; (3) the function of the introduced gene is known and does not cause plant disease; (4) the GM plant is not toxic to nontarget organisms; (5) the introduced gene will not cause the creation of new plant viruses; and (6) the GM plant cannot contain genetic material from animal or human pathogens (see http://www.aphis.usda.gov:80/bbep/bp/7cfr340.html).

The current FDA policy was developed in 1992 (Federal Register Docket No. 92N-0139) and states the agribiotech companies may voluntarily ask the FDA for a consultation. Companies working to create new GM foods are neither required to consult the FDA nor required to follow the FDA's recommendations after the consultation. Consumer interest groups want this process to be mandatory, so that all GM food products, whole foods or otherwise, must be approved by the FDA before being released for commercialization. The FDA counters that the agency currently does not have the time, money, or resources to carry out exhaustive health and safety studies of every proposed GM food product. Moreover, the FDA policy as it exists currently does not allow for this type of intervention.

GMO Foods and Labeling

Labeling of GM foods and food products is also a contentious issue. On the whole, agribusiness industries believe that labeling should be voluntary and influenced by the demands of the free market. If consumers prefer labeled foods to nonlabeled foods, then the industry will have the incentive to regulate itself or risk alienating the customer. Consumer interest groups, on the other hand, are demanding mandatory labeling. People have the right to know what they are eating, argue the interest groups, and historically the industry has proven itself to be unreliable at self-compliance with existing safety regulations. The FDA's current position on food labeling is governed by the Food, Drug and Cosmetic Act, which is only concerned with food additives and not whole foods or food products that are generally recognized as safe (GRAS). The FDA contends that GM foods are substantially equivalent to non-GM foods, and therefore not subject to more stringent labeling. If all GM foods and food products are to be labeled, the Congress must enact sweeping changes in the existing food-labeling policy.

Many questions must be answered if labeling of GM foods becomes mandatory. First, are consumers willing to absorb the cost of such an initiative? If the food production industry is required to label GM foods, factories will need to construct two separate processing streams and monitor the production lines accordingly. Farmers must be able to keep GM crops and non-GM crops from mixing during planting, harvesting, and shipping. It is almost assured that the industry will pass along these additional costs to consumers in the form of higher prices. Second, what are the acceptable limits of GM contamination in non-GM products? The EC has determined that 1% is an acceptable limit of cross-contamination, yet many consumer interest groups argue that only 0% is acceptable. Some companies such as Gerber, which makes baby foods, and Frito-Lay have pledged to avoid use of GM foods in any of their products.

Scientists agree that current technology is unable to detect minute quantities of contamination, and hence 0% contamination using existing methodologies is not guaranteed. Yet researchers disagree on what level of contamination really is detectable, especially in highly processed food products such as vegetable oils or breakfast cereals, wherein the vegetables used to make these products have been pooled from many different sources. A 1% threshold may already be below current levels of detectability.

Food labels must be designed to clearly convey accurate information about the product in simple language that everyone can understand. This may be the greatest challenge faced by a new food-labeling policy: how to educate and inform the public without damaging public trust and causing alarm or fear of GM food products.

In January 2000, an international trade agreement for labeling GM foods was established. More than 130 countries, including the U.S., the world's largest producer of GM foods, signed the agreement. The policy states that exporters must be required to label all GM foods and that importing countries have the right to judge for themselves the potential risks and reject GM foods, if they so choose. This new agreement will likely spur the U.S. government to resolve the domestic food-labeling dilemma more rapidly.

Conclusion

GM foods have the potential to solve many of the world's hunger and malnutrition problems and to help protect and preserve the environment by increasing yield and reducing reliance on chemical pesticides and herbicides. Yet there are many challenges ahead for governments, especially in the areas of safety testing, regulation, international policy, and food labeling. Many people feel that genetic engineering is the inevitable wave of the future and that we cannot afford to ignore a technology that has such enormous potential benefits. However, we must proceed not only with caution to avoid causing unintended harm to human health and the environment as a result of our enthusiasm for this powerful technology but also with better education and information to the public about the usefulness of GM.

STUDY QUESTIONS AND EXERCISES

1. Design an HACCP plan for elementary-school children who want to make chocolate chip cookies for sale at their annual fundraiser.
2. Describe the pitfalls of the nonjudicious use of antibiotics for the common cold. What are the problems associated with overuse of antibiotics in animal feeds?
3. What are the science-based concerns regarding the development of new foods using genetic techniques?
4. How are the GM foods regulated?
5. What are the relationships between SOPs, GMPs, HACCP, and food production or service?

RECOMMENDED READINGS

Bower, C.K. and Daeschel, M.A., Resistance response of microorganisms in food environments, *Int. J .Food Microbiol.,* 50, 33-44, 1999.
Bryan, F.L., Hazard analysis critical control point (HACCP) systems for retail food and restaurant operations, *J. Food Prot.,* 53(11), 978-983, 1990.
Buchanan, R.L., HACCP: A re-emerging approach to food safety, in *Trends in Food Science & Technology,* Elsevier, Amsterdam, 1990.
Corlett, D.A. Jr., Regulatory verification of industrial HACCP systems, *Food Technol.,* 45(5),144-146, 1991.
Hilleman, M.R., Overview: cause and prevention in biowarfare and bioterrorism, *Vaccine,* 2, 3055-3067, 2002.
Khan, A.S., Swerdlow, D.L., and Juranek, D.D., Precautions against biological and chemical terrorism directed at food and water supplies, *Pub. Hlth. Rep.,* 116, 3-14, 2001.
Kuiper, H.A., Kleter, G.A., Noteborn, H.P., and Kok, E.J., Substantial equivalence: an appropriate paradigm for the safety assessment of genetically modified foods?, *Toxicology,* 181/182, 427-431, 2002.
Martens, M.A., Safety evaluation of genetically modified foods, *Int. Arch. Occup. Environ. Hlth.,* 73, S14-S18, 2000.
Society of Toxicology, The safety of genetically modified foods produced through biotechnology, *Toxicol. Sci.,* 71, 2-8, 2003.
Stevenson, K.E., Implementing HACCP in the food industry, *Food Technol.,* 42(5),179-180, 1990.
van den Bogaard, A.E., Human health aspects of antibiotic use in food animals: a review, *Tijdschr. Diergeneeskd.,* 126, 590-605, 2001.
U.S. Food Code, http://vm.cfsan.fda.gov/~dms/fc01-toc.html.

Index

A

Acceptable daily intakes (ADIs), 77, 89
Acesulfame, 255
Acetylcholine, 234
Acinetobacter, 294
Acute promyelocytic leukemia (APL), 247
Acute toxicity testing, 41, 42
ADA, *see* American Dietetic Association
Adenosine diphosphate (ADP), 111
Adenosine triphosphate (ATP), 111
S-Adenosyl-L-homocysteine (SAH), 133
ADIs, *see* Acceptable daily intakes
ADP, *see* Adenosine diphosphate
Affect modifications, 101
Aflatoxin, 30, 95, 97–198
Agent Orange, 242
Agreement on the Application of Sanitary and Phytosanitary Measures (SPS), 77
Agreement on Technical Barriers to Trade (TBT), 77
Agricultural Marketing Service (AMS), 74
Agricultural Research Service (ARS), 75
Alcohol dehydrogenase, 126, 129
Aldehyde dehydrogenases, 129
Alimentary toxic aleukia (ATA), 199
Alitame, 256
Allergens, 152
Allergic reaction(s)
 food colors and, 95
 IgE-mediated, 154
Allergy, *see* Food intolerance and allergy
Alteromonas, 184
Alzheimer's disease, 226
Amanita muscaria, 7
American Dietetic Association (ADA), 270
Ames assay, 52, 53
Amino acid(s)
 imbalances, 27
 protein synthesis and, 26
 pyrolysis, 276
Amphetamines, 15
AMS, *see* Agricultural Marketing Service
Amylase, 105
Analytical studies, 97
Anaphylactic episodes, 151

Anaphylactoid reactions, definition of, 155
Anaphylaxis, 154, 158
Animal enzyme systems, categories of, 123
Animal and Plant Health Inspection Service (APHIS), 74, 303
Animal supply facilities, 63
Animal toxins, marine animals, 180–185
 ciguatoxin, 184–185
 pyropheophorbide-A, 183
 saxitoxin, 182–183
 scombroid poisoning, 181–182
 tetrodotoxin, 183–184
Anthrax, 164
Antibiotic resistance, 163, 293–296
Antibody systems, 153
Anticancer agents, phytochemicals acting as, 9
Anticholinesterase toxicant, 192
Antihistamines, 20, 159, 182
Antiminerals, 212
Antinutrients, 211–213
 antiminerals, 212
 antiproteins, 211
 antivitamins, 212
Antioxidant(s), 138, 252–254
 ascorbic acid, 252
 BHT and BHA, 253–254
 intakes of, 99
 phytochemicals acting as, 9
 propyl gallate, 253
 systems, enzymatic, 139
 tocopherol, 253
Antivitamins, 212
APHIS, *see* Animal and Plant Health Inspection Service
APL, *see* Acute promyelocytic leukemia
Arochlor®, 239
ARS, *see* Agricultural Research Service
Artificial kidney, 141
Ascorbic acid, 252
Aspartame, 255
Aspergillus, 195
 flavus, 197
 ochraceus, 202
Asthma, 154, 157
Astroviruses, 220, 222
ATA, *see* Alimentary toxic aleukia
ATP, *see* Adenosine triphosphate

Autopsy, animal, 47
Avidin, 213

B

Bacillus
  anthracis, 164
  cereus, 164–165
  thuringiensis, 297
Bacterial toxins, 163–178
  infections, 168–177
    Campylobacter jejuni, 170–171
    Clostridium perfringens, 171
    Escherichia coli, 171–175
    Listeria monocytogens, 175
    Salmonella, 168–170
    Shigella, 175–176
    Vibrio, 176–177
    Yersinia enterocolitica, 177
  intoxications, 164–168
    Bacillus cereus, 164–165
    Clostridium botulinum, 165–167
    staphylococci, 167–168
BALT, see Bronchus-associated lymphoid tissue
Barbiturate
  metabolism of, 30
  sleeping times, 27
Benzoic acid, 251
BHA, see Butylated hydroxyanisole
BHT, see Butylated hydroxytoluene
Bias
  information, 101, 102
  selection, 101
Biliary excretion, 142
Bioaccumulation factor, 12, 13
Bioactivation, metabolite, 13
Biogenic amines, 193
Biohazard protection, 66
Biomarker(s)
  stability of, 102
  use of in epidemiological studies, 101
Biomembrane structure, 26
Biotoxification, 58
Biotransformation
  enzymology, 123
  scenarios, 122
  xenobiotic, 121
Bipyridyliums, 238
Blood perfusion rates, 115
Body lice, 215
Botulinum toxins, 3
Botulism
  first food associated with, 166
  infant, 167
  wound, 167
Bovine spongiform encephalopathy (BSE), 223
  diagnosis, 225, 226
  form of CJD associated with, 224
Brassica species, 185
Breast-feeding, 159
Bronchus-associated lymphoid tissue (BALT), 153
BSE, see Bovine spongiform encephalopathy
Butylated hydroxyanisole (BHA), 157
Butylated hydroxytoluene (BHT), 8, 157

C

Cadaverine, 181
Caffeine, toxicity of, 25
Caliciviruses, 220, 222
Campylobacter jejuni, 170–171
Cancer(s)
  genetic toxicity and, 51
  high-fat diets and, 28
  -producing substances, testing for, 50
Carbamates, 235
Carbaryl, 236
Carbohydrates, classes of, 206
Carbon monoxide poisoning, 143
Carcinogenesis, 22
Carotenoids, prevention of lung cancer by, 95
Case control studies, 100, 103
Case reports, 97
Catalytic specificity, 124
Catechol-O-methyltransferase (COMT), 133
CCPs, see Critical control points
CDC, see Centers for Disease Control and Prevention
Celiac disease, 155
Cellular reductants, antioxidants and, 138
Center for Food Safety and Applied Nutrition (CFSAN), 37, 74
Centers for Disease Control and Prevention (CDC), 74, 103, 245
Ceresan, 239
CFSAN, see Center for Food Safety and Applied Nutrition
Chemical preservatives, 8
Chemophobia, 81, 82
Chinese hamster cells, forward mutations in, 54
Chloramphenicol, 170
Chlordane, accumulation of in fat depots, 117
Chlorophyll, 192
Chlorphenoxy acid esters, 237
Cholesterol, 26, 28, 112
Chronic toxicity testing, 50

Ciguatoxin, 184–185
Cipro®, 165
CJD, see Creutzfeldt–Jakob disease
Claviceps purpurea, 196
Clostridium
  botulinum, 165–167, 263, 279
  perfringens, 171
Codex Alimentarius, 76, 77, 270
Color Additives Amendment, 79
Coloring agents, 256–259
  methyl anthranilate, 258
  monosodium glutamate, 259
  Red No. 2, 257–258
  Red No. 3, 258
  safrole, 258
  Yellow No. 4, 258
COMT, see Catechol-*O*-methyltransferase
Confounding, definition of, 101
CO poisoning, see Carbon monoxide poisoning
Copper toxicity, 210
Coumarin, 189, 191
COX, see Cyclooxygenases
Creatine, 276
Creutzfeldt–Jakob disease (CJD), 223, 224, 225
Critical control points (CCPs), 286
  definition of, 288
  documented, 289
  establishment of procedures to monitor, 289
Cross-contamination, potential for, 163
Cross-sectional studies, 98
Cyanide metabolism, 187
Cyanogenic glycosides, 186
Cyclodiene insecticides, 236
Cyclooxygenases (COX), 28
Cystic fibrosis, 51
Cytochrome P450
  enzyme system, 127
  expression, 33
  microsomal monooxygenase reactions, 126
  systems, oxidation reactions and, 134

D

Dairy products, contaminated, 195
Data storage facilities, 64
DBPCFC, see Double-blind placebo-controlled food challenge
DDT, see Dichloro diphenyl trichloroethane
Deep freezing, 261
Dehydration, 119
Delaney Clause, 78, 79, 92, 250
Dermatitis, 143
Detoxification, enzymatic mechanisms of, 26

Diarrhea
  fluid balance and, 118
  nutritional deficiencies during chronic, 120
Diazinon, 235
Dichloro diphenyl trichloroethane (DDT), 25, 117, 231, 232
Dietary fiber, 212
Dietary reference intake (DRI), 6, 31, 89, 205
Dietary Supplement Health and Education Act, 79
Dioxins, 241
Diphyllobothrium latum, 218
Diquat, 238
Diseases, preferred method to study, 100
DNA
  aflatoxin binding to, 30
  damage, 53, 140
  repair, 51, 53
  viruses and, 218
Dose–response assessment, 86
Dose–response curve
  lethality, 47
  sigmoidal, 16
  threshold assumption and, 91
Dose–response relationship, 14
Dose–response symptoms, 47
Double-blind placebo-controlled food challenge (DBPCFC), 158
Down's syndrome, 51
DRI, see Dietary reference intake
Drosophila melanogaster, 54
Dursban, 235

E

Ecological studies, 96
ED, see Effective dose
EDB, see Ethylene dibromide
Effective dose (ED), 15
Egg product inspection, AMS and, 75
EIEC, see Enteroinvasive *Escherichia coli*
ELEM, see Equine leukoencephalomalacia
Elimination diet, allergy and, 159
Endocytosis, 111
Entamoeba histolytica, 215
Enterocyte metabolism, 110
Enterohepatic circulation, 41
Enteroinvasive *Escherichia coli* (EIEC), 172
Enteropathogenic *Escherichia coli* (EPEC), 172
Enterotoxigenic *Escherichia coli* (ETEC), 173
Enterotoxin, 167
Environmental contaminants, 239–247
  halogenated hydrocarbons, 239–242
  heavy metals, 242–247

Environmental Protection Agency (EPA), 73
　Office of Pesticides and Toxic Substances, 75
　regulations, costs of, 84
　standards promulgated by, 73
Enzyme(s)
　antioxidant systems, 139
　degradation, age-associated, 30
　drug-metabolizing, 30
　efficiency of, 124
　induction, teratogenesis and, 55
　lipid-digesting, 105
　microsomal, 126
　nonmicrosomal, 128
　system, cytochrome P450, 127
EPA, *see* Environmental Protection Agency
EPEC, *see* Enteropathogenic *Escherichia coli*
Epicatechin, 191
Epidemiological research, gold standard of, 99
Epidemiology, 95–104
　analytical strategies, 97–100
　　cross-sectional studies, 98
　　meta-analysis, 100
　　prospective studies, 98–99
　　retrospective studies, 99–100
　descriptive strategies, 96–97
　　case reports, 97
　　ecological studies, 96–97
　foodborne diseases and epidemiology, 103
　molecular epidemiology, 100–103
　　exposure–dose studies, 102
　　gene–environment interactions, 102–103
　　physiological studies, 102
Equine leukoencephalomalacia (ELEM), 201
Ergonovine, 197
Ergotamine, 197
Escherichia coli, 118, 171–175, 264, 294
ETEC, *see* Enterotoxigenic *Escherichia coli*
Ethylene dibromide (EDB), 92
Euphorbia pulcherrima, 185
Exocytosis, 111
Exposure
　assessment, 85
　–disease continuum, 102
Extracorporeal dialysis, 141

F

Fad diets, 207
Fair Packaging and Labeling Act, 79
FAO, *see* Food and Agricultural Organization
Fasting, drug metabolism and, 25
Fat-soluble vitamins, 209
Fatty acids, oxygenation products of, 29
FDA, *see* Food and Drug Administration

Fecal excretion, 142
Federal Food, Drug, and Cosmetic Act, 79
Federal Insecticide, Fungicide, and Rodenticide
　Act (FIFRA), 59, 78, 79
Federal Meat Inspection law, 79
Federal Poultry Product Inspection Act, 79
FIFRA, *see* Federal Insecticide, Fungicide, and
　Rodenticide Act
Fish poisoning, common forms of, 181
Flavin-containing monooxygenase (FMO), 126,
　128, 132
Flavonoids, 188, 190, 191
Fluid balance, diarrhea and, 118
FMO, *see* Flavin-containing monooxygenase
Folacin, 209
Folate deficiency, 31
Food(s)
　allergens, definitions of, 152
　allergies, IgE-mediated, 158
　anaphylactic episodes due to, 151
　cyanide in, 187
　handling practices, 163
　industry, start of governmental controls on, 5
　sensitivities, 152, 155
Food additives, 7, 8, 249–260
　antioxidants, 252–254
　　ascorbic acid, 252
　　BHT and BHA, 253–254
　　propyl gallate, 253
　　tocopherol, 253
　coloring agents, 256–259
　　methyl anthranilate, 258
　　monosodium glutamate, 259
　　Red No. 2, 257–258
　　Red No. 3, 258
　　safrole, 258
　　Yellow No. 4, 258
　preservatives, 251–252
　　benzoic acid and sodium benzoate, 251
　　hydrogen peroxide, 252
　　nitrite and nitrate, 252
　　sorbate, 251
　sweeteners, 254–256
　　acesulfame, 255
　　alitame, 256
　　aspartame, 255
　　saccharin, 254
　　sodium cyclamate, 254–255
　　sucralose, 256
　　sugar alcohols, 256
　　D-tagatose, 256
Food Additives Amendment, 77, 79
Food allergy, *see* Food intolerance and allergy
Food and Agricultural Organization (FAO), 76,
　263

Index   311

Foodborne disease(s), 95, 220
  microbial-related, 163
  outbreak investigations, 103
Food Code, 293
Food and Drug Administration (FDA), 261
  ability of to ensure food safety, 77
  Center for Food Safety and Applied Nutrition, 74
  HACCP plan development and, 287
  inspection of testing facility by, 60
  standards promulgated by, 73
Food, Drug, and Cosmetic Act, 78
  Food Additives Amendment to, 250
  questions with passage of, 262
Food and Drugs Act, 77
Food intolerance and allergy, 151–160
  allergy and types of hypersensitivity, 152–157
    primary food sensitivity, 152–157
    secondary food sensitivity, 157
  symptoms and diagnosis, 157–158
  treatment, 158–159
Food irradiation, 261–271
  by-products of, 268–269
  effectiveness of, 267–268
  history of, 262–265
  misconceptions, 269
  regulations, 269–271
  study questions and exercises, 271
  types of, 265–267
Food poisoning
  botulinum-induced, 166
  outbreaks of, 193
Food processing
  advantages of, 249
  drawbacks, 250
  materials used in, 3
  objectives of, 249
  use of additives in, 250
Food safety assessment, compliance with regulations, 59–80
  good laboratory practices, 59–72
    equipment, 65
    facility, 63–64
    general provisions, 60
    organization and personnel, 60–63
    protocol for and conduct of nonclinical laboratory study, 68–69
    records and reports, 69–72
    test and control articles, 67–68
    testing facilities operation, 65–67
  good manufacturing practices, 73
  regulatory agencies, 73–77
    Centers for Disease Control and Prevention, 74

Food and Drug Administration, 74
  international agencies, 76–77
  local and state agencies, 76
  National Marine Fisheries Service, 76
  Occupational Safety and Health Administration, 75–76
  U.S. Department of Agriculture, 74–75
  U.S. Environmental Protection Agency, 75
study questions and exercises, 80
U.S. food laws, 77–79
Food safety assessment, laboratory methods, 37–58
  analysis of toxicants in foods, 38–40
  genetic toxicity, 51–55
    Ames tests, 52
    eukaryotic cells *in vitro*, 53–54
    eukaryotic cells *in vivo*, 54–55
    host-mediated assays, 52–53
  oral ingestion studies, 40–51
    acute toxicity testing, 41–48
    chronic toxicity testing, 50–51
    subchronic toxicity testing, 48–50
  specialized oral ingestion studies, 55–58
    developmental toxicity, 55–56
    metabolic, 56–58
    reproductive, 56
  study questions and exercises, 58
Food Safety Council Scientific Committee, 37
Food safety issues, 285–305
  antibiotic resistance, 293–296
  GMOs, 296–305
    cold tolerance, 298
    disease resistance, 298
    drought tolerance and salinity tolerance, 298
    economic concerns, 301–303
    environmental hazards, 300–301
    GMO foods and labeling, 303–304
    herbicide tolerance, 298
    human health risks, 301
    nutrition, 299
    pest resistance, 298
    pharmaceuticals, 299
    phytoremediation, 299–300
  HACCP, 285–293
    corrective action when critical limit is exceeded, 290–291
    critical control points, 288–289
    critical limits for preventive measures, 89
    development of HACCP plan, 287–288
    hazard analysis, 288
    procedures to monitor CCPs, 289–290
    record-keeping systems, 291
    verification procedures, 291–293

study questions and exercises, 305
Foods Safety and Inspection Service (FSIS), 74
Force-air drying, 195
Free fatty acids, 28
Frequency–response
  curve, 16
  mortality, 17
Fructose intolerance, 180
FSIS, see Foods Safety and Inspection Service
Fugu rubripes, 7
Fungal mycotoxins, 195–203
  aflatoxin, 197–198
  ergot alkaloids and ergotism, 196–197
  other mycotoxins, 202
  penicillia mycotoxins, 201–202
    patulin, 202
    rubratoxin, 201–202
    yellow rice toxins, 202
  trichothecenes, 198–201
Fungicides, 238–239
Fusarium, 195, 199

G

Galactosemia, 180
Gallic acid, 191
GALT, see Gut-associated lymphoid tissue
Gastroenteritis, Norwalk, 222
Gastrointestinal (GI) tract, 105
  anatomy and digestive functions, 105–110
  fluid balance and diarrhea, 118–120
  functions of, 106
  gut absorption and enterocyte metabolism, 110–114
    carrier-mediated, 111
    endocytosis and exocytosis, 111–112
    movement of substances across cellular membranes, 112–114
    passive diffusion, 110–111
  physiology and biochemistry of, 105–120
  organs of, 105
  sections of, 106
  transport into circulation, 114–118
    bone, 116–117
    delivery of toxicant from systemic circulation to tissues, 114–115
    lipid depots, 117
    liver and kidney, 116
    physiologic barriers to toxicants, 117–118
    storage sites, 115–116
Gene–environment interactions, 102
Generally recognized as safe (GRAS), 8, 77, 304

Genetically modified organisms (GMOs), 285
  cold tolerance, 298
  disease resistance, 298
  drought tolerance and salinity tolerance, 298
  economic concerns, 301–303
  environmental hazards, 300
  foods and labeling, 303
  herbicide tolerance, 298
  human health risks, 301
  nutrition, 299
  pest resistance, 298
  pharmaceuticals, 299
  phytoremediation, 299
Genetic engineering, 297
Genetic screen, 226
Genetic toxicity, 51
GH, see Growth hormone
Giardia lamblia, 215
Giardiasis, 215
GI tract, see Gastrointestinal tract
GI tract
Gliadin, 155
GLPs, see Good laboratory practices
Glucosides, sulfur-containing, 186
Glucosinolates, 212
Glucuronidation, 132, 133
Glutathione (GSH), 156
  peroxidase system, 139
  reductase, 126
Glutathione-S-transferases (GSTs), 134
Glycophosphatidyl inositol (GPI), 223
Glycoproteins, acid-resistant, 153
Glycosides, cyanogenic, 186
GMOs, see Genetically modified organisms
GMPs, see Good manufacturing practices
Goitrin formation, 186
Goitrogens, 185
Gonorrhea, 283
Good laboratory practices (GLPs), 59
  guidelines, 72
  studies, humane treatment of animals in, 66
Good manufacturing practices (GMPs), 73, 79, 286
Gossypol, 212
GPI, see Glycophosphatidyl inositol
GRAS, see Generally recognized as safe
Green revolution, 231
Growth
  hormone (GH), 33
  retardation, 55
GSH, see Glutathione
GSTs, see Glutathione-S-transferases
Guillain–Barre syndrome, 170
Gut absorption, 110
Gut-associated lymphoid tissue (GALT), 153

Index

H

Haber–Weiss reaction, 135
HACCP, *see* Hazard Analysis of Critical Control Points
Haliotis, 183
Hallucinogen, 196
Halogenated hydrocarbons, 239–242
Hazard
    analysis, 288
    definition of, 85
    identification, 85
        definition of, 84
        major issues of animal studies in, 86
Hazard Analysis of Critical Control Points (HACCP), 285
    -based inspection program, 76
    plan, development of, 287
    principles, 286
    record-keeping systems, 291
    verification reports, 292
HCAs, *see* Heterocyclic amines
HCN, *see* Hydrocyanic acid
HDLs, *see* High-density lipoproteins
Health maintenance organizations (HMOs), 296
Heavy metals, 242–247
    arsenic, 246–247
    cadmium, 245–246
    lead, 244–245
    mercury, 242–244
Hemagglutinins, 211
Heme synthesis, 32
Hemlock, 4
Henderson–Hasselbalch equations, 113
Hepatitis, 220, 221
Hepatitis A, 220
Hepatitis B, 221
Hepatitis E
    common source of, 220
    transmission of, 221
Herbicides, 186, 237–238
HERP, *see* Human exposure/rodent potency
Heterocyclic amines (HCAs), 273, 275
    activation of, 276
    formation, factors influencing, 278
High-density lipoproteins (HDLs), 116, 210
High-fat diets, cancer and, 28
High-protein diets, 207
Hippocratic screen, 43, 44–46
Histamine poisoning, 193
HMOs, *see* Health maintenance organizations
Home economics classes, 163
Human epidemiological studies, examples of use in food toxicology, 95
Human exposure/rodent potency (HERP), 92

Hydrocyanic acid (HCN), 186
Hydrogen peroxide, 252
Hydrolysis, 131
Hydrolytic reactions, characteristics of, 126
Hypersensitivity, hyposensitivity vs., 22
Hyperthyroidism, 33

I

IACUC, *see* Institutional Animal Care and Use Committee
IAEA, *see* International Atomic Energy Agency
IDEs, *see* Investigational device exemptions
Idiosyncratic reactions, 156
IgE, *see* Immunoglobulin E
IgG antibodies, 219
Immunoglobulin E (IgE), 152
    -mediated allergic reaction, 154, 157
    role of in fighting parasitic infections, 153
INDs, *see* Investigational new drug applications
Industrial contaminants, 239–247
    halogenated hydrocarbons, 239–242
    heavy metals, 242–247
Infant botulism, 167
Information bias, 101, 102
Inorganic phosphate (Pi), 111
Insecticides, 231–237
    carbamates, 235
    cyclodiene, 236
    DDT, 231
    organophosphates, 234
Institutional Animal Care and Use Committee (IACUC), 66
International Atomic Energy Agency (IAEA), 263
International food trade, 76
Intervention study, 99
Intestinal motility, 119
Investigational device exemptions (IDEs), 71
Investigational new drug applications (INDs), 71
Iron overloads, 210

K

Kidney dialysis machine, 141

L

Laboratory
    animals, use of in nonclinical research, 59
    operation areas, 64
Laboratory study, nonclinical
    conduct of, 69
    protocol for, 68

reporting results of, 70
LD, *see* Lethal dose
LDLs, *see* Low-density lipoproteins
Lectins, 211
Lethal dose (LD), 15
Lethality, dose-response curve for, 47
Lingual lipase, 105
Lipid(s)
    depots, 117
    peroxidation, 32, 137
    primary toxicity issue for, 207
    solubility, 124
    -to-water partition coefficient, 112
Listeria monocytogens, 175
Listeriosis, 175
Livona pica, 184
LOAEL, *see* Lowest observed adverse effect level
LOEL, *see* Lowest observed effect level
Low-density lipoproteins (LDLs), 116
Low-dose response, models used in determination of, 91
Lowest observed adverse effect level (LOAEL), 89
Lowest observed effect level (LOEL), 89
Lung cancer, prevention of by carotenoids, 95
Lysergic acid, 197

M

Macronutrients, 205–207
    carbohydrates, 205–206
    lipids, 206–207
    protein, 207
Mad cow disease, 223
Magnesium, renal failure and, 210
Maillard reaction, 281, 282
Malabsorption syndrome, severe, 155
Malaria, 233, 293
Malathion, 235
Manganese, airborne, 211
MAO, *see* Monoamine oxidase
Margin of safety (MOS), 20, 90
Mathematical models, 58
Maximum contaminant levels (MCLs), 275
MCls, *see* Maximum contaminant levels
Meat products, effects of heating nitrite-cured, 281
Medical surveillance, 61
Melanoidins, 281
Membrane structure, 112
Metabolic food disorders, 156
Methyl parathion, 235
Micronucleus test, 55
Micronutrients, 207–211

Microsomal enzymes, 126
Mixed-function oxidase enzymes, 27
Models
    low-dose response, 91
    mathematical, 58
    multicompartment, 149
Molecular epidemiology, 100
Molybdenum hydroxylases, 126, 130
Monitoring equipment design, 65
Monoamine oxidase (MAO), 129, 193
Monosodium glutamate (MSG), 157
Morning sickness, 14
Morphine, 20
MOS, *see* Margin of safety
Motor activity, decrease of, 43
Mouse lymphoma cell assay, 54
MSG, *see* Monosodium glutamate
Multicompartment models, 149
Mutagenesis, 22
Mutations, frameshift, 52
Mycobacterium tuberculosis, 294
Mycotoxicoses, 195
Mycotoxins, 202
    adverse effects of, 196
    processes for reducing, 196
    see also Fungal mycotoxins
Myristicin, 191

N

National Bladder Cancer Study, 100
National Institute for Occupational Safety and Health (NIOSH), 241
National Marine Fisheries Service (NMFS), 76
NEDs, *see* Normal equivalent deviations
Neurodegenerative diseases, 226
Neurospora crassa, 53
Neurotoxicity, 236
Niacin, 209
Nicotinamide, 209
NIOSH, *see* National Institute for Occupational Safety and Health
Nitrate, 252, 279
Nitric oxide (NO), 136
Nitrite, 252, 279
Nitrosamines, 279, 280
NMFS, *see* National Marine Fisheries Service
NO, *see* Nitric oxide
NOAEL, *see* No observed adverse effect levels
NOEL, *see* No observable effect level
Nonclinical laboratory study
    conduct of, 69
    protocol for, 68
    reporting results of, 70

Index

Nonimmunological reactions, 155
Nonmicrosomal enzymes, 128
Nonthreshold
    observation vs., 91
    relationships, 90
No observable effect level (NOEL), 50, 88
No observed adverse effect levels (NOAEL), 85, 89
Normal equivalent deviations (NEDS), 18
Norwalk-like virus, 220, 221
Nucleic acid(s)
    metabolism, 7
    oxidation, 140
    polymer alterations and, 140
Nutrient
    absorption, 111
    deficiency, 5
Nutrients, toxicity of, 205–213
    antinutrients, 211–213
        antiminerals, 212
        antiproteins, 211
        antivitamins, 212–213
    macronutrients, 205–207
        carbohydrates, 205–206
        lipids, 206–207
        protein, 207
    micronutrients, 207–211
        minerals and trace elements, 209–211
        vitamins, 207–209
Nutritional Labeling and Education Act, 79
Nutritional toxicology, definition of, 3

O

Occupational Health and Safety Administration (OSHA), 61
    irradiation facility requirements of, 266
    occupational safety and health standards mandated by, 75
    regulations, 61
    requirements, 66
OPs, *see* Organophosphates
Oral ingestion studies, 40
Organic Foods Product, The, 79
Organophosphates (OPs), 21, 234
OSHA, *see* Occupational Health and Safety Administration
Osmosis, definition of, 111
Oxalate, 180, 212
Oxidation, 131, 140
Oxidative reactions, 125
Oxidative stress, 134, 139
Oxygen consumption, calorie restriction and, 30
Ozone, 137

P

PAHs, *see* Polycyclic aromatic hydrocarbons
Pancreatitis, 211
Paralytic shellfish poisoning (PSP), 182
Paraquat, 238
Parasites
    protozoa, 215–216
        Entamoeba histolytica, 215–216
        Giardia lamblia, 216
        Toxoplasma gondii, 216
    see also Prions; Viruses
    worms, 216–218
        roundworms, 216–218
        tapeworms, 218
Parasitic infection, role of IgE in fighting, 153
Parkinson's disease, 211
Passive diffusion, definition of, 110
Pathogen, heat-resistant, 289
Pathogen Reduction Act, 79
Patulin, 202
PCB, *see* Polychlorinated biphenyl
PELs, *see* Permissible exposure levels
Penicillium, 195
Penicillium notatum, 201
Peristalsis, 108
Permissible exposure levels (PELs), 83, 84
Pest control measures, 67
Pesticide(s)
    contamination of groundwater by, 231
    residues, Food, Drug, and Cosmetic Act and, 78
Pesticide Chemical Amendment, The, 79
PGS, *see* Prostaglandin synthetase
Pharmacokinetics (PK), 40, 143
Phenolic substances, 188
Phenylketonuria, 180
Phenylmercury acetate (PMA), 239
Photosynthesis, 7
Physiological compartments, compounds used to measure, 148
Physiological studies, 102
Physostigmine, 185, 192
Phytochemicals, as anticancer agents, 9
Pi, *see* Inorganic phosphate
Pillsbury Company, 285
PK, *see* Pharmacokinetics
Plant(s)
    natural weapons of, 8
    toxicants, 185–193
        biogenic amines, 193
        cholinesterase inhibitors, 192–193
        cyanogenic glycosides, 186–188
        goitrogens, 185–186
        phenolic substances, 188–192

Plasma proteins, 115
PMA, see Phenylmercury acetate
Poisonous animals, 179
Polychlorinated biphenyl (PCB), 8, 82
  accumulation of in fat depots, 117
  fish exposed to, 241
  molecular structure of, 240
Polycyclic aromatic hydrocarbons (PAHs), 273
Polycyclic aromatic hydrocarbons and other processing products, 273–283
  benzo(α)pyrene and polycyclic aromatic hydrocarbons, 273–275
  heterocyclic amines, 275–278
  nitrates, nitrites, and nitrosamines, 279–281
  products of Maillard reaction, 281–283
  study questions and exercises, 283
Polymer alterations, 140
Polymorphonuclear leukocyte phagocytosis, 164
Polyunsaturated fatty acids (PUFAs), 134, 137, 140, 206
Preservatives, 251–252
  benzoic acid and sodium benzoate, 251
  hydrogen peroxide, 252
  nitrite and nitrate, 252
  sorbate, 251
Prions, 223–226; see also Parasites; Viruses
Processing products, see Polycyclic aromatic hydrocarbons and other processing products
Prolonged toxicity tests, 49
Propyl gallate, 253
Prospective studies, 98
Prostaglandin synthetase (PGS), 126
Protein(s)
  -binding, 116
  metal-binding sites of, 140
  synthesis, amino acids and, 26
Protozoa, 215–216
  Entamoeba histolytica, 215–216
  Giardia lamblia, 216
  Toxoplasma gondii, 216
Pseudomonas, 294
Psoralen, 180
PSP, see Paralytic shellfish poisoning
PUFAs, see Polyunsaturated fatty acids
Pulmonary gases, 142
Pure Food and Drug Act, 79
Putrescine, 181
Pyridoxine, 209
Pyrolytic decomposition, 273
Pyropheophorbine-a, 183

Q

QA unit, see Quality assurance unit
Quality assurance (QA) unit, 60
  FDA representative and, 63
  monitoring of study by, 62
  role of, 61

R

Radioallergosorbent test (RAST), 159
RAST, see Radioallergosorbent test
Raw food material, contamination of, 166
RCRA, see Resource Conservation and Recovery Act
RDAs, see Recommended dietary allowances
Reactive oxygen species (ROS), 25, 134, 135
  generation of, 25
  selenium and, 32
Recommended dietary allowances (RDAs), 6, 205
Reductive reactions, 126, 130
Reproductive tests, 56
Residues in foods, 231–248
  fungicides, 238–239
  herbicides, 237–238
  industrial and environmental contaminants, 239–247
    halogenated hydrocarbons, 239–242
    heavy metals, 242–247
  insecticides, 231–237
    carbamates, 235–236
    cyclodiene insecticides, 236–237
    DDT, 232–234
    organophosphates, 234–235
Resource Conservation and Recovery Act (RCRA), 66
Respiratory depression, 20
Respiratory paralysis, 167
Retinols, 32
Retrospective studies, 99
Rheumatoid arthritis, 105
Rhodenase, 187
Rhubarb, oxalate in, 180
Riboflavin deficiency, 31
Risk, 81–93
  –benefit, 81–85
  characterization, 87–92
    nonthreshold relationships, 90–91
    risk put into perspective, 91–92
    threshold relationships, 88–90
  dose–response assessment, 86
  exposure assessment, 86–87
  hazard identification, 85–87

Index

ROS, *see* Reactive oxygen species
Rotavirus, 220, 222
Roundup®, 298
Rubratoxin, 201–202

S

Saccharin, 254
Saccharomyces forward-mutation assay, 53
Safe, misuse of the term, 81
Safety decision tree protocol, food additive, 38
Safrole, 189, 191
SAH, see *S*-Adenosyl-L-homocysteine
Salmonella, 118, 168–170, 264
    gallinarum, 168
    pullorum, 168
    sensitivity of to acid, 107
    typhimurium, 52, 169
Salmonellosis, 168, 169
SALT, *see* Skin-associated lymphoid tissue
Saurine, 181
Saxitoxin, 182–183
Scombroid poisoning, 181–182
    clinical symptoms, 181–182
    mode of action, 181
SD, *see* Study director
Seafood poisons, categories of, 180
Selection bias, 101
Selenium
    deficiency, lipid peroxidation and, 32
    toxicity, 211
September 11, 2001, 164
Shewanella, 184
Shiga-toxin-producing *E. coli* (STEC), 173
Shigella, 175–176
Shigellosis, transmission of, 175
Short-term exposure limits (STELs), 83, 84
Siberia, 1913 food shortage in, 198
Sickle-cell anemia, 51
Silent Spring, 232
Sister chromatid exchanges, 54
Skin-associated lymphoid tissue (SALT), 153
Skin prick test, 158
Society of Quality Assurance (SQA), 60
Sodium benzoate, 251
Sodium cyclamate, 254–255
Solanine, 179, 192
Solanum
    intrusum, 185
    nigrum, 185
Solute absorption, diseases of, 119
SOPs, *see* Standard operating procedures
Sorbate, 251
Species population differences, 16

SPS, *see* Agreement on the Application of Sanitary and Phytosanitary Measures
SQA, *see* Society of Quality Assurance
Standard operating procedures (SOPs), 65, 286
Staphylococcus aureus, 118, 167, 294
STEC, *see* Shiga-toxin-producing *E. coli*
STELs, *see* Short-term exposure limits
Steroid hormones, 27
Stomach, cells and glands of, 107
Study(ies)
    analytical, 97
    case control, 100, 103
    cross-sectional, 98
    director (SD), 61
    ecological, 96
    intervention, 99
    large-scale epidemiological, 101
    physiological, 102
    prospective, 98
    retrospective, 99
    transitional, 101
Subchronic toxicity testing, 48
Sucralose, 256
Sucrase deficiency, 180
Sudden infant death syndrome, 167
Sugar alcohols, 256
Sulfite sensitivity, 157
Superoxide
    anion, formation of, 135
    dismutase, 135
Susceptibility gene analysis, 103
Sweeteners, 254–256
    acesulfame, 255
    alitame, 256
    aspartame, 255
    saccharin, 254
    sodium cyclamate, 254–255
    sucralose, 256
    sugar alcohols, 256
    D-tagatose, 256
Swine pulmonary edema, 201
Syphilis, 247

T

Taenia solium, 218
D-Tagatose, 256
Tannins
    condensed, 189
    liver injury and, 188
Taricha torosa, 183–184
Tartrazine sensitivity, 157
TD, *see* Toxicodynamics

Teratogenesis, 22, 55
Test article characterization, 67
Testing facilities operation, 65
Tetrodotoxin, 183–184
Thalidomide, 14
Thermonuclease (TNase), 167
Thiamin deficiency, 31
Third World countries, common problem in, 299
Threshold
　assumption, dose–response curve and, 91
　limit values (TLVs), 83
　relationships, 88
Time-weighted averages (TWAs), 83, 84
Tissue tropism, 219
TK, see Toxicokinetics
TLVs, see Threshold limit values
TNase, see Thermonuclease
TNT, see Agreement on Technical Barriers to Trade
Tocopherol, 138, 253
Tomatine, 180
Toxicant(s), 3
　anticholinesterase, 192
　bioactivity of, 41
　delivery of from systems circulation to tissues, 114
　excretion of, 140–143
　　biliary and fecal excretion, 142
　　pulmonary gases, 142
　　routes of, 140, 143
　　urinary excretion, 141–142
　impact of diet on effects of, 8–9
　in foods and their effects on nutrition, 5–8
　　food additives and contaminants, 7–8
　　naturally occurring toxicants, 7
　　nutrients, 5–7
　in vivo distribution of, 122
　metabolism of, 121–140
　　biotransformation enzymology, 123–134
　　conversion with intent to excrete, 121–123
　　oxidative stress, 134–140
　naturally occurring, 7, 180
　physiologic barriers to, 117
　relationship between time and bolus dose of, 146
　removal of, 141, 142
　uptake and elimination of, 11
　metabolism of toxicants,
　principles of toxicokinetics, 143–150
　　design of TK study, 144–145
　　multicompartment models, 149–150
　　one-compartment TK, 145–148
Toxicity
　caffeine, 25
　categories of, 20, 21

　genetic, 51
　organophosphate, 21
　response, reversibility of, 21
　screening, decision tree approach for, 51
　testing
　　acute, 41, 42
　　chronic, 50
　　rodent used for, 39
　　subchronic, 48
　ultimate extreme in, 20
Toxicodietetics, 25
Toxicodynamics (TD), 57, 143
Toxicokinetics (TK), 143
　definition of, 40
　multicompartment models, 149–150
　one-compartment, 145–148
　principles of, 143–150
　studies, 58, 62, 144
　　design of, 144–145
Toxicological effects, phases of, 11, 12
Toxicology
　factors that influence, 25–35
　　diet and biotransformation, 25–32
　　　macronutrient changes, 26–30
　　　micronutrient changes, 30–32
　　gender and age, 32–34
　　species, 34
　fundamental concept of, 4
　general principles of, 11–23
　　dose–response relationship, 14–22
　　categories of toxicity, 20–21
　　frequency response, 15–19
　　hypersensitivity vs. hyposensitivity, 22
　　potency and toxicity, 19–20
　　reversibility of toxicity response, 21–22
　phases of toxicological effects, 11–14
　　exposure phase, 11–13
　　toxicodynamic phase, 14
　　toxicokinetic phase, 13
　screen, 42
　testing, regulations governing, 72
Toxic Substance Control Act (TSCA), 59, 78
Toxin(s)
　botulinum, 3
　Shiga, 173
　yellow rice, 202
Toxoplasma gondii, 215
Toxoplasmosis, 215
Transitional studies, 101
Transmissible spongiform encephalopathies (TSEs), 223
Trichothecenes, 198–201
Triglycerides, 28
Tryptophan, 276

Index

TSCA, see Toxic Substance Control Act
TSEs, see Transmissible spongiform encephalopathies
Tuberculosis, 293
TWAs, see Time-weighted averages
Typhoid Mary, 170

U

UDP-glucuronosyl transferases (UGTs), 133
UGTs, see UDP-glucuronosyl transferases
UL, see Upper level
Undercooked hamburger, 174
Upper level (UL), 6
    definition of, 6
    determination of in dietary reference intakes, 89
    objective of, 7
U.S. food laws, 79
U.S. Food Safety Council, 37

V

Venomous animals, 179
Very-low-density lipoproteins (VLDLs), 116
Veterinary pharmaceuticals, 8
Vibrio, 176–177
Vietnam veterans, exposure of to Agent Orange, 242
Viruses, 218–223
    enteric, 220
    foodborne, 220
    replication of, 219, 220
    transmission of, 220
    see also Parasites; Prions
Vitamin(s)
    fat-soluble, 208
    intakes, insufficient, 207
    toxicity, 208
    water-soluble, 209

Vitamin B6, 209
Vitamin C deficiency, 31
Vitamin D intakes, excessive, 208
Vitamin E deficiency, reversal of, 138
VLDLs, see Very-low-density lipoproteins
Volume of distribution, estimation of, 148
Vomitoxin, 200

W

Water-soluble vitamins, 209
WHO, see World Health Organization
Wholesome Meat Act, 79
Woolsorters' disease, 164
World Health Organization (WHO), 76, 89, 263
Worms, 216–218
    roundworms, 216–218
    tapeworms, 218
Wound botulism, 167

X

Xenobiotic(s)
    exposure to, 22
    metabolism, 123
    transformation, products of, 121

Y

Yellow rice toxins, 202
Yersinia enterocolitica, 177

Z

Zinc
    deficiency, 32
    toxicity, 210